The Johns Hopkins
Handbook of Obstetrics and Gynecology

Notice

Medicine is an ever-changing science. As new research and clinical experience broaden our knowledge, changes in treatment and drug therapy are required. The authors and the publisher of this work have checked with sources believed to be reliable in their efforts to provide information that is complete and generally in accord with the standards accepted at the time of publication. However, in view of the possibility of human error or changes in medical sciences, neither the authors nor the publisher nor any other party who has been involved in the preparation or publication of this work warrants that the information contained herein is in every respect accurate or complete, and they disclaim all responsibility for any errors or omissions or for the results obtained from use of the information contained in this work. Readers are encouraged to confirm the information contained herein with other sources. For example and in particular, readers are advised to check the product information sheet included in the package of each drug they plan to administer to be certain that the information contained in this work is accurate and that changes have not been made in the recommended dose or in the contraindications for administration. This recommendation is of particular importance in connection with new or infrequently used drugs.

The Johns Hopkins
Handbook of Obstetrics and Gynecology

Linda M. Szymanski, MD, PhD
The Johns Hopkins School of Medicine
Department of Gynecology and Obstetrics
Baltimore, Maryland

Jessica L. Bienstock, MD, MPH
The Johns Hopkins School of Medicine
Department of Gynecology and Obstetrics
Baltimore, Maryland

New York   Chicago   San Francisco   Athens   London   Madrid   Mexico City
Milan   New Delhi   Singapore   Sydney   Toronto

The Johns Hopkins Handbook of Obstetrics and Gynecology

1 2 3 4 5 6 7 8 9 0   DOC/DOC   19 18 17 16 15

ISBN 978-0-07-177272-3
MHID 0-07-177272-3

This book was set in Sabon LT Std-Roman by MPS Limited.
The editors were Alyssa Fried and Brian Kearns
The production supervisor was Catherine Saggesse.
Project management was provided by Ruchika Abrol of MPS Limited.
RR Donnelley was printer and binder.

This book is printed on acid-free paper.

Library of Congress Cataloging-in-Publication Data

Szymanski, Linda Marie, author.
The Johns Hopkins handbook of obstetrics and gynecology / Linda M.
    Szymanski, Jessica Bienstock.
        p. ; cm.
    Handbook of obstetrics and gynecology
    Obstetrics and gynecology
    Includes bibliographical references.
    ISBN 978-0-07-177272-3 (pbk. : alk. paper) — ISBN 0-07-177272-3 (pbk. : alk. paper)
  I. Bienstock, Jessica L., author.   II. Title.   III. Title: Handbook of obstetrics and gynecology.
IV. Title: Obstetrics and gynecology.
    [DNLM: 1. Genital Diseases, Female.   2. Gynecology—methods.
3. Pregnancy Complications.   4. Urologic Diseases. WP 140]
    RG110
    618—dc23
                                                            2015021052

Contents

Contributors

Obstetrics:
Linda M. Szymanski, MD, PhD
Maternal-Fetal Medicine
Department of Gynecology and
Obstetrics
Johns Hopkins University School of
Medicine
Medical Director of Labor &
Delivery, Johns Hopkins Hospital
Baltimore, Maryland

Maureen Grundy, MD
Clinical Fellow
Maternal-Fetal Medicine
Department of Gynecology and
Obstetrics
Johns Hopkins University School of
Medicine
Baltimore, Maryland

Gynecology:
Dayna Burrell, MD
Assistant Professor
Department of Gynecology and
Obstetrics
Johns Hopkins University School
of Medicine
Baltimore, Maryland

Dipa Joshi, MD
Resident Physician
Department of Gynecology and
Obstetrics
Johns Hopkins University School
of Medicine
Baltimore, Maryland

Gynecologic Oncology:
Kara Long Roche, MD, MSc
Gynecology Service, Department of
Surgery
Memorial Sloan Kettering Cancer
Center
New York, New York

Diana Cholakian, MD
Resident Physician
Department of Gynecology and
Obstetrics
Johns Hopkins University School
of Medicine
Baltimore, Maryland

Reproductive Endocrinology
and Infertility:
Mindy S. Christianson, MD
Assistant Professor
Reproductive Endocrinology and
Infertility
Department of Gynecology and
Obstetrics
Johns Hopkins University School of
Medicine
Baltimore, Maryland

Irene Woo, MD
Fellow
Reproductive Endocrinology and
Infertility
University of Southern California
Los Angeles, California

Urogynecology:
Chi Chiung Grace Chen, MD
Assistant Professor
Female Pelvic Medicine and
Reconstructive Surgery
Department of Gynecology and
Obstetrics
Johns Hopkins University School of
Medicine
Baltimore, Maryland

Jennifer L. Hallock, MD
Fellow
Female Pelvic Medicine &
Reconstructive Surgery
Department of Gynecology and
Obstetrics
Johns Hopkins University School of
Medicine
Baltimore, Maryland

Roxanne Jamshidi, MD, MPH
Assistant Professor
Department of Gynecology and
Obstetrics
Johns Hopkins University School of
Medicine
Baltimore, Maryland

Preface

The origin of the *Johns Hopkins Handbook of Obstetrics and Gynecology* goes back nearly 20 years ago to a group of dedicated senior residents. These residents wanted to both educate their junior residents using the best available evidence and standardize, as much as possible, the way we cared for our patients. What started as a few dozen spiral bound pages has grown into the book you now have in your hands. Over the years our handbook has been used by hundreds of medical students, residents, fellows, faculty members, midwives, physician assistants, nurse practitioners, and nurses at Johns Hopkins. Every new member of our team quickly finds their copy of the *Handbook* to be indispensable. Our goal in offering our book for use by care providers outside of Johns Hopkins is that we want to make it as easy as possible for all patients to benefit from the best obstetric and gynecologic care available. The *Johns Hopkins Handbook of Obstetrics and Gynecology* is a compact and user-friendly resource for how to care for your patients. It is not meant to be used as a stand-alone textbook teaching you everything you need to know about a disease. Rather, it is a guidebook for how to care for the patient in front of you now. We are grateful to our numerous past and current residents and faculty who have contributed to making the *Johns Hopkins Handbook of Obstetrics and Gynecology* a remarkably concise and useful resource.

Jessica Bienstock, MD, MPH
Linda M. Szymanski, MD, PhD

Obstetrics

PREGNANCY DATING

β-hCG (mIU/mL)

- Produced by cytotrophoblasts and syncytiotrophoblasts (primarily)
- Ninety-two amino acid alpha subunit (identical to leutinizing hormone, follicle stimulating hormone, thyroid stimulating hormone (TSH)); 145 amino acid β-subunit (unique to hCG)
- Serum/urine pregnancy tests are sensitive to levels of 1–20 mIU/mL (varies by test)
- Within 24 hours of implantation (about 3 weeks after last menstrual period (LMP)), β-hCG is detectable in maternal serum. A sensitive pregnancy test can be (+) 1–2 days after implantation
- Peak maternal levels reach about 100 000 mIU/mL (60–80 days after LMP); then decline; nadir about 16 weeks, and stay at this level for remainder of pregnancy (Figure 1-1)
- After pregnancy (delivery or loss), it takes approximately 6–70 days for β-hCG to return to undetectable levels
- Elevated levels also in molar pregnancy, renal failure with impaired hCG clearance, physiological pituitary hCG, and hCG-producing tumors (GI, ovary, bladder, lung)

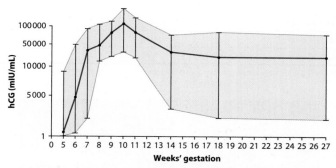

Figure 1-1 Mean concentration (95% CI) of human chorionic gonadotropin (hCG) in serum of women throughout normal pregnancy. (Used with permission from Cunningham F, Leveno KJ, Bloom SL, et al. Chapter 9. Prenatal care. In: Cunningham F, Leveno KJ, Bloom SL, et al., eds. *Williams Obstetrics*. 24th ed. New York, NY: McGraw-Hill; 2013.)

Ultrasound

See Table 1-1, Guidelines for Transvaginal Ultrasonographic Diagnosis of Pregnancy Failure in a Woman with an Intrauterine Pregnancy of Uncertain Viability

Establishing Estimated Date of Delivery (EDD)

- EDD is 280 days after the first day of the LMP (assumes regular, 28-day cycles, ovulation occurring at day 14, accurate recall)
- Ultrasound in the first trimester (up to 13-6/7 weeks) is the most accurate method to establish/confirm gestational age (GA)—accuracy of ±5–7 days
- If IVF pregnancy, age of the embryo, and date of transfer are used (day 5 transfer, EDD is 261 days from transfer date; day 3 transfer, EDD is 263 days from transfer date)
- Average fetal heart rate (FHR) 90–110 bpm at 6 weeks. Poor prognosis if less than 90 bpm
- See Table 1-2 for LMP vs ultrasound for establishing EDD

First Trimester Ultrasound (up to and including 13-6/7 weeks)

- Most accurate method to establish/confirm EDD
- Crown-Rump Length (CRL) (Figure 1-2)
  - Use if GA is less than 14-0/7 weeks
  - Accurate ±5–7 days
  - Midsagittal plane
  - Maximum length as a straight line from cranium to caudal rump
  - Average of three discrete measures
  - If CRL >84 mm (corresponding to about 14-0/7 weeks), accuracy of CRL decreases. Use other parameters

TABLE 1-1 DIAGNOSTIC CRITERIA FOR NONVIABLE PREGNANCY USING TRANSVAGINAL ULTRASONOGRAPHY

Diagnostic Findings for Nonviable Pregnancy*
• CRL of ≥7 mm and no heartbeat
• Mean sac diameter of ≥25 mm; no embryo
• Absence of embryo with heartbeat ≥2 weeks after ultrasound showed a gestational sac without yolk sac
• Absence of embryo with heartbeat ≥11 days after ultrasound showed a gestational sac with yolk sac

CRL, crown rump length.
*If findings are suspicious for, but do not meet these criteria for nonviable pregnancy, repeat ultrasound in 7-10 days.
Data from Doubilet PM, Benson CB, Bourne T, et al. Diagnostic criteria for nonviable pregnancy early in the first trimester. *NEJM* 369;15:1443-1451.

TABLE 1-2 LMP VS ULTRASOUND FOR ESTABLISHING EDD

Gestational Age by LMP (weeks)	Redate by Ultrasound if Discrepancy:
≤8-6/7	>5 days
9-0/7–15-6/7	>7 days
16-0/7–21-6/7	>10 days
22-0/7–27-6/7	>14 days
≥28-0/7	>21 days

Data from ACOG: Method for estimating due date. Committee Opinion no. 611; *Obstet Gynecol.* 2014;124:863–866

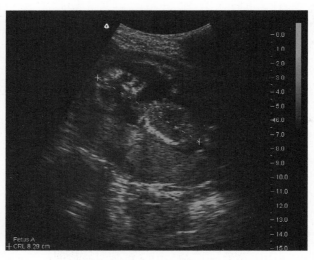

Figure 1-2 Crown rump length. (Used with permission from Usatine RP, et al. Chapter 4. Pregnancy and birth. In: Usatine RP, et al., eds. *The Color Atlas of Family Medicine*, 2nd ed. New York, NY: McGraw-Hill; 2013.)

Second Trimester Ultrasound (14-0/7–27-6/7 weeks)

• For dating, typically use BPD, HC, FL, and AC. See Figure 1-3
• Accuracy
  • Weeks 14-0/7–21-6/7: ±7–10 days
  • Weeks 22-0/7–27-6/7: ±10–14 days
• Biometry

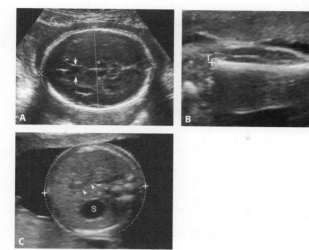

Figure 1-3 Fetal biometry. **A.** Biparietal diameter, and head circumference. **B.** Femur length. **C.** Abdominal circumference. Used with permission from Cunningham F, Leveno KJ, Bloom SL, et al. Chapter 10. Fetal imaging. In: Cunningham F, Leveno KJ, Bloom SL, et al., eds. Williams Obstetrics, 24th ed. New York, NY: McGraw-Hill; 2013.

Biparietal Diameter (BPD)
- Transverse view, transthalamic view
- Visualize thalami (*) and cavum septum pellucidum (arrows)
- Cerebellar hemispheres should not be visible
- Outer edge of skull to inner edge

Head Circumference (HC)
- Same view as BPD; measure outer edges of calvarium

Femur Length (FL)
- Measured from blunt end to blunt end, parallel to shaft

Abdominal Circumference (AC)
- Landmarks: Fetal stomach (S), spine, umbilical vein joining portal vein (forms a "J"). Most variability among measures

Third Trimester Ultrasound (28-0/7+ weeks)

- Least reliable method; accuracy ±21–30 days
- DATING BY THIRD TRIMESTER ULTRASOUND ALONE IS PROBLEMATIC
- Must use clinical picture to guide as a small fetus may have intrauterine growth restriction (IUGR)
- Adjust EDD if this is first ultrasound and discrepancy from LMP is >21 days
- May need repeat ultrasound to evaluate interval growth

LABOR AND DELIVERY

Labor

Definitions
- Three Stages of Labor
  - First stage: Onset of contractions until complete cervical dilation
  - Second stage: Complete cervical dilatation to expulsion of the fetus
  - Third stage: Expulsion of the fetus to expulsion of the placenta

Historical Perspective (Friedman's Work)
- First stage of labor
  - **Latent phase:** Begins with maternal perception of labor.
  - "Prolonged" when >20 hours in nulliparas and >14 hours in multiparas
  - **Active phase:** Point where rate of cervical dilation significantly increases
- Active-phase labor abnormalities

- **Protraction disorder:** Slower progress than normal
  - Cervical dilatation of <1.2 cm/h for nulliparous and <1.5 cm/h for multiparous
- **Arrest disorders:** Complete cessation of progress
  - Absence of cervical change for ≥2 hours if adequate uterine contractions and cervical exam at least 4 cm

Contemporary Perspective (Table 1-3 and Figure 1-4)
- More gradual increase in rate of cervical dilation as labor progresses
- No clear transition from "latent" to "active"
- Rates of cervical dilation less than 1 cm/h before 5–6 cm
- From 4 to 6 cm, nulliparous and multiparous women dilate at essentially same rate (more slowly than historical definitions)
- Beyond 6 cm, multiparous women have a slightly faster labor
- Active phase may not start until at least 6 cm dilated
- Median duration from 6 cm to complete dilation was 2.1 hours in nulliparas and 1.5 hours in multiparas
- NOTE: these data excluded all women with cesarean delivery (CD) and compromised neonates. Only women who achieved vaginal birth with a normal infant outcome were included
- Table 1-3 shows duration of labor from one cm of dilation to the next

TABLE 1-3 DURATION OF LABOR (IN HOURS*) BY PARITY— SPONTANEOUS LABOR

Cervical Dilation (cm)	Para 0	Para 1	Para 2+
3–4	1.8 (8.1)	–	–
4–5	1.3 (6.4)	1.4 (7.3)	1.4 (7.0)
5–6	0.8 (3.2)	0.8 (3.4)	0.8 (3.4)
6–7	0.6 (2.2)	0.5 (1.9)	0.5 (1.8)
7–8	0.5 (1.6)	0.4 (1.3)	0.4 (1.2)
8–9	0.5 (1.4)	0.3 (1.0)	0.3 (0.9)
9–10	0.5 (1.8)	0.3 (0.9)	0.3 (0.8)
Second stage—with epidural	1.1 (3.6)	0.4 (2.0)	0.3 (1.6)
Second stage—NO epidural	0.6 (2.8)	0.2 (1.3)	0.1 (1.1)

* Data are median (95th percentile)
Used with permission from Zhang J, Landy HJ, Branch DW, et al. Contemporary patterns of spontaneous labor with normal neonatal outcomes. *Obstet Gynecol.* 2010;116(6):1281–1287. Copyright © 2010 Lippincott Williams & Wilkins.

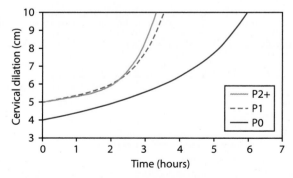

Figure 1-4 Contemporary labor curve. Average labor curves by parity in singleton term pregnancies with spontaneous onset of labor, vaginal delivery, and normal neonatal outcomes. P0, nulliparous women; P1, women of parity 1; P2+, women of parity 2 or higher. (Used with permission from Zhang J, Landy H, Branch DW, et al. Contenporary patterns of spontaneous labor with normal neonatel outcomes. *Obstet Gynecol.* 2010;116(6):1281. Copyright © 2010 Lippincott Williams & Wilkins.)

Definitions—using contemporary data

- **Failed induction of labor:** Failure to generate regular contractions and cervical change after at least 24 hours of oxytocin administration, with artificial membrane rupture if feasible
- **First-stage arrest:** 6 cm or greater dilation with membrane rupture and no cervical change for
  - ≥4 hours of adequate contractions (>200 Montevideo units (MVUs))
  - ≥6 hours if contractions are inadequate
- **Second-stage arrest:** No progress (descent or rotation) for
  - ≥4 hours in nulliparous women with an epidural
  - ≥3 hours in nulliparous women without an epidural
  - ≥3 hours in multiparous women with an epidural
  - ≥2 hours in multiparous women without an epidural
- **Bandl's ring:** Pathological retraction ring or constriction of uterus that develops with prolonged obstructed labors. Associated with thinning of lower uterine segment. May also occur between delivery of first and second twin

Important Points from ACOG/SMFM Consensus Statement*

- Prolonged first stage has been associated with increased risk of chorioamnionitis, but this is not an indication for CD
- Duration of second stage and association with
  - *Neonatal outcomes:* Results are conflicting. Some studies show no relationship between adverse outcomes and longer pushing duration; however, others have shown adverse outcomes (5 min Apgar <7, neonatal intensive care unit (NICU) admission, increased neonatal morbidity)
  - *Maternal outcomes:* More adverse outcomes with longer duration, such as higher rates of puerperal infection, third/fourth degree perineal lacerations, and postpartum hemorrhage. Also decreased probability of spontaneous vaginal delivery as time increases. After a ≥3 hour second stage, one of four nulliparas and one of three multiparas women deliver spontaneously
- Performing low or outlet operative deliveries in fetuses not believed to be macrosomic may reduce risk of CD

  *ACOG/SMFM obstetric care consensus. Safe prevention of the primary cesarean delivery. Obstet Gynecol. 2014;123:693–711.

Cesarean Delivery (CD)

- Most common indications
  - Labor arrest (34%)
  - Abnormal or indeterminate (formerly nonreassuring) FHR (23%)
  - Fetal malpresentation (17%)
  - Multiple gestation (7%)
  - Suspected fetal macrosomia (4%)
- See Table 1-4 for ACOG/SMFM Recommendations for Safe Prevention of Primary Cesarean Delivery

TABLE 1-4 ACOG/SMFM RECOMMENDATIONS FOR SAFE PREVENTION OF PRIMARY CESAREAN DELIVERY

Recommendations: Safe Prevention of the Primary Cesarean Delivery (CD)
First Stage of Labor
Prolonged latent phase (>20 hours in nulliparas; >14 hours in multiparas) is not an indication for CD
Cervical dilation of 6 cm should be threshold for active phase in labor
CD for active-phase arrest in first stage if: • ≥6 cm dilated with ruptured membranes with no progress despite 4 hours of adequate uterine activity **OR** • At least 6 hours of oxytocin administration with inadequate uterine activity and no cervical change
Second Stage of Labor
Before diagnosing arrest of labor (*if maternal/fetal status allows*): • Allow at least 3 hours of pushing in nulliparas • Allow at least 2 hours of pushing in multiparas • Longer duration may be considered on individualized basis if progress is documented • Consider adding 1 additional hour if epidural
Operative vaginal delivery (by experienced/trained physicians) is a safe alternative to CD
Manual rotation of fetal occiput (if malposition) is reasonable prior to performing operative vaginal delivery/CD. Assess fetal position

(Continued)

TABLE 1-4 ACOG/SMFM RECOMMENDATIONS FOR SAFE PREVENTION
OF PRIMARY CESAREAN DELIVERY (*Continued*)

Recommendations: Safe Prevention of the Primary Cesarean Delivery (CD)
Fetal Heart Rate Monitoring
Consider amnioinfusion for repetitive variable fetal heart rate decelerations
Scalp stimulation can assess fetal acid-base status
Induction of Labor (IOL)
If <41-0/7 weeks, IOL generally performed for maternal/fetal indications
If ≥41-0/7 weeks, IOL generally performed to reduce risk of CD/perinatal morbidity and mortality
Cervical ripening methods should be utilized if cervix is unfavorable
Before diagnosing failed IOL (*if maternal/fetal status allows*): • Allow longer latent phase (up to ≥24 hours) • Require oxytocin use for at least 12-18 hours after membrane rupture
Other
Assess fetal presentation beginning at 36-0/7 weeks to allow for external cephalic version
Limit offering CD for suspected fetal macrosomia unless estimated fetal weight is: • ≥5000 g in diabetics • ≥4500 g in nondiabetics
Counsel patients on Institute of Medicine weight guidelines to avoid excessive weight gain
In twin gestation, if presentation is either cephalic/cephalic or cephalic/noncephalic, women should be counseled to attempt vaginal delivery. Outcomes are not improved with CD

Used with permission from ACOG/SMFM Obstetric Care Consensus No. 1: Safe Prevention of the Primary Cesarean Delivery. *Obstet Gynecol*. 2014;123:693–711. Copyright © 2014 Lippincott Williams & Wilkins.

Timing of Delivery

Terminology

Preterm	20-0/7–36-6/7
Late preterm	34-0/7–36-6/7
Early term	37-0/7–38-6/7
Full term	39-0/7–40-6/7
Late term	41-0/7–41-6/7
Post term	≥42-0/7

Background/Recommendations
- Medically Indicated *Late Preterm* and *Early Term* Delivery (Table 1-5)
  - *Early Term* Delivery
    - Non-medically indicated delivery before full term (39 weeks) is not appropriate
    - Differences in morbidity and mortality between neonates delivered at 37 (and 38) weeks compared with 39 weeks are consistent across multiple studies
    - Adverse neonatal outcomes in *Early Term* deliveries:

• Respiratory distress syndrome (RDS)	• NICU admission
• Transient tachypnea of the newborn	• Hypoglycemia
• Ventilator use	• 5-minute Apgar <7
• Pneumonia	• Neonatal mortality

  - Although greatest risks of *Early Term* delivery are respiratory, nonrespiratory morbidity is also increased. Documenting fetal lung maturity does NOT justify early nonindicated delivery
- *A reduction of nonindicated deliveries before 39 weeks should not be accompanied by an increase in expectant management of those with maternal or fetal indications for delivery before 39 weeks*
- *Late Term* and *Post Term*
  - Risk factors for *Post Term* (about 5% of pregnancies): Nulliparity, prior post term pregnancy, male fetus, maternal obesity, possible genetic predisposition, fetal disorders (anencephaly, placental sulfatase deficiency)

TABLE 1-5 MEDICALLY INDICATED LATE PRETERM AND EARLY TERM DELIVERIES

Condition	Delivery Timing
Placenta previa	36-0/7–37-6/7
Placenta previa and suspected accreta, increta, percreta	34-0/7–35-6/7
Prior classical CD	36-0/7–37-6/7
Prior myomectomy	37-0/7–38-6/7
IUGR (singleton) – otherwise uncomplicated	38-0/7–39-6/7
IUGR (singleton), with oligohydramnios, abnormal Dopplers, maternal co-morbidity (eg, preeclampsia, chronic hypertension)	34-0/7–37-6/7
Oligohydramnios	36-0/7–37-6/7
Preterm premature rupture of membranes	34-0/7
Maternal Hypertension	
• Chronic, controlled on no medications	38-0/7–39-6/7
• Chronic, controlled on medications	37-0/7–39-6/7
• Chronic, difficult to control	36-0/7–37-6/7
• Gestational	37-0/7–38-6/7
• Preeclampsia – severe	At diagnosis after 34-0/7
• Preeclampsia – mild	At diagnosis after 37-0/7
Maternal Diabetes	
• Pregestational, well controlled and no other complications	39-0/7–40-0/7
• Pregestational with vascular complications	37-0/7–39-6/7
• Pregestational, poorly controlled	Individualized
• Gestational, well controlled on diet or medications	39-0/7–41-0/7
• Gestational, poorly controlled	Individualized
Twins:	
• Di-Di twins	38-0/7–38-6/7
• Mono-Di twins	34-0/7–37-6/7
• Di-Di, isolated IUGR	36-0/7–37-6/7
• Di-Di, IUGR with abnormal Dopplers, maternal co-morbidity (eg, preeclampsia, chronic hypertension)	32-0/7–34-6/7
• Mono-Di, isolated IUGR	32-0/7–34-6/7

Data from ACOG Committee Opinion No. 560. Medically indicated late-preterm and early-term deliveries. April 2013. *Obstet Gynecol.* 2013;121:908–10.

- *Post Term* associated with increased perinatal morbidity and mortality
  - Neonatal convulsions, meconium aspiration syndrome, 5-minute Apgars <4, NICU admission
  - Increased risk of macrosomia (twofold), increasing risk of operative and CD, and shoulder dystocia
  - More frequent oligohydramnios (increasing risk of FHR abnormalities, meconium, umbilical cord pH <7)
  - Increased fetal mortality compared to 40 weeks
    41 weeks—1.5 fold; 42 weeks—1.8 fold; 43 weeks—2.9 fold
- *Post Term* associated with increased maternal risks:
  - Severe perineal lacerations, infection, postpartum hemorrhage, CD
- Trial of labor after cesarean (TOLAC) failure rate increases with GA
  - Before 40 weeks: 22.2% failure rate
  - After 41 weeks: 35.4% failure rate

- *Management*
  - Fetal testing: Start at 41-0/7 weeks. Insufficient data to define optimal type/frequency. Twice weekly modified biophysical profiles (BPPs) [Nonstress test (NST) + amniotic fluid index (AFI)] or BPPs are reasonable
  - Membrane sweeping reduces risk of *late term* and *post term*
  - Induce labor after 42-0/7 weeks

Induction of Labor (IOL)

- Although often stated that IOL increases rate of CD, the relationship between IOL and CD is controversial. Data are insufficient!
- When IOL is compared to expectant management, either NO difference in CD or a decreased risk of CD has been reported in women undergoing IOL
- Predictors of successful vaginal delivery: Multiparity, favorable cervix
- Cervical ripening methods should be used with an unfavorable cervix as they are associated with a lower rate of CD
- Latent phase is longer in IOL
- Elective IOL should not be performed before 39-0/7 weeks (increased neonatal morbidity and mortality)
- No consensus on IOL versus expectant management at full term (39-0/7–40-6/7 weeks)

Cervical Ripening
- No single definition to differentiate favorable from unfavorable
- *Bishop Scoring System* has been used (Table 1-6). Originally developed to predict likelihood of multiparous women at term to enter spontaneous labor. Generally
  - Favorable: Bishop's score >8 has same likelihood of vaginal delivery with IOL as spontaneous labor
  - Unfavorable: Bishop's score ≤6

TABLE 1-6 BISHOP SCORING SYSTEM

Score	Dilation (cm)	Effacement (%)	Station*	Consistency	Position
0	Closed	0–30	−3	Firm	Posterior
1	1–2	40–50	−2	Medium	Midposition
2	3–4	60–70	−1,0	Soft	Anterior
3	5–6	80	+1,+2	–	–

*Station reflects a −3 to +3 scale.
Used with permission from Bishop EH. Pelvic scoring for elective induction. *Obstet Gynecol* 1964;24:266–268.
Copyright © 1964 Lippincott Williams & Wilkins.

Methods of Cervical Ripening

Cervical Ripening Agents (ie, prostaglandins)

PGE₁–Misoprostol (Cytotec®)
- Effective for ripening and induction
- Most common complication is tachysystole (with or without FHR changes)
- Optimal dose and dosing interval not known
- *Contraindications*
  - Previous uterine scar
- *Administration*
  - Misoprostol 25 µg is placed in the **posterior fornix** of the vagina
  - Frequency of administration: Every 3–6 hours
  - Higher dose (50 µg) may be appropriate in certain cases; however, there is a greater risk of tachysystole
  - Oral dosing is possible (buccal, sublingual); however, limited data are available
  - Oxytocin should not be administered <4 hours after last misoprostol dose

PGE₂ – dinoprostone (Cervidil®, Prepidil®)
- **Cervidil®:** Dinoprostone 10 mg, timed-release vaginal insert, leave in up to 12 hours. Can remove if tachysystole or FHR abnormalities. Oxytocin may be started 30 minutes after removal
- **Prepidil®:** Dinoprostone 0.5 mg in 2.5 mL gel for endocervical administration. Repeat dose in 6–12 hours. Maximum dose 1.5 mg in 24 hours. Oxytocin should not be started prior to 6–12 hours after final dose
- *Contraindications*
  - Previous uterine scar
  - Caution if glaucoma, severe hepatic or renal dysfunction, or asthma

Mechanical Methods

- Directly dilate cervix
- Cause release of prostaglandins

Advantages	**Disadvantages**
• Low cost	• Possible increased risk of infection
• Lower risk of tachysystole	• Possible disruption of low-lying placenta
• Few systemic side effects	• Maternal discomfort

Balloon Catheters (Foley Bulb)

- *Contraindications*:
  - Placenta previa, vasa previa, low-lying placenta
- *Procedure*
  - Place using aseptic technique. Insert either under direct visualization (use ring forcep and pass through cervical os) or place similar to an intrauterine pressure catheter (IUPC)
  - Instill 30–60 mL saline into balloon; apply traction (tape to inner thigh)
  - If bleeding or resistance, discontinue
  - No consensus on management of Foley bulb in setting of ruptured membranes
  - Foley bulb *plus* oxytocin does not appear to shorten time to delivery when compared to Foley bulb alone

Osmotic Dilators

- *Laminaria Tents*
  - Absorb moisture and gradually expand
  - Removed after 12–24 hours
  - Designed for first and second trimester termination
  - No large-scale trials for term cervical ripening

Other Methods

Membrane Sweeping

- Increases likelihood of spontaneous labor within 48 hours. Insufficient data for recommendations if GBS (+)

Amniotomy

- Insufficient evidence on amniotomy alone for IOL; however, with oxytocin, may be shorter interval to delivery

Oxytocin Induction/Augmentation (at term)

- Gradual increase in uterine response to oxytocin from 20 to 30 weeks, then plateaus from 34 weeks until term. Sensitivity then increases with spontaneous labor
- Uterus responds within 3–5 minutes; steady level in plasma by 40 minutes
- Various protocols exist; institutions typically standardize their own protocols
  - Low-dose oxytocin protocols typically involve increases of 1–2 mU/min every 15–40 minutes.
  - High-dose oxytocin protocols may involve increases of 3–6 mU/min every 15–40 minutes
  - At Johns Hopkins, our high-dose protocol is 4 mU/min increases every 15 minutes
  - 40 mU/min is usually maximum dose
- Increase oxytocin per protocol until an adequate contraction pattern is achieved
- **Adequate labor in MVUs: 200**

SECOND TRIMESTER TERMINATIONS

- Dilation and evacuation (D&E) is associated with fewer complications than IOL
- Rare complications of both D&E and IOL include hemorrhage, cervical laceration, retained products of conception, infection; uterine perforation in D&E; and uterine rupture in IOL
- IOL may be preferable at times (fetal anomalies, genetic disorders)—intact fetus
- Adding mifepristone, a progesterone receptor antagonist that primes the uterus and cervix, appears to shorten expulsion time
- With IOL, consider premedicating for fever/nausea/vomiting/diarrhea. IV PCA or epidural for pain management
- See Table 1-7 for IOL regimens for second trimester termination of pregnancy

TABLE 1-7 REGIMENS FOR SECOND TRIMESTER MEDICAL ABORTION

	ACOG (up to 26 weeks)	Society of Family Planning (24–28 weeks)
Mifepristone **Plus** **Misoprostol**	• Mifepristone 200 mg orally *24–48 hours later administer either:* • Misoprostol 800 μg PV, then 400 μg PV or SL every 3 hours (maximum 5 doses)[1] • Misoprostol 400 μg buccally every 3 hours (maximum 5 doses)	• Mifepristone 200 mg or 600 mg orally *36–48 hours later*[4]: Misoprostol 200 μg or 400 μg every 4 hours[3] (24-hour expulsion rate of 80–97%; mean expulsion time 8.5–13.6 hours]
Misoprostol	• Misoprostol 400 ug PV or SL[2] every 3 hours (maximum 5 doses)[1] • Vaginal loading dose of misoprostol 600–800 μg followed by 400 μg PV or SL every 3 hours may be more effective	• Misoprostol 100 μg or 200 μg PV every 4 hours[3] (24-hour expulsion rate of 84–100%; mean expulsion time 10–11 hours)
Oxytocin (if misoprostol not available)	• Oxytocin 20–100 units IV over 3 hours, followed by 1 hour without oxytocin to allow diuresis. Slowly increase to a maximum of 300 units over 3 hours[5]	

PV = per vagina
SL = sublingual
[1]If not complete after five doses, allow patient to rest for 12 hours before restarting cycle.
[2]Vaginal dosage is superior to sublingual for nulliparous women.
[3]Higher doses of misoprostol (400 μg with misoprostol alone and 600 μg with mifepristone-misoprostol) appear safe but do not clearly decrease expulsion time. Most studies used vaginal administration.
Consider 200 μg or less per dose of misoprostol if prior uterine scar.
[4]May consider a shorter interval, such as 24 hours.
[5]High-dose oxytocin is not commonly used because of inefficient uterine response in second trimester.
Data from ACOG Second-trimester abortion. Practice Bulletin no. 135, June 2013; Society of Family Planning interruption of nonviable pregnancies of 24–28 weeks' gestation using medical methods. SFP Guideline #20133. *Contraception* 2013:88:341–349.

Examples of High-Dose Oxytocin Protocols (may be used in women with prior uterine scar)

- 14-0/7–26-0/7 weeks: Oxytocin 200 units in 500 mL NS at 50 mL/h (20 units/h)
  - Place laminaria prior to starting oxytocin
  - High doses for prolonged periods of time can lead to water retention and hyponatremia
  - Check electrolytes after 7–12 hours
- 26-1/7–28-0/7: Oxytocin 200 units in 500 mL NS at 25 mL/h (10 units/h)

After Fetus Delivers

- If placenta has NOT delivered: Can start Oxytocin 40 units in 100 mL NS at 50 mL/h
- If D&C, *antibiotic prophylaxis* with doxycycline (100 mg IV) or cefazolin (2 g IV)

OPERATIVE VAGINAL DELIVERIES

- Rates are declining
- Account for approximately 3.6% of births in the United States (vacuum:forceps is 4:1)
- Failure to result in delivery: Forceps 0.4%; vacuum 0.8%
- Fetal (nonreassuring fetal status) and maternal (exhaustion, prolonged second stage, maternal comorbidities such as heart disease) indications
- Do not switch from vacuum to forceps or vice-versa due to increased neonatal morbidity

Prior to performing, ensure
- Fetal position and station
- Adequate maternal anesthesia
- Empty maternal bladder
- Personnel for neonatal resuscitation are available if needed

Vacuum-Assisted Deliveries

- Contraindicated if under 34 weeks gestation or estimated fetal weight is <2500 g
- A maximum of three "pop-offs," three sets of pulls, and/or a total vacuum application time of 15–30 minutes is commonly recommended. No data-based guidelines are available

- *Application* (Figure 1-5)
  - Apply at "flexion point"—center of cup approximately 3 cm in front of posterior fontanelle and 6 cm from anterior fontanelle
  - Avoid placing over fontanelles
  - Palpate around entire cup after placement to verify maternal tissue is not under cup
  - Consider lowering suction level between contractions
  - Do not attempt to rotate the fetal head or use rocking movements
  - Maximum suction pressure should not exceed 600 mm Hg
- *Fetal risks* (Figure 1-6)
  - Retinal hemorrhages (20–40%)
  - Superficial abrasions (10%)
  - Cephalohematoma (delineated by suture lines, limited in size) (14–16%)
- *Clinically significant fetal risks*
  - Subgaleal hemorrhage (2.6–4.5%). Bleeding not contained by sutures
  - Intracranial hemorrhage (<0.5%)
  - Skull fracture (<0.5%)

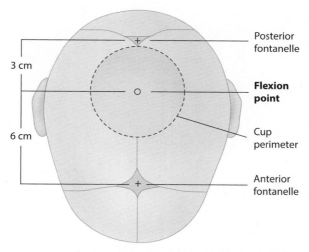

Figure 1-5 Application of vacuum. (Used with permission from Cunningham F, Leveno KJ, Bloom SL, et al. Chapter 29. Operative vaginal delivery. In: Cunningham F, Leveno KJ, Bloom SL, et al., eds. *Williams Obstetrics*. 24th ed. New York, NY: McGraw-Hill; 2013.)

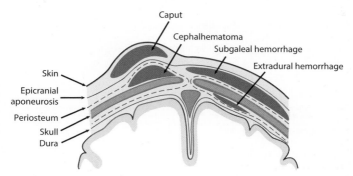

Figure 1-6 Sites of extracranial bleeding in the newborn. (Used with permission from Rosenberg AA, Grover T. Chapter 2. The newborn infant. In: Hay WW, Jr., Levin MJ, Deterding RR, Abzug MJ, eds. *Current Diagnosis & Treatment: Pediatrics*. 22nd ed. New York, NY: McGraw-Hill; 2013.)

Forceps-Assisted Deliveries

Application (Figure 1-7)

- Sagittal suture should be perpendicular to the plane of the forcep shanks
- Posterior fontanelle should be midway between blades and one finger's breadth above plane of shanks
- With fenestrated blades, a small but equal amount of fenestration should be felt on each blade

Risks

- Facial nerve injury (<0.5%)
- Cephalohematoma (2%)
- Depressed skull fracture
- Maternal: Third and fourth degree lacerations (13–44%)

A

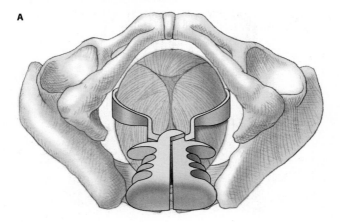

B

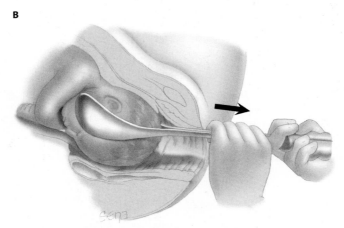

Figure 1-7 Forceps placement. **A.** The forceps are symmetrically placed and articulated. **B.** The direction of gentle traction for delivery of the head is indicated (*arrow*). (Used with permission from Cunningham F, Leveno KJ, Bloom SL, et al. Chapter 29. Operative vaginal delivery. In: Cunningham F, Leveno KJ, Bloom SL, et al., eds. *Williams Obstetrics*. 24th ed. New York, NY: McGraw-Hill; 2013.)

Classification of Forceps Deliveries (Table 1-8)

- *Classical instruments*
  - **Elliot type**
    - Overlapping shanks
    - Short, rounder cephalic curve

- Best for round, unmolded heads, no caput
- Examples: Tucker–McLane, Elliot
- **Simpson type**
  - Parallel, separated shanks
  - Long, tapering cephalic curve
  - Fit better on longer, molded heads
  - Examples: DeLee, Irving

TABLE 1-8 CLASSIFICATION OF FORCEPS DELIVERIES ACCORDING TO STATION AND ROTATION

Type	Classification
Outlet	• Scalp is visible at the introitus without separating labia • Fetal skull has reached pelvic floor • Sagittal suture is in anteroposterior diameter, ROA, LOA, ROP, LOP • Fetal head is at or on perineum • Rotation does not exceed 45 degrees
Low	• Leading point of fetal skull at station ≥ +2 cm, and not on pelvic floor, and • Rotation ≤45 degrees (LOA or ROA to OA, or LOP or ROP to OP) OR • Rotation >45 degrees
Mid	• Station above +2 cm but head engaged • Station is between 0 and +2 cm
High	• Not in classification

OA = occiput anterior; OP = occiput posterior; R = right; L = left.
Used with permission from Cunningham F, et al. Chapter 29. Operative Vaginal Delivery. In: Cunningham F, et al., eds. *Williams Obstetrics*, 24th ed. New York, NY: McGraw-Hill; 2013.

EPISIOTOMY/LACERATION

Perineal Laceration Definitions

First degree	Superficial laceration of vaginal mucosa. May extend into skin at introitus
Second degree	Laceration that involves the vaginal mucosa and perineal body. May extend to the transverse perineal muscles and requires repair
Third degree	Laceration that extends into the muscle of the perineum and may involve the transverse perineal muscles and external anal sphincter. Does not involve rectal mucosa
Fourth degree	Involves rectal mucosa

Episiotomy

- Per ACOG, "The best available data do not support liberal or routine use of episiotomy ... there is a place for episiotomy for maternal or fetal indications, such as avoiding severe maternal lacerations or facilitating or expediting difficult deliveries"
- *Types*
  - **Median: "Midline"** (Figure 1-8)
    - Place fingers between fetal head and perineum. Incise 2–3 cm aiming at 6:00
    - Extends to the transverse perineal muscles
    - Easier repair; better healing
    - Greater risk of extension into a third or fourth degree
  - **Mediolateral: 45 degrees from midline**
    - Similar technique with scissors aimed at 5:00 or 7:00, toward ipsilateral ischial tuberosity
    - Bulbospongiosus is main muscle that is incised
    - More difficult to repair
    - Increased blood loss
    - Increased pain

Laceration Repair

- **Antibiotic** prophylaxis should be considered with third and fourth degree repairs—single dose of a second-generation cephalosporin or clindamycin if allergic to penicillin

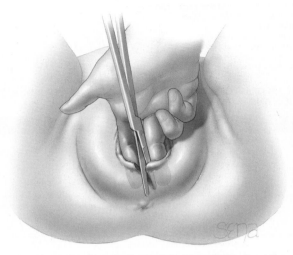

Figure 1-8 Midline episiotomy. (Used with permission from Cunningham F, Leveno KJ, Bloom SL, et al. Chapter 27. Vaginal delivery. In: Cunningham F, Leveno KJ, Bloom SL, et al., eds. *Williams Obstetrics*. 24th ed. New York, NY: McGraw-Hill; 2013.)

Third Degree Laceration Repair - See Figure 1-9

- *End-End Repair*
  - Grasp ends of the external anal sphincter muscle and capsule with Allis clamps
  - Place interrupted sutures at the 3:00, 6:00, 9:00, and 12:00 positions through the capsule of the sphincter. Place the inferior and posterior sutures first
  - Repair second degree in typical fashion
  - *Overlapping Repair*
  - Alternative method
  - Current data do not suggest this repair provides superior results compared to end-end

Fourth Degree Laceration Repair - See Figure 1-9

- Identify apex
  - For rectal mucosa, use 4-0 suture in running or locking fashion. Should not penetrate mucosal layer. Place reinforcing layer through rectal muscularis (3-0 suture) in running or interrupted fashion
  - Repair third degree as above

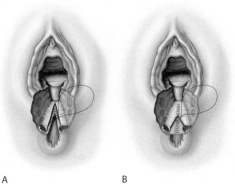

A   B

Figure 1-9 Laceration repair. **A.** Reapproximate anorectal mucosa and submucosa in a running or interrupted fashion using 4–0 chromic or Vicryl. Place sutures approximately 0.5 cm apart down to the anal verge. **B.** A second layer is placed through the rectal muscularis using 3–0 Vicryl in a running or interrupted fashion. This "reinforcing layer" should incorporate the torn ends of the internal anal sphincter, the glistening white fibrous structure between the anal canal submucosa and the fibers of the external anal sphincter (EAS). The internal sphincter may retract laterally.

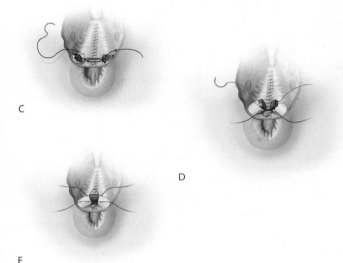

Figure 1-9 (*Continued*) C. End-to-end approximation of the EAS: a suture is placed through the EAS muscle, and four to six interrupted 2–0 or 3–0 Vicryl sutures are placed at the 3, 6, 9, and 12 o'clock positions through the connective tissue capsule of the sphincter. Grasp EAS tissue with Allis clamps. Place posterior then inferior sutures first. D. Sutures through the EAS (*blue suture*) and inferior capsule wall. E. Sutures to reapproximate the anterior and superior walls of the EAS capsule. Complete repair as typical second degree laceration (not shown). Place anchor stitch above the wound apex using 2–0 or 3–0 suture (Vicryl) and reapproximate vaginal mucosa with interlocking stitches. After reapproximating the hymenal ring, the needle and suture are positioned to close the perineal incision and a continuous closure with absorbable 2–0 or 3–0 suture is used to close the fascia and muscles of the incised perineum. The continuous suture is then carried upward as a subcuticular stitch. The final knot is tied proximal to the hymenal ring. (Used with permission from Cunningham F, Leveno KJ, Bloom SL, et al. Chapter 27. Vaginal Delivery. In: Cunningham F, Leveno KJ, Bloom SL, et al., eds. *Williams Obstetrics*. 24th ed. New York, NY: McGraw-Hill; 2013.

VAGINAL BIRTH AFTER CESAREAN (VBAC)

Terminology

- *Trial of labor (TOL) or trial of labor after cesarean (TOLAC):* A planned attempt to labor by a woman with a previous CD
- *VBAC:* Vaginal birth after cesarean; successful trial of labor
- *Unsuccessful or failed TOL:* CD after a TOL
- *Elective repeat CD:* Planned CD in woman with one or more prior CDs

Success Rates

- Evidence suggests that women with at least a 60–70% chance of VBAC have equal or less maternal morbidity when they undergo TOLAC than women undergoing repeat CD. If less than 60% chance of success, more chance of morbidity with TOLAC
- **Success rates** for trials of labor are consistently high (*overall: 60–80%*)
- *VBAC Calculator:* https://mfmunetwork.bsc.gwu.edu/PublicBSC/MFMU/VGBirthCalc/vagbirth.html
- Factors Associated with Increased Success
  - Prior vaginal birth
  - Spontaneous labor
  - Nonrecurring indication (ie, breech)
  - Birth weight <4000 g
  - Prior successful VBAC. *Rate of VBAC increases with each prior VBAC.*
    - No prior SVD: 63% VBAC
    - Prior SVD before CD: 83% VBAC
    - Prior VBAC: 94% VBAC
- Factors Associated with Decreased Success
  - Recurrent indication for initial CD (ie, second stage arrest)
  - Increased maternal age
  - Nonwhite ethnicity
  - GA >40 weeks

- Maternal obesity
- Preeclampsia
- Short interpregnancy interval
- Increased neonatal birth weight
- Labor augmentation/induction

Uterine Rupture

- *Uterine rupture*: Complete separation of all uterine layers leading to possible fetal or maternal compromise
- *Uterine scar dehiscence*: Often an occult scar separation with intact uterine serosa; does not lead to fetal or maternal compromise
- Rate of *symptomatic* uterine rupture for women who undergo TOL: 0.7–0.8%. See Table 1-9 for Rates of Uterine Rupture according to prior uterine incision type
- Low vertical uterine incision: LIMITED DATA. ACOG says likely same success rate as low transverse; NIH says "increased" risk of rupture
- *Unknown* scar: Only a problem if high clinical suspicion of previous classical CD
- Women with **more than one prior CD**
  - *Per ACOG:* Limited data; however, it is reasonable to attempt TOLAC in patients with two previous CDs. One large study showed no increase in uterine rupture rates with multiple prior CDs (0.9% versus 0.7% with one CD); another found increase from 0.9% with one prior CD to 1.8% with two prior CDs
- **Labor augmentation/induction**
  - Oxytocin: Possible increase in risk of rupture (up to 1.5% versus 0.8% with spontaneous labor)
  - Misoprostol: Increased risk of rupture
- **Single versus double layer uterine closure:** conflicting data; studies suggest possible decreased uterine rupture in 2 layer closure versus 1 layer closure
- **Twins:** Similar outcomes to singletons. No increased risk

Signs of Uterine Rupture
  - *Nonreassuring* FHR pattern with decelerations or bradycardia
  - Loss of station
  - Hypovolemia
  - New onset intense uterine pain
  - Vaginal bleeding

Miscellaneous

- No data suggest monitoring with IUPC is superior to external monitoring to prevent uterine rupture
- External cephalic version (ECV) is not contraindicated in women with prior CD if appropriate candidate for TOLAC and ECV
- Effective regional anesthesia may be used and will not mask signs and symptoms of uterine rupture
- TOLAC should be undertaken at facilities equipped to perform immediate emergency deliveries

TABLE 1-9 RATES OF UTERINE RUPTURE

Prior Incision Type	Rupture Rate (%)
Low transverse	0.5–1.0
Low vertical	0.8–1.1
Classical or "T"	4–9

PLACENTA PREVIA

- Terminology
  - **Low-Lying Placenta**
    - Placental edge within 2 cm of internal os
    - Follow-up ultrasound recommended at 32 weeks gestation
    - Vaginal delivery more likely if placental edge is 10–20 mm from os
  - **Placenta Previa**
    - Placenta covers internal os
    - Follow-up ultrasound recommended at 32 weeks gestation
    - Incidence of placenta previa: 1:200 births

- Risk factors for placenta previa: **Previous CD**, maternal age, smoking, multiples, multiparity, previous uterine curettage
- Placenta covers os in about 5% of pregnancies midpregnancy; the majority resolve when the upper third of cervix develops into lower uterine segment; placenta "migrates" away
- Presentation: Painless vaginal bleeding (most commonly around 34 weeks)
- On 32 week follow-up ultrasound: If still low-lying or previa, follow-up transvaginal ultrasound recommended at 36 weeks

PLACENTA ACCRETA

- **Definitions:** Abnormal attachment of the placenta to the uterine wall. See Figure 1-10
  - *Accreta:* General term used to describe condition when placenta invades and is inseparable from uterine wall
  - *Increta:* Invasion into myometrium
  - *Percreta:* Invasion through myometrium and serosa, occasionally into adjacent organs such as the **bladder**
- Occurs in approximately 3:1000 deliveries
- *Risk Factors*
  - Placenta previa, especially if prior CD (Table 1-10)
  - Prior uterine surgery
  - Increasing parity
  - Maternal age >35
- *Diagnosis*
  - Ultrasound
    - Sensitivity: 77%
    - Specificity: 96%
    - Positive predictive value: 65%
    - Negative predictive value: 98%
  - MRI
    - Sensitivity and specificity are comparable with ultrasound
    - May be useful to determine extent of invasion and involvement of abdominal/adnexal structures or when ultrasound is nondiagnostic

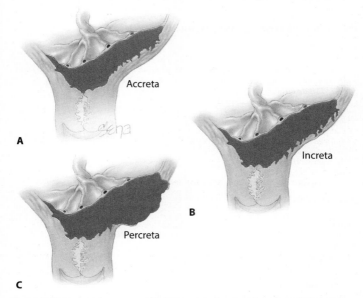

Figure 1-10 Placenta accreta, increta, percreta. (Used with permission from Cunningham F, Leveno KJ, Bloom SL, et al. Chapter 41. Obstetrical hemorrhage. In: Cunningham F, Leveno KJ, Bloom SL, et al., eds. *Williams Obstetrics.* 24th ed. New York, NY: McGraw-Hill; 2013.)

TABLE 1-10 PRIOR CESAREAN DELIVERIES AND ACCRETA RISK

Number of Prior Cesarean Deliveries	Accreta Risk (%)	
	Previa	No Previa
1	3.3	0.03
2	11	0.2
3	40	0.1
4	61	0.8
5	67	0.8
≥6	67	4.7

Data from Silver RM, Landon MB, Rouse DJ, et al. Maternal morbidity associated with multiple repeat cesarean deliveries. *Obstet Gynecol.* 2006;107:1226; ACOG Committee Opinion #529. Placenta accreta, July 2012.

- **Prognosis**
  - Average blood loss at delivery is 3–5 L
  - 90% require blood transfusion
  - 40% require more than 10 units of packed red blood cells
  - About two-thirds require cesarean hysterectomy
  - Maternal mortality is as high as 7%
- **Management of suspected placenta accreta**
  - Timing of delivery must be individualized. PLANNED delivery is associated with fewer complications and less blood loss
  - Multidisciplinary team, including pelvic surgeon (eg, gynecologic oncologist)
  - **Maternal and neonatal outcome is optimized in stable patients with planned delivery at 34 weeks without amniocentesis for FLM**
  - Avoid manual removal of placenta. Leave placenta in situ → hysterectomy

GROUP B STREPTOCOCCUS (GBS) PROPHYLAXIS

Early-Onset GBS

- Infection in newborn within first week of life. (*Late Onset* GBS—infant older than 6 days)
- *Leading infectious cause of morbidity and mortality in infants in the United States*
- Mortality higher among preterm (about 20–30% if ≤33 weeks versus 2–3% in full term)
- Risk factors for early-onset GBS disease in infants
  - Maternal genital tract colonization (10–30% of pregnant women)
  - GBS UTI any time during pregnancy (2–7% of women). Surrogate for heavy maternal colonization (even if vaginal-rectal swab is negative)
  - GA less than 37-0/7 weeks
  - Prolonged rupture of membranes (≥18 hours)
  - Intra-amniotic infection (≥38.0 C)
  - Young maternal age
  - Black race
  - Previous delivery of infant with invasive GBS disease

Testing for GBS

- *Collect at 35–37 weeks* GA in all women unless diagnosed with GBS bacteriuria in this pregnancy or previous infant with invasive GBS disease
  - Swab lower vagina (introitus), followed by the rectum (through anal sphincter)
- If planned CD
  - Patients should still undergo routine screening for GBS at 35–37 weeks. Onset of labor or rupture of membranes (ROM) may occur before the planned CD
  - Administer antibiotics *IF* labor/ROM
- Results good for 5 weeks

Neonatal Perspective

- Appropriate antibiotics ≥4 hours before delivery highly effective. Shorter duration (≥2 hours) may provide some protection
- No *medically indicated* obstetric procedure should be delayed to achieve 4 hours of prophylaxis prior to delivery

Antibiotics for GBS Prophylaxis (Table 1-11)

- Indications for prophylaxis (Table 1-11)
- Antibiotic recommendations (Figure 1-11)
  - Penicillin is the agent of choice; ampicillin is an acceptable alternative
  - Increasing resistance to erythromycin (25–32%) and clindamycin (13–20%)
    - Erythromycin NO LONGER recommended
- Algorithm for GBS Prophylaxis in Preterm Labor (Figure 1-12)

TABLE 1-11 ANTIBIOTIC PROPHYLAXIS FOR GBS

Intrapartum GBS Prophylaxis Indicated	Intrapartum GBS Prophylaxis Not Indicated

• Previous infant with invasive GBS disease
• GBS bacteriuria in current pregnancy
• Positive GBS screening culture during current pregnancy
• Unknown GBS status (culture not done, incomplete, results unknown) AND any of
  • Delivery at less than 37 weeks
  • Membrane rupture ≥18 hours
  • Intrapartum temperature ≥100.4 (38.0°C)*
  • Intrapartum NAAT† positive for GBS
	• GBS colonization or bacteriuria during previous pregnancy, unless positive in this pregnancy
	• Negative vaginal/rectal GBS culture at 35–37 weeks, regardless of intrapartum risk factors
	• CD performed before onset of labor or membrane rupture (regardless of maternal GBS status or GA)

*If amnionitis suspected, broad-spectrum antibiotics that include an agent known to treat GBS should replace GBS prophylaxis.
†NAAT (nucleic acid amplification tests) testing is optional and may not be available in all settings. If result is negative, but any other intrapartum risk factor is present then *antibiotic prophylaxis is indicated.*

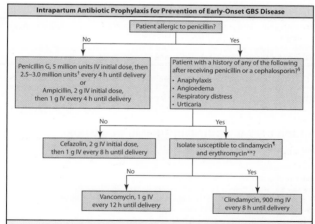

Figure 1-11 Antibiotics for GBS prophylaxis. (Used with permission from Ogle JW, Anderson MS. Chapter 42. Infections: Bacterial & Spirochetal. In: Hay WW, Jr., Levin MJ, Deterding RR, Abzug MJ, eds. *Current Diagnosis & Treatment: Pediatrics.* 22nd ed. New York, NY: McGraw-Hill; 2013.)

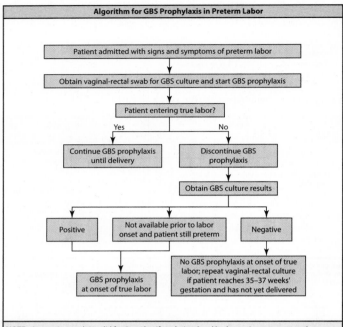

Figure 1-12 GBS prophylaxis in preterm labor—algorithm. (Used with permission from Ogle JW, Anderson MS. Chapter 42. Infections: Bacterial & Spirochetal. In: Hay WW, Jr., Levin MJ, Deterding RR, Abzug MJ, eds. *Current Diagnosis & Treatment: Pediatrics*. 22nd ed. New York, NY: McGraw-Hill; 2013.)

ELECTRONIC FETAL MONITORING (NICHD WORKSHOP)

Definitions

Uterine Contractions

- Number of contractions in a 10-minute window, averaged over 30 minutes
  - *Normal:* ≤5 contractions in 10 minutes, averaged over a 30-minute window
  - *Tachysystole:* >5 contractions in 10 minutes averaged over a 30-minute window
    - Always note presence/absence of associated FHR decelerations
    - Applies to both spontaneous and induced labor
  - The terms *hyperstimulation* and *hypercontractility* are not defined and should be abandoned!

Fetal Heart Rate Patterns

Baseline: Mean FHR (rounded to 5 bpm) in 10-minute window, excluding accels, decels, and periods of marked variability (>25 bpm). Baseline must be for at least 2 (not necessarily contiguous) minutes in any 10-minute segment

- Normal: 110–160 bpm
- Tachycardia: >160 bpm for 10 minutes or longer
- Bradycardia: <110 bpm for 10 minutes or longer

Variability: Fluctuations in baseline FHR that are irregular in amplitude and frequency

- Absent: Amplitude from peak to trough undetectable
- Minimal: Amplitude from peak to trough detectable but ≤5 bpm
- Moderate: Amplitude from peak to trough 6–25 bpm
- Marked: Amplitude from peak to trough >25

Accelerations: Abrupt increase (onset to peak <30 seconds) in the FHR

- At ≥32 weeks, acceleration has peak of ≥15 bpm above baseline, with a duration of ≥15 seconds but <2 minutes from onset to return
- Before 32 weeks, acceleration has peak of ≥10 bpm above baseline, with a duration of ≥10 seconds but <2 minutes from onset to return
- *Prolonged acceleration*: ≥2 minutes and <10 minutes
- If an acceleration lasts >10 minutes it is a baseline change

Decelerations: Decrease in FHR associated with contractions or other physiologic events. Periodic decelerations are abrupt (peak <30 seconds) or gradual (peak >30 seconds); *recurrent* if occur with ≥50% of contractions in any 20-minute window; *intermittent* if occur in less than 50% of contractions (see Figure 1-13)

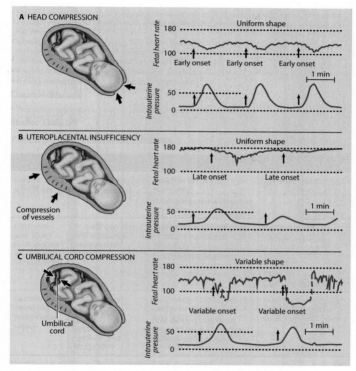

Figure 1-13 Fetal heart rate decelerations. (Used with permission from Frölich MA. Chapter 41. Obstetric anesthesia. In: Butterworth JF, IV, Mackey DC, Wasnick JD, eds. *Morgan & Mikhail's Clinical Anesthesiology*. 5th ed. New York, NY: McGraw-Hill; 2013.)

Early Deceleration
- Usually symmetrical, **gradual** decrease and return of FHR associated with a contraction
- From the onset to the FHR nadir of ≥30 seconds
- Nadir of deceleration occurs at the same time as peak of contraction
- Decrease ≤15 bpm below FHR baseline
- In most cases, onset, nadir, and recovery are coincident with the beginning, peak, and end of contraction
- Due to head compression

Late Deceleration
- Usually symmetrical, **gradual** decrease and return of FHR associated with a contraction
- From the onset to FHR nadir reached of ≥30 seconds
- Deceleration is delayed in timing—nadir occurs after peak of contraction
- In most cases, onset, nadir, and recovery occur after the beginning, peak, and end of contraction
- Reflect transient or chronic uteroplacental insufficiency

Variable Deceleration
- **Abrupt** decrease in FHR—from the onset to FHR nadir of <30 seconds
- Decrease in FHR is ≥15 bpm, lasting ≥15 seconds, and <2 minutes duration
- If progress to greater depth and longer duration, more indicative of impending fetal acidemia
- Due to cord or head compression. Can occur at any time
- When associated with contractions, onset, depth, and duration may vary

Prolonged Deceleration
- Visually apparent decrease in FHR below the baseline
- Decrease in FHR is ≥15 bpm, lasting ≥2 minutes, but <10 minutes
- If lasts ≥10 minutes or longer, it is a baseline change

Sinusoidal Pattern: Smooth, sine wave–like undulating pattern with a cycle frequency of 3–5 per minute which persists for ≥20 minutes
- Ominous pattern; seen with chronic fetal anemia
- Actual FHR baseline is indeterminable and baseline variability is absent/minimal
- Pseudosinusoidal pattern seen when narcotics given in labor

Fetal Tachycardia: Potential causes: Chorioamnionitis, pyelonephritis, other maternal infections, medications (terbutaline, cocaine, stimulants), hyperthyroidism, placental abruption, fetal bleeding, fetal tachyarrhythmias

Prolonged Decelerations/Fetal Bradycardia: Potential causes: Maternal hypotension (post-epidural), umbilical cord prolapse/occlusion, rapid fetal descent, tachysystole, placental abruption, uterine rupture, congenital heart abnormalities

Minimal Variability: Potential causes: Maternal medications (opioids, magnesium sulfate), fetal sleep cycle (20–60 minutes), fetal acidemia

INTERPRETATION OF FETAL HEART RATE TRACINGS

Three-Tier System (Table 1-12)

TABLE 1-12 FETAL HEART RATE INTERPRETATION SYSTEM

Category I	Baseline: 110–160 bpm
	Baseline FHR variability: moderate
	Late or variable decelerations: absent
	Early decelerations: present or absent
	Accelerations: present or absent
Category II	Baseline rate
	• Bradycardia not accompanied by absent variability
	• Tachycardia
	Baseline FHR variability
	• Minimal baseline variability
	• Absent baseline variability not accompanied by recurrent decelerations
	• Marked baseline variability
	Accelerations
	• Absence of induced accelerations after fetal stimulation
	Periodic or episodic decelerations
	• Recurrent variable decelerations accompanied by minimal or moderate variability
	• Prolonged decelerations ≥2 minutes but <10 minutes
	• Recurrent late decelerations with moderate baseline variability
	• Variable decelerations with other characteristics, ie, slow return to baseline, "overshoots," or "shoulders"
Category III	Absent baseline FHR variability and any of the following:
	• Recurrent late decelerations
	• Recurrent variable decelerations
	• Bradycardia
	Sinusoidal pattern

Management of Fetal Heart Rate Tracings
Category I
- Reassuring
- Continue expectant management

Category II

- Require evaluation, continued surveillance, initiation of appropriate corrective measures, and reevaluation.
- FHR accelerations and/or moderate variability are highly predictive of normal fetal acid–base status

Category III

- Abnormal; increased risk for fetal acidemia
- Associated with increased risk for neonatal encephalopathy, cerebral palsy (CP), neonatal acidosis
- Predictive value for abnormal neurologic outcome is poor
- If unresolved by intrauterine resuscitative measures (Table 1-13), typically requires expeditious delivery

TABLE 1-13 RESUSCITATIVE MEASURES FOR CATEGORY II OR CATEGORY III TRACINGS

Goal	Associated Fetal Heart Rate Abnormality[a]	Potential Intervention(s)[b]
Improve fetal oxygenation and uteroplacental blood flow	• Recurrent late decelerations • Prolonged decelerations or bradycardia • Minimal or absent FHR variability	• Initial lateral decubitus positioning • Administer maternal oxygen • Administer IV fluid bolus • Reduce uterine contraction frequency
Take steps to diminish uterine activity	• Tachysystole with category II or III tracing	• Discontinue oxytocin or prostaglandins • Tocolytics, e.g., terbutaline
Relieve umbilical cord compression	• Recurrent variable decelerations • Prolonged decelerations or bradycardia	• Reposition mother • Amnioinfusion • With prolapse of cord, manually elevate the presenting part while preparing for immediate delivery

[a]Simultaneous evaluation of the suspected cause(s) is also an important step in management of abnormal FHR tracings.
[b]The combination of multiple interventions simultaneously may be appropriate and potentially more effective than doing them individually or serially.
FHR = fetal heart rate.
Used with permission from Cunningham F, et al. Chapter 24. Intrapartum Assessment. In: Cunningham F, et al., eds. *Williams Obstetrics*, 24th ed. New York, NY: McGraw-Hill; 2013.

Miscellaneous

- Vibroacoustic stimulation (VAS): Position on maternal abdomen. Apply stimulus for 1–2 seconds. If response is not elicited, may repeat up to three times for progressively longer durations of up to 3 seconds. If acceleration of 10 beats for 10 seconds, scalp pH is at least 7.20
- When fetal scalp stimulation is followed by an acceleration of 15 bpm lasting 15 seconds, the fetal pH value is at least 7.20

NEWBORN ASSESSMENT/COMPLICATIONS

Apgar Scores (Table 1-14)

- Clinical tool to assess clinical status of newborn and response to resuscitative measures
- Affected by many factors: Maternal sedation, anesthesia, congenital malformations, trauma, interobserver variability, infection, cardiorespiratory conditions
- Five-minute Apgar has prognostic significance for survival. A score of 0–3 at 5 minutes correlates with neonatal mortality but does not predict later neurologic dysfunction

TABLE 1-14 APGAR SCORES

Sign	Apgar Score		
	0 Point	1 Point	2 Points
Heart rate	Absent	<100 bpm	≥100 bpm
Respiratory effort	Absent	Weak cry, hypoventilation	Good, crying
Muscle tone	Limp	Some extremity flexion	Active motion
Reflex irritability	No response	Grimace	Cry or active withdrawal
Color	Blue, pale	Acrocyanotic (body pink, extremities blue)	Completely pink

- Not intended to define asphyxia injury or predict neurological outcome; however, low Apgar scores at 5 and 10 minutes confer an increased relative risk of CP. Yet most infants with low Apgar scores will not develop CP
- If 5-minute Apgar is $\geq$7, unlikely that peripartum hypoxia-ischemia played a major role in causing neonatal encephalopathy

Umbilical Cord Blood Gases

- Umbilical cord artery metabolic acidemia has a relatively weak predictive value for longer-term complications, such as neonatal encephalopathy or CP
- Neonatal arterial blood gases obtained within 1 hour after birth can be interpreted in a similar fashion to umbilical cord arterial blood gas samples
- *Obtaining Umbilical Cord Gases*
  - Both arterial and venous should be sampled to ensure artery has been sampled
  - Doubly clamp cord. If delay in obtaining is more than 20 minutes, store on ice. Interpret base deficit with caution
  - pH, Po_2, and Pco_2 values remain essentially unchanged for up to 60 minutes in clamped vessels
- If umbilical artery pH >7.2, unlikely that intrapartum hypoxia played a role in causing neonatal encephalopathy
- **Umbilical artery pH <7.0 or base deficit $\geq$12.0 mmol/L** increases chances that neonatal encephalopathy (if present) had an intrapartum hypoxic component
- **Base deficit 12–16 mmol/L:** 10% with moderate-severe complications
- **Base deficit >16 mmol/L:** 40% with moderate to severe complications
- Is a continuum of increasing risk of neonatal encephalopathy with worsening acidemia. Even with significant acidemia, most newborns will be neurologically normal

Respiratory Distress Syndrome (RDS)

- Primarily from a deficiency of pulmonary surfactant (produced by Type II pneumocytes), which increases surface tension, causing collapse of small alveoli and overinflation of large alveoli
- Major cause of morbidity and mortality in preterm infants
- *Incidence* (Table 1-15)
  - Increased risk if male or Caucasian (compared with Asian, Black, Hispanic)
  - Increased risk if delivered by CD
  - **Elective CD at term**
    - Compared to delivery at 39 weeks, the Odds Ratio of RDS with delivery at
      - 37 weeks is 4.2
      - 38 weeks is 2.1
- Administration of *antenatal corticosteroids* reduces risk of RDS by enhancing maturational changes. (See Preterm Labor (PTL) section for more information)
  - Reduction in RDS (relative risk: 0.66; thus 34% reduction)
  - Reduction in moderate to severe RDS (relative risk: 0.55)
  - In original study, maximum benefit occurred when delivered more than 48 hours but less than 7 days after administration
  - Minimal interval between administering steroids and delivery needed to achieve benefit is not yet known
  - Some studies suggest benefits may be seen after several hours

TABLE 1-15 INCIDENCE OF RDS BY GESTATIONAL AGE

Gestational Age (weeks)	% with RDS
22–26	94–98
27–28	86–90
30–31	<30
34	10.5
35	6.0
36	2.8
37	1.0
38–40	0.3

Numbers depend on population studied, etc.
Data from Stoll BJ, Hansen ni, Bell eF, et al. neonatal outcomes of extremely preterm infants from the nicHD neonatal Research network. *Pediatrics*. 2010;126:443–456; the consortium on Safe Labor. Respiratory morbidity in late preterm births. *JAMA*. 2010;304:419–425.

Fetal Lung Maturity (FLM) Testing

- Few indications
- May help identify a fetus at risk of RDS; however, a positive FLM test does not reliably predict other adverse outcomes
- Even if FLM testing is mature before 39 weeks, neonate is still at higher risk of adverse outcomes than neonate delivered after 39 weeks without FLM testing
- FLM testing should *not* be performed when delivery is mandated for fetal or maternal indications
- Various tests have been used
  - Lecithin-to-sphingomyelin (L/S) ratio
  - Phosphatidyl-glycerol (PG)—Detection
  - Lamellar body count

MALPRESENTATION

Breech Presentation (Figures 1-14 and 1-15)

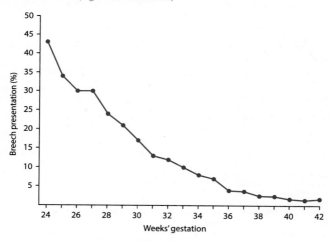

Figure 1-14 Breech presentation by gestational age. (Used with permission from Cunningham F, Leveno KJ, Bloom SL, et al. Chapter 28. Breech delivery. In: Cunningham F, Leveno KJ, Bloom SL, et al., eds. *Williams Obstetrics*. 24th ed. New York, NY: McGraw-Hill; 2013.)

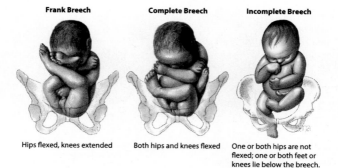

Figure 1-15 Types of breech presentations. (Used with permission from Cunningham F, Leveno KJ, Bloom SL, et al. Chapter 28. Breech delivery. In: Cunningham F, Leveno KJ, Bloom SL, et al., eds. *Williams Obstetrics*. 24th ed. New York, NY: McGraw-Hill; 2013.)

Incidence

- 3–4% of term pregnancies
- Decreases with increasing GA
- Earlier GA with higher percentage of footling breech compared to later GA when most are frank breech

Delivery

- "The decision regarding the mode of delivery should depend on the experience of the health care provider .... Planned vaginal delivery of a term singleton breech fetus may be reasonable under hospital-specific protocol guidelines for both eligibility and labor management" [ACOG Committee Opinion No. 340, July 2006]

Risk Factors

· Uterine anomalies (bicornuate, septate)	· Contracted maternal pelvis
· Space occupying lesions (fibroids)	· Fetal anomaly (anencephaly, hydrocephaly, sacrococcygeal teratoma)
· Placental abnormalities (previa)	· Neurologic impairment
· Multiparity	· Short umbilical cord
· Amniotic fluid abnormalities (poly/oligo)	· Fundal placenta
· Prior breech delivery	

Breech Delivery Definitions

- ***Spontaneous delivery***: No traction or manipulation of fetus. Often occurs in very preterm, previable, deliveries
- ***Assisted breech delivery (partial breech extraction):*** Most common type of vaginal breech. Fetus delivers spontaneously up to umbilicus. Maneuvers used to assist in the delivery of the remainder of the body, arms, and head
- ***Total breech extraction:*** Feet grasped; entire fetus extracted. Ideally, it should be used only for second twin; not singleton as cervix may not be dilated to allow passage of head

Maneuvers for Breech Delivery

- Leave fetal membranes intact as long as possible to act as dilating wedge and prevent cord prolapse
- Do not exert traction until fetal umbilicus is past perineum
- ***Pinard maneuver*** may be needed to deliver legs (after fetal umbilicus reached). Exert pressure in popliteal space of knee and flex knee; guide thigh away from trunk as trunk is rotated in opposite direction (Figure 1-16)
- With thumbs over sacrum and fingers resting on anterior superior iliac crests (to minimize soft tissue injury), apply gentle, steady downward/outward traction until scapulae are visible (Figure 1-17)
- Maternal expulsive efforts will assist
- ***Lovsett maneuver*** to deliver extended or nuchal arms. Slide 2 fingers along humerus until elbow is reached. Sweep forearm across chest and out of vagina

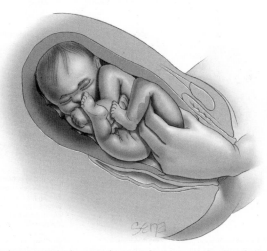

Figure 1-16 Pinard maneuver. (Used with permission from Cunningham F, Leveno KJ, Bloom SL, et al. Chapter 28. Breech delivery. In: Cunningham F, Leveno KJ, Bloom SL, et al., eds. *Williams Obstetrics.* 24th ed. New York, NY: McGraw-Hill; 2013.)

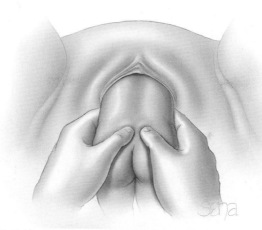

Figure 1-17 Breech delivery. (Used with permission from Cunningham F, Leveno KJ, Bloom SL, et al. Chapter 28. Breech delivery. In: Cunningham F, Leveno KJ, Bloom SL, et al., eds. *Williams Obstetrics*. 24th ed. New York, NY: McGraw-Hill; 2013.)

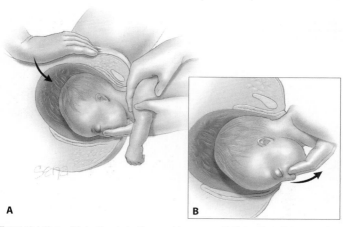

A   **B**

Figure 1-18 **A.** Flexion of the head is maintained by suprapubic pressure provided by an assistant. **B.** Pressure on the maxilla is applied simultaneously by the operator as upward and outward traction is exerted. (Used with permission from Cunningham F, Leveno KJ, Bloom SL, et al. Chapter 28. Breech delivery. In: Cunningham F, Leveno KJ, Bloom SL, et al., eds. *Williams Obstetrics*. 24th ed. New York, NY: McGraw-Hill; 2013.)

- *Mauriceau-Smellie-Veit maneuver:* May be needed to deliver fetal head.
  - Principle is traction down the axis of the birth canal and flexion of the fetal head (Figure 1-18)
  - Index and middle finger on fetal maxilla
- During delivery of the head, avoid extreme elevation of the body, which may result in hyperextension of the cervical spine and potential neurologic injury

Entrapment of the Aftercoming Head

- Consider IV nitroglycerin (50–100 μg)
- **Dührssen Incisions:** See Figure 1-19. Bandage scissors used to make one to three incisions extending the full length of the cervical lip, typically at 2 and 10 o'clock, possibly 6 o'clock also. Incisions may extend into lower uterine segment or broad ligament and may injure uterine vessels, ureter, and bladder
- **Piper Forceps:** Designed to deliver the aftercoming head. See Figure 1-20

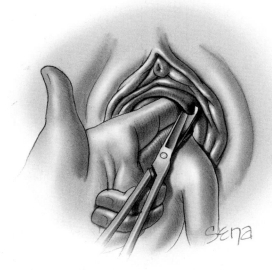

Figure 1-19 Duhrssen incisions. (Used with permission from Cunningham F, Leveno KJ, Bloom SL, et al. Chapter 28. Breech delivery. In: Cunningham F, Leveno KJ, Bloom SL, et al., eds. *Williams Obstetrics*. 24th ed. New York, NY: McGraw-Hill; 2013.)

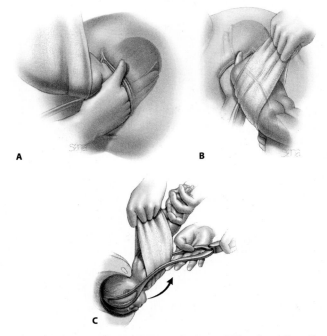

Figure 1-20 Piper forceps. (Used with permission from Cunningham F, Leveno KJ, Bloom SL, et al. Chapter 28. Breech delivery. In: Cunningham F, Leveno KJ, Bloom SL, et al., eds. *Williams Obstetrics*. 24th ed. New York, NY: McGraw-Hill; 2013.)

Complete Breech Extraction
- Grasp one or both (preferably) feet (Figure 1-21)
- Apply traction on feet and ankles
- Gentle downward traction until hips are delivered
- Deliver with typical breech maneuvers

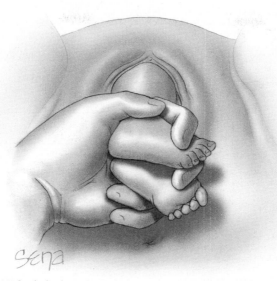

Figure 1-21 Complete breech extraction. (Used with permission from Cunningham F, Leveno KJ, Bloom SL, et al. Chapter 28. Breech delivery. In: Cunningham F, Leveno KJ, Bloom SL, et al., eds. *Williams Obstetrics*. 24th ed. New York, NY: McGraw-Hill; 2013.)

Face/Brow Presentation

Associated with multiparity, cephalopelvic disproportion, fetal anomalies (anencephaly, anterior neck mass), macrosomia, platypelloid pelvis, prematurity, and PPROM.

Face Presentation
- Occurs in 1:500 live births
- Majority in mentum anterior position (about 60%)
- Approximately 26% will be in mentum posterior position
- Nearly one-third to one-half in mentum transverse and mentum posterior positions will spontaneously convert to mentum anterior position during labor
- **Only *mentum anterior* are likely to deliver vaginally.** As chin passes under symphysis, slight flexion may occur
- Persistent *mentum posterior* will not deliver vaginally (unless very preterm). CD is indicated

Brow Presentation
- Occurs in about 1:500 to 1:1500 deliveries
- If persistent, not compatible with vaginal birth unless fetus is very small
  - 50% will spontaneously convert to face or vertex presentation. Labor may progress with careful monitoring. Deliver by CD if arrest of progress

External Cephalic Version (ECV)

- Women near term with breech presentation should be offered version attempt
- Best GA to perform: Most common GA in trials is about 36 weeks. *Per ACOG* (Practice Bulletin No. 13, 2000), preferred candidates have completed 36 weeks of gestation (ie, may do at 36-0/7)
- Needs to be performed in a facility with access to CD
- **Successful in 35–86%; average 58%**
- Short-term fetal bradycardia may be seen in more than 20%, but urgent CD for nonreassuring FHR occurs in less than 1% (1:600)
- **Tocolysis:** *Terbutaline* 0.25 mg subcutaneously 5–10 minutes prior to procedure may increase success

- **Anesthesia**: Conflicting evidence. A meta-analysis suggested success rates were higher with regional anesthesia (59.7% compared with 37.6%)
- NST should be performed before and after procedure
- No evidence is available to support immediate IOL after successful ECV
- Contraindications: The usual contraindications to vaginal birth (ie, placenta previa, prior classical CD vasa previa)
- Relative contraindications: Ruptured membranes, oligohydramnios, known uterine or fetal anomaly, unexplained uterine bleeding, active labor
- Previous low segment transverse CD is NOT a contraindication. Similar success rates, but limited data on safety of procedure

Possibly linked to increased success	*Possibly* linked to decreased success
• Parity • Transverse or oblique lie • Normal or increased amniotic fluid • Anterior placenta	• Fetal weight less than 2500 g • Advanced dilatation • Low station • Maternal obesity

PRETERM LABOR (PTL)

- Preterm birth: 20-0/7–36-6/7 weeks
- Diagnosis of PTL: Regular contractions with cervical change (dilation or effacement) or initial presentation of contractions and dilation of at least 2 cm
- Less than 10% of those with the clinical diagnosis of PTL deliver within 7 days of presentation
- Approximately 30% of PTL spontaneously resolves
- 50% of patients hospitalized for PTL deliver at term

Evaluation

- Do a STERILE speculum exam/send following labs:
  - Fetal fibronectin (fFN) **before** any other portion of exam (Table 1-16)
  - Test for PPROM (pooling, nitrazine, ferning)
  - GC/CT/GBS, wet prep for trichomonas/bacterial vaginosis, urinalysis, and culture
  - Consider transvaginal cervical length
  - DO NOT DIGITALIZE if slightest suspicion of ruptured membranes. Assess cervix visually

TABLE 1-16 FETAL FIBRONECTIN (fFN)

A major component of the extracellular matrix of the membranes of the amniotic sac. Glycoprotein ("trophoblast glue") that promotes cellular adhesion at uterine-placental and decidual-fetal membrane interfaces; released into cervicovaginal secretions when chorionic/decidual interface is disrupted. Not usually present during weeks 22–34

Technique
- Collect prior to any other vaginal/cervical specimens. Gel may interfere
- During speculum* exam, rotate swab across posterior fornix for about 10 seconds

Cannot do if
- Ruptured membranes, moderate vaginal bleeding, cervical dilation >3 cm
- Cervical manipulation in last 24 hours (intercourse, exam, TV sono)
- **Cerclage:** Data show fFN *is* valid if cerclage in place

High *negative predictive value* in symptomatic women. *If negative*:
- About 99.5% with signs and symptoms of PTL fail to deliver within 7 days
- About 99.2% remain undelivered for 14 days

*The manufacturer and FDA currently recommend using speculum—method used in most research studies.

Tocolysis

- *Primary purpose*: To prolong pregnancy to administer steroids and magnesium sulfate for neuroprotection (or maternal transport)
- NO evidence that it has direct favorable effect on neonatal outcome
- Generally not indicated before neonatal viability (may be appropriate after event known to cause PTL, such as intra-abdominal surgery)
- Generally not indicated after 34 weeks

- If PPROM, in absence of maternal infection, may tocolyze for purposes of maternal transport or steroids (depends on GA)
- **Maintenance Tocolysis:** No data available at this time supporting its use to prevent preterm delivery

Tocolytic Drugs

Nifedipine 10–20 mg orally every 4–6 hours
- Hold for blood pressure <90/40
- Use caution if using with magnesium sulfate
  - *Possible* interaction between magnesium and nifedipine leading to pulmonary edema and/ or severe neuromuscular blockade with resultant severe hypotension. This interaction *has not* been confirmed in large randomized trials. Data from one randomized clinical trial did not find hypotension with combination of magnesium and nifedipine. Another study: nifedipine with magnesium did not increase serious magnesium-related side effects

Indomethacin (*Indocin*) 50 (to 100) mg oral load, then 25–50 mg orally every 4 hours for 48–72 hours
- Fetal concerns
  - Constriction of the ductus arteriosus
    - Depends on GA and duration of exposure
    - Limit use to **<32 weeks** GA
  - May affect fetal kidneys. If continued for more than 72 hours, consider ultrasound for amniotic fluid assessment ductus arteriosus evaluation

Terbutaline 0.25 mg SQ every 15–20 minutes × 3 doses
- May use for preterm contractions; however, not generally useful in PTL
- Hold for maternal pulse over 120
- Caution in: Diabetics (causes hyperglycemia); cardiac disease; hyperthyroid

Magnesium sulfate 6 g bolus, then 3–4 g/h; titrate down to lowest effective dose
- Therapeutic levels: 4–7 mEq/L (4.8–8.4 mg/dL)
- If renal insufficiency/failure, consider lower dose (4 g bolus; 0.5–1 g/h)
- Check level after 6 hours if patient has a renal history, low urine output, or appears toxic
- **Magnesium is not currently used as a first line therapy**

Antenatal Corticosteroid Administration (also see RDS section)

- Most beneficial intervention to improve neonatal outcome. Lower risk of
  - RDS (RR 0.66)
  - Intracranial hemorrhage (RR 0.54)
  - Necrotizing enterocolitis (RR 0.46)
  - Death (RR 0.69)
- If delivery prior to 23 weeks, not recommended
- If 24–34 weeks, steroids ASAP if at risk for delivery within 7 days
- *Newer data suggests benefit if delivery expected at 23 weeks*
- Treatment for less than 24 hours is still associated with improved neonatal outcomes. Still administer even if you are unsure you will be able to complete the course prior to delivery
- No benefit shown with shorter dosing intervals
- Possible maternal side effects
  - Transient hyperglycemia (starts in about 12 hours and lasts up to 5 days)
  - Leukocyte increase: Within 24 hours (about 30%); typically returns to baseline in 3 days

Antenatal Corticosteroids

- **Betamethasone** 12 mg IM every 24 hours × 2 doses

OR

- **Dexamethasone** 6 mg IM every 12 hours × 4 doses

"Rescue" Steroids

- A rescue course of steroids should be considered for women who previously received a course of steroids at least 7–14 days earlier (but did not deliver), yet may still deliver before 34 weeks GA
- This has been shown to decrease respiratory complications without apparent adverse effects

Magnesium Sulfate for Fetal Neuroprotection (before 32 weeks GA)

- There are three large, randomized, placebo-controlled trials supporting reduction in risk of CP in early preterm birth. (Treating 63 patients threatening to deliver before 32 weeks will prevent 1 case of moderate/severe CP). NO SPECIFIC PROTOCOL RECOMMENDED Examples:
  - 6-g load, then 2 g/h for up to 12 hours. If after 12 hours, delivery is not imminent, discontinue magnesium and restart if delivery threatens. Re-bolus if 6 hours have elapsed
  - 4-g bolus, then 1 g/h for up to 24 hours
  - 4-g load only within 24 hours of expected delivery

Prematurity Calculator

- NIH Web site for outcomes using Extremely Preterm Birth Outcome Data: http://www.nichd.nih.gov/about/org/der/branches/ppb/programs/epbo/pages/epbo_case.aspx

Cerclage

- Cervical insufficiency is defined as the inability of the cervix to retain a pregnancy in the absence of the signs and symptoms of clinical contractions or labor or both in the second trimester
- Short cervical length in the second trimester is associated with increased risk of preterm delivery, but is not diagnostic for cervical insufficiency
- Indications for cerclage (singleton pregnancies)
  - **History**
    - History of one or more second trimester loss related to painless cervical dilation in the absence of labor or placental abruption
    - Prior cerclage due to painless cervical dilation in the second trimester
    - Place at 13–14 weeks
  - **Physical Examination ("emergency" or "rescue" cerclage)**
    - Painless cervical dilation in the second trimester
  - **Ultrasonographic Finding with History of Prior Preterm Birth ("ultrasound indicated")**
    - Prior spontaneous birth less than 34 weeks and *cervical length less than 25 mm* before 24 weeks gestation

Progesterone for Prevention of Preterm Delivery (Table 1-17 and Figure 1-22)

TABLE 1-17 SMFM RECOMMENDATIONS—PROGESTOGENS FOR PREVENTION OF PRETERM BIRTH

Population	Recommendation
Asymptomatic	
· Singletons without prior spontaneous PTB and unknown or normal TVUS CL	No evidence of effectiveness
· Singletons with prior spontaneous PTB	*17P 250 mg IM weekly* from 16–20 to 36 weeks*
· Singletons without prior spontaneous PTB but CL ≤20 mm at ≤24 weeks	*Vaginal progesterone 90 mg gel or 200 mg suppository daily* from diagnosis of short cervical length until 36 weeks
· Multiple gestations	No evidence of effectiveness
Symptomatic	
· PTL	No evidence of effectiveness
· PPROM	No evidence of effectiveness

PTB, preterm birth; CL, cervical length; TVUS, transvaginal ultrasound; 17P: 17α-hydroxyprogesterone caproate
*Best evidence is to use 17P and to start before 21 weeks; however, beneficial effects seen when started at ≤27 weeks. Progesterone suppository 100 mg vaginally has also been shown to reduce preterm birth in women with a prior preterm delivery; however, evidence for 17P is stronger. May consider suppository if *unable* to use 17P.
Used with permission from SMFM, Berghella V. Progesterone and preterm birth prevention: translating clinical trials data into clinical practice. *Am J Obstet Gynecol.* 2011;206:376–386.

Algorithm for use of progestogens in prevention of PTB in clinical care

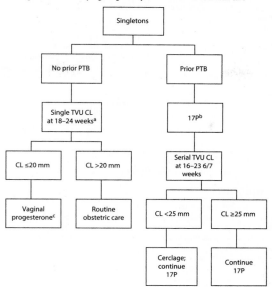

^aIf TVU CL screening is performed; ^b17P 250 mg intramuscularly every week from
16–20 weeks to 36 weeks; ^ceg, daily 200-mg suppository or 90-mg gel from time of
diagnosis of short CL to 36 weeks.
CL, cervical length; *PTB*, preterm birth; *17P*, 17-alpha-hydroxyprogesterone caproate;
TVU, transvaginal ultrasound.

Figure 1-22 Algorithm for use of progestogens in prevention of PTB in clinical care. (Used with permission from Progesterone and preterm birth prevention: translating clinical trials data into clinical practice. *Am J Obstet Gynecol.* 2012;206(5):376–386.)

PRETERM PREMATURE RUPTURE OF MEMBRANES (PPROM)

- *Terminology*
  - *Premature:* Rupture before the onset of labor
  - *Preterm:* Before 37 weeks
  - *Prolonged:* Longer than 24 hours
- In women with PPROM, clinically evident antepartum infection occurs in 15–25%; postpartum infection in 15–20%. Incidence of infection is higher at earlier GA
- *Risks of PPROM*
  - Complications of prematurity
  - RDS, sepsis, intraventricular hemorrhage, necrotizing enterocolitis, neurodevelopmental impairment
  - Infection and umbilical cord accident: 1–2% risk of fetal demise after PPROM
  - Placental abruption occurs in 2–5% of pregnancies with PPROM

Diagnosis

- History and physical examination
- Avoid digital exams unless in active labor or imminent delivery
- Sterile speculum exam: Inspect for cord prolapse, cervical dilation, obtain cultures including GBS
- Pooling, nitrazine positive, ferning present
- Ultrasound examination for presentation and assessment of amniotic fluid (not diagnostic)
- Fetal fibronectin is sensitive but nonspecific (if negative, suggests intact membranes)
- Commercially available tests (*AmniSure*)
- Amniocentesis with blue dye test (indigo carmine)

Management

- Manage expectantly if PPROM before 34-0/7 weeks, if possible
- Close observation for infection, abruption, fetal well-being, labor
- Administer antenatal corticosteroids between 24-0/7 and 34-0/7 weeks (in some cases as early as 23-0/7 weeks). NOT linked with increased maternal or neonatal infection

- Administer magnesium sulfate for neuroprotection if delivery anticipated before 32-0/7 weeks
- Tocolysis is generally not recommended. In certain situations, it may be considered to complete corticosteroid course
- Administer latency antibiotics

IV for 48 hours:	Ampicillin 2 g IV every 6 hours
	Erythromycin* 250 mg IV every 6 hours
	* If no erythromycin, use azithromycin 500 mg IV daily
THEN	
Orally for 5 days:	Amoxicillin 250 mg orally every 8 hours
	Erythromycin 250 mg orally every 6 hours

If penicillin allergy: Reasonable to administer erythromycin alone. Use GBS prophylaxis per guidelines.

- Deliver if nonreassuring fetal status or clinical chorioamnionitis
- Deliver at 34-0/7 weeks even if otherwise stable
- *With conservative management, 50–60% with PPROM will deliver within 1 week*

CHORIOAMNIONITIS

- Inflammation of the fetal membranes
- Frequently associated with prolonged membrane rupture and long labor
- *Funisitis:* Inflammation of the umbilical cord
- Most commonly, an ascending infection of organisms that are part of the normal vaginal flora (bacteroides, *Escherichia coli*, anaerobic streptococci, and GBS)
- Incidence is greater in earlier gestations with PROM
- *Management*: Antibiotics and expedient delivery (not an indication for CD)

Risk Factors

- Young age
- Low socioeconomic status
- Internal monitors
- Preexisting lower genital tract infections
- Extended duration of labor
- Multiple vaginal exams
- Nulliparity

Clinical Features

- Fetal tachycardia
- Maternal fever
- Fundal tenderness
- Leukocytosis
- Maternal tachycardia
- Foul-smelling vaginal discharge

Treatment

Ampicillin 2 g IV every 6 hours
   *[If penicillin allergic, **clindamycin** 600 mg IV every 8 hours]*
      PLUS
Gentamicin 2 mg/kg IV load, then 1.5 mg/kg every 8 hours
Tylenol 650 mg rectally/orally for temperature ≥38.0°C every 4–6 hours as needed

POSTPARTUM ENDOMYOMETRITIS (OR ENDOMETRITIS)

- Mainly a clinical diagnosis (tender uterus and fever)
  - Temperature >39°C once or two temperatures ≥38°C 2–4 hours apart
  - Fundal tenderness
  - Negative evaluation for other sources of fever
  - May also have foul smelling lochia, elevated WBC count, and left shift

- **Blood cultures:** If clinical picture is consistent with endometritis, do NOT need to obtain secondary to low yield. Blood cultures *should* be drawn if patient is experiencing shaking chills or rigors (obtain at time of fever spike) or if continues to spike fever after adequate antibiotic therapy
- Endometrial cultures tend to be unhelpful because they are usually contaminated by vaginal or cervical flora, and generally endometritis is a polymicrobial infection

Treatment

- Treat with triple antibiotic therapy (IV) until 48 hours afebrile. No oral antibiotics necessary

---

Ampicillin 2 g IV every 6 hours
Gentamicin 5–7 mg/kg every 24 hours (actual body weight) *(or continue every 8 hours dosing)*
Clindamycin 600–900 mg IV every 8 hours
   OR
Metronidazole (*Flagyl*) 500 mg IV every 8 hours
   *If penicillin allergy, only give gentamicin/clindamycin or add **vancomycin***

OBSTETRIC EMERGENCIES

Postpartum Hemorrhage (PPH)

Definitions
- *Early/Primary:* First 24 hours post-delivery; occurs in 4–6% of pregnancies
- *Late/Secondary:* Between 24 hours and 6–12 weeks postpartum
- ≥500 mL blood loss for vaginal delivery
- ≥1000 mL blood loss for CD

Risk Factors

• Placenta previa, low-lying placenta	• Multiple gestation
• Suspected placenta accreta/percreta	• Known coagulopathy
• More than four prior vaginal births	• Morbid obesity
• Chorioamnionitis	• Prior CD or uterine surgery
• History of PPH	• Prolonged oxytocin use
• Estimated fetal weight >4000 g	• Prolonged second stage of labor
• Large uterine fibroids	• Magnesium sulfate administration

Etiologies

Early PPH	Late PPH
• Uterine **atony**	• Subinvolution of placental site
• Retained placenta (eg, accreta)	• Retained products of conception
• Laceration (cervical, vaginal)	• Infection
• Defects in coagulation	• Inherited coagulation defects
• Uterine inversion	
• Uterine rupture	

Management
- Type and cross on admission if considered high risk
- Notify anesthesia team
- Bimanual uterine compression—vigorous uterine massage (Figure 1-23)
- Call for help, including blood products
- Secure two large bore IVs (#18 gauge) if not in place
- Volume resuscitation with crystalloid
- Evaluate for cause of bleeding
- Quantitate blood loss—graduated containers, weigh materials (1 g = 1 mL)
- KEEP TRACK of cumulative blood loss
- **DO NOT DELAY TRANSFER TO THE OPERATING ROOM for further management**

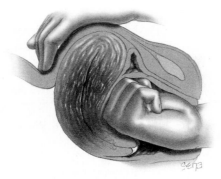

Figure 1-23 Bimanual uterine massage. (Used with permission from Cunningham F, Leveno KJ, Bloom SL, et al. Chapter 41. Obstetrical hemorrhage. In: Cunningham F, Leveno KJ, Bloom SL, et al., eds. *Williams Obstetrics*. 24th ed. New York, NY: McGraw-Hill; 2013.)

Medications for Uterine Atony (Table 1-18)

TABLE 1-18 MEDICATIONS FOR UTERINE ATONY

Medications for Uterine Atony		
Medication	**Dosage**	**Cautions**
Oxytocin (*Pitocin*)	• 10–40 units per liter • Run at 10 mL/min initially, then 1–2 mL/min • 10 units IM if no IV	• Do not give as large bolus as it can result in profound hypotension
Methylergonovine maleate (*Methergine*) Semi-synthetic ergot alkaloid	• 0.2 mg IM (preferred) or IV every 2–4 hours (maximum 5 doses) • May give additional doses of 0.2 mg orally every 6 hours. **Do not start orally until 4 hours after the last IM or IV dose**	• Hypertension • Raynaud's phenomenon • On protease inhibitor • May cause fevers
Carboprost tromethamine (*Hemabate*) (15-methyl PGF$_{2\alpha}$)	• 250 µg IM (skeletal or myometrium) every 15–90 minutes, not to exceed 8 doses in 24 hours	• Asthma • Cardiac, renal, hepatic disease • Also causes nausea, vomiting, diarrhea, fever
Misoprostol (*Cytotec*®); PGE$_1$	• 800–1000 µg per rectum • 600 µg sublingual	• Renal or cardiac disease

Transfusion
• Transfuse based on clinical signs—initiate massive transfusion protocol if needed
  • Packed red blood cells (pRBCs): 1 unit increases hematocrit by 3%
  • Fresh frozen plasma (FFP): Consider if transfusing > 2 units pRBCs
  • Platelets: Six pack provides 40 000–50 000 transient increase in platelets
  • Cryoprecipitate: 10 unit pack raises fibrinogen approximately 80–100 mg/dL
  • Consider the following ratios
    • *6:4:1 (pRBC:FFP:Platelet)* OR *4:4:1 (pRBC:FFP:Platelet)*

Surgical Management
• Uterine tamponade: Intrauterine balloons, such as the *Bakri* Tamponade Balloon Catheter (instill 300–500 mL saline), packing (gauze, can soak with thrombin 5000 units in 5 mL saline), Foley bulb (instill 60–80 mL saline)
• Hemostatic sutures
  • Uterine Artery Ligation (Figure 1-24)
  • B-Lynch compression suture. Use large needle and suture (#2 Chromic or Vicryl) (Figure 1-25)
  • Hypogastric (internal iliac) artery ligation (to decrease pulse pressure)
• Arterial embolization via interventional radiology
• Hysterectomy

Uterine Inversion

- Collapse of uterine fundus toward cervix and vagina
- Occurs in approximately 1:2000 to 1:20 000 deliveries
- Avoid aggressive traction on the umbilical cord when delivering placenta
- Must promptly recognize and treat. Can lead to severe hemorrhage and maternal death

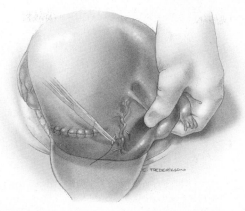

Figure 1-24 Uterine artery ligation. Ligate uterine artery and vein at lower uterine segment, 2–3 cm below level of uterine incision. Place 2–3 cm medial to uterine vessels through myometrium and then lateral to vessels through broad ligament. Palpate ureter medial to lower uterine segment. For hemorrhage, need **bilateral** sutures—decreases pulse pressure. (Used with permission from Cunningham F, Leveno KJ, Bloom SL, et al. Chapter 41. Obstetrical hemorrhage. In: Cunningham F, Leveno KJ, Bloom SL, et al., eds. *Williams Obstetrics*. 24th ed. New York, NY: McGraw-Hill; 2013.)

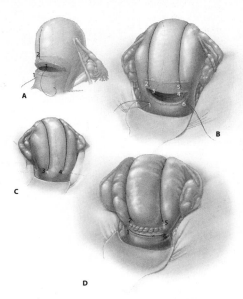

Figure 1-25 B-Lynch (uterine compression suture). **Step 1.** Beginning below the incision, the needle pierces the lower uterine segment to enter the uterine cavity. **Step 2.** The needle exits the cavity above the incision. The suture then loops up and around the fundus to the posterior uterine surface. **Step 3.** The needle pierces the posterior uterine wall to reenter the uterine cavity. The suture then traverses from left to right within the cavity. **Step 4.** The needle exits the uterine cavity through the posterior uterine wall. From the back of the uterus, the suture loops up and around the fundus to the front of the uterus. **Step 5.** The needle pierces the myometrium above the incision to reenter the uterine cavity. **Step 6.** The needle exits below the incision and the sutures at points 1 and 6 are tied below the incision. The hysterotomy incision (if not already closed) is then closed in the usual fashion. (Used with permission from Cunningham F, Leveno KJ, Bloom SL, et al. Chapter 41. Obstetrical hemorrhage. In: Cunningham F, Leveno KJ, Bloom SL, et al., eds. *Williams Obstetrics*. 24th ed. New York, NY: McGraw-Hill; 2013.)

Degrees of Uterine Inversion (Figure 1-26)

- First: Fundus remains within endometrial cavity
- Second: Fundus protrudes through cervical os
- Third: Fundus protrudes to or beyond introitus
- Fourth: Uterus and vagina are completely inverted

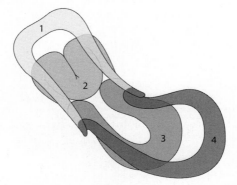

Figure 1-26 Degrees of uterine inversion. (Used with permission from Cunningham F, Leveno KJ, Bloom SL, et al. Chapter 41. Obstetrical hemorrhage. In: Cunningham F, Leveno KJ, Bloom SL, et al., eds. *Williams Obstetrics.* 24th ed. New York, NY: McGraw-Hill; 2013.)

Principles of Management

- Rapid replacement of uterus to correct position, manage hemorrhage, prevent recurrence

Interventions Once Inversion Is Identified

- Stop all uterotonic medications
- Call for help: Nursing, obstetric, anesthesia
- Consider transfer to operating room
- Establish two large bore IVs, administer IV fluids and blood products as needed
- Do not remove placenta to minimize blood loss
- Attempt to manually reduce the uterine fundus to its proper position
- If constriction of lower uterine segment, give 50–100 µg nitroglycerin IV
- Consider terbutaline or magnesium sulfate for additional uterine relaxation
- If manual reduction fails, perform laparotomy for additional surgical techniques
- Once successfully reduced, keep hand in place until uterine tone optimized
- Restart uterotonics

Amniotic Fluid Embolism

- Anaphylactoid syndrome of pregnancy
- Very rare (1–12:100 000 deliveries)
- Amniotic fluid enters maternal circulation triggering severe inflammatory response, cardiogenic shock, respiratory failure, and coagulopathy
- Presents during or immediately following labor and delivery with abrupt onset of hypotension, hypoxemia, and disseminated intravascular coagulation (DIC)
- Rapid cardiovascular collapse
- High maternal morbidity and mortality

Possible Associated Factors

- Precipitous delivery
- Advanced maternal age
- Operative delivery
- Placenta previa
- Placenta abruption
- Grand multiparity
- Eclampsia

Management

- Aggressive supportive care
- Intubation and mechanical ventilation
- Vascular access
- Volume support, inotropic agents and vasopressors to maintain blood pressure
- Blood products

Maternal Cardiac Arrest

Potential Causes of Cardiac Arrest in Pregnancy

- Pulmonary: Pulmonary embolism, amniotic fluid embolism, asthma
- Cardiovascular: MI, arrhythmia, cardiomyopathy, stroke, preeclampsia/eclampsia
- Hematologic: Atony or abnormal placentation causing hemorrhage, DIC
- Infectious: Sepsis
- Medication: Drug toxicity (think about magnesium toxicity), illicit drug use, anaphylaxis
- Trauma

Maternal Code

- Follow ACLS recommendations for administration of medications
- Defibrillate using standard ACLS protocol—remove uterine or fetal monitors before defibrillating
- Calcium gluconate (1 amp)
- If gravid uterus is greater than 20 weeks size, uterus should be manually and laterally displaced toward the left
- Hands should be more cephalad above the sternum to perform compressions effectively
- A dedicated timer should indicate when 4 minutes have passed after the onset of cardiac arrest
- AHA guidelines recommend beginning a **perimortem CD** at 4 minutes of resuscitative efforts with delivery of the newborn by 5 minutes in a pregnant woman who is suspected to be of a viable gestation
- If the fundus extends above the level of the umbilicus, aorto-caval compression may occur. Emergency CD should be performed regardless of GA
- Success rates of resuscitation improve with delivery early within the resuscitation process
- Do NOT move the patient to the operating room to perform the CD

Seizure

Differential Diagnosis

- Eclampsia, epilepsy, trauma, substance use, hypoglycemia, electrolyte imbalance, infection

Immediate Assessments and Interventions

- Supportive care: Maintain airway ± mechanical ventilation, assess neurologic, pulmonary, and circulatory status
- IVs, hydration, ECG, and bed padding for safety
- Obtain history from family members
- Labs: CBC, CMP, uric acid, coagulation studies, LDH, toxicology screen, urine culture, glucose
- Contact anesthesia and neurology services
- Avoid delivery until maternal stabilization and reevaluation of fetal well-being after patient recovers from seizure

Medication Options

- Magnesium 4–6 g IV bolus or 5 g IM in each buttock
- Lorazepam 0.1 mg/kg (typical 4–8 mg dose) or diazepam 10 mg IV over 1 minute
- Phenytoin 1000–1500 mg (weight based) load with goal level at 2 hours of 12–20 µg/mL; once therapeutic, monitor levels every 12 hours

Sepsis

- Pertinent physiologic changes of pregnancy
  - Increased heart rate and cardiac output
  - Increased tidal volume and decreased P_{CO_2}
  - Mild leukocytosis
- Systemic Inflammatory Response Syndrome (SIRS) (requires at least two of the following)
  - Temperature >38°C or <36°C
  - Heart rate >90 beats/min
  - Respiratory rate >20 breaths/min or Pa_{CO_2} <32
  - WBC >12 000, WBC <4000 or >10% bands

Definition

- Sepsis: SIRS in setting of an infection
- Severe Sepsis: Sepsis with end organ dysfunction (Table 1-19)

Septic Shock Management

- Fluid resuscitation with crystalloid
- Add pressors after aggressive fluid resuscitation depending on patient's response
  - Norepinephrine first line (0.1 µg/kg/min, titrate to MAP of 65)
- Try to obtain blood cultures, but goal for antibiotics within 45 minutes

- Consider need for imaging
- Start broad with antibiotics and tailor them as more information is gathered
- Think about all potential sites of infection and get source control!

Antimicrobials
- Resistant Gram-Positive Organisms: Vancomycin, Daptomycin, Linezolid
- Resistant Gram-Negative Organisms: Piperacillin/Tazobactam, Carbapenemases
- CMV: Valgancyclovir
- Fungal: Micafungin, Caspofungin, Amphotericin B

Surviving Sepsis Campaign Bundles (Table 1-20)

TABLE 1-19 SEVERE SEPSIS WITH EVIDENCE OF END-ORGAN DYSFUNCTION

System	Dysfunction
Neurologic	Confusion, encephalopathy
Pulmonary	Hypoxemia, acute lung injury, ARDS
Cardiovascular	Hypotension
GI	Transaminitis, coagulopathy, hyperbilirubinemia
Renal	Acute kidney injury, oliguria
Hematologic	Thrombocytopenia
Metabolic	Lactic acidosis

TABLE 1-20 SURVIVING SEPSIS CAMPAIGN BUNDLES

To Be Completed Within 3 Hours

- Measure lactate level
- Obtain blood cultures prior to administration of antibiotics
- Administer broad spectrum antibiotics
- Administer 30 mL/kg crystalloid for hypotension or lactate ≥4 mmol/L

To Be Completed Within 6 Hours

- Administer vasopressors (for hypotension that does not respond to initial fluid resuscitation) to maintain a mean arterial pressure (MAP) of ≥65 mm Hg
- In the event of persistent arterial hypotension despite volume resuscitation (septic shock) or initial lactate ≥4 mmol/L (36 mg/dL)
  - Measure central venous pressure (CVP)*
  - Measure central venous oxygen saturation (SCVO$_2$)*
  - Re-measure lactate if initial lactate was elevated*

*Targets for quantitative resuscitation included in the guidelines are CVP ≥8 mm Hg, SVCO$_2$ ≥70%, and normalization of lactate. Used with permission from Dellinger RP, Levy MM, Rhodes A, et al. Surviving sepsis campaign: international guidelines for management of severe sepsis and septic shock: 2012. *Crit Care Med*. 2013;41:580–637.

Shoulder Dystocia

Risk Factors
- Macrosomia
- Pregestational and gestational diabetes
- Previous shoulder dystocia (up to 25% recurrence risk)
- Abnormal second stage of labor—prolonged or precipitous
- Maternal obesity
- Operative vaginal delivery
- Post term pregnancy
- Excess gestational weight gain

Diagnosis
- Retraction of fetal head toward perineum (Turtle Sign)
- Failure to deliver the anterior shoulder after restitution and gentle, downward guidance of the fetal head

Management
- Communicate to team once shoulder dystocia has been identified
- Call support teams (nursing, anesthesia, pediatric, obstetric) to room to provide assistance

- Note the time of shoulder dystocia
- Instruct patient to stop pushing and ensure maternal positioning at end of bed is optimal
- Empty bladder, if needed
- Consider episiotomy
- *Maneuvers:* (no particular order after McRoberts and suprapubic pressure)
  - **McRoberts:** Sharp flexion of maternal thighs against the abdomen
  - **Suprapubic Pressure:** Pressure exerted just above pubic symphysis and onto posterior aspect of the baby's anterior shoulder to rotate the shoulder beneath the pubic bone. Do not apply direct downward pressure or fundal pressure
  - **Posterior Arm:** Insert hand along the posterior arm to the elbow. Flex elbow and bring baby's forearm across the chest to bring the hand and forearm out of the vagina (see Figure 1-27)
  - **Rubin Maneuver:** Place hand on the posterior aspect of either the anterior or posterior shoulder of baby to adduct the baby's shoulder and rotate it anteriorly toward the fetal chest (Figure 1-28)
  - **Woods Corkscrew:** Place hand on the anterior surface of the posterior shoulder. Rotate the shoulder clockwise (if baby facing toward maternal left) or counterclockwise (if baby facing toward maternal right) 180 degrees so the posterior shoulder now becomes the anterior shoulder. Can be repeated again in opposite direction to try to release the shoulder

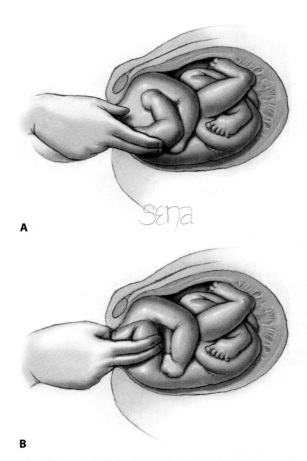

A

B

Figure 1-27 Delivery of the posterior shoulder for relief of shoulder dystocia. **A.** Palpate fetal posterior humerus. **B.** The arm is splinted and swept across the chest, keeping the arm flexed at the elbow.

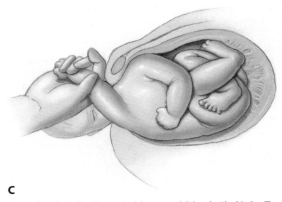

C

Figure 1-27 (*Continued*) **C.** The fetal hand is grasped and the arm extended along the side of the face. The posterior arm is delivered from the vagina. (Used with permission from Cunningham F, Leveno KJ, Bloom SL, et al. Chapter 27. Vaginal delivery. In: Cunningham F, Leveno KJ, Bloom SL, et al., eds. *Williams Obstetrics*. 24th ed. New York, NY: McGraw-Hill; 2013.)

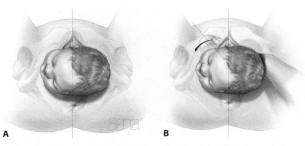

A   **B**

Figure 1-28 Rubin maneuver. **A.** The shoulder-to-shoulder diameter is aligned vertically. **B.** The more easily accessible fetal shoulder (the anterior is shown here) is pushed toward the anterior chest wall of the fetus (*arrow*). Most often, this results in adduction of both shoulders, which reduces the shoulder-to-shoulder diameter and frees the impacted anterior shoulder. (Used with permission from Cunningham F, Leveno KJ, Bloom SL, et al. Chapter 27. Vaginal delivery. In: Cunningham F, Leveno KJ, Bloom SL, et al., eds. *Williams Obstetrics*. 24th ed. New York, NY: McGraw-Hill; 2013.)

- *Less common maneuvers*
  - Clavicle fracture: One or both clavicles is fractured by pulling clavicle in an outward direction from the chest to avoid fetal lung or vascular injury
  - Gaskins: Place patient on hands and knees to deliver posterior shoulder by applying gentle, downward pressure
  - Symphysiotomy: Displace bladder and urethra laterally and incise symphysis cartilage
  - Zavanelli: Replacement of the fetal head into the pelvis followed by CD

MATERNAL COMPLICATIONS OF PREGNANCY

Hypertensive Disorders

- *Hypertension:* Systolic blood pressure (BP) of ≥140 mm Hg, diastolic BP of ≥90 mm Hg, or both
- Diagnosis requires at least two determinations at least 4 hours apart; however, with severe hypertension, diagnosis can be confirmed within a shorter interval to facilitate timely antihypertensive therapy
- Postpartum hypertension: Preeclampsia (PEC) can first develop postpartum. At time of discharge, women must be made aware of symptoms (severe headache, visual disturbances, epigastric pain) that they should report to their provider

Classification of Hypertensive Disorders of Pregnancy (Table 1-24)

TABLE 1-21 CLASSIFICATION OF HYPERTENSIVE DISORDERS OF PREGNANCY

Hypertensive Disorders of Pregnancy	
Gestational hypertension	• New-onset hypertension after 20 weeks GA; absence of proteinuria; often near term • If BP does not return to normal postpartum, diagnosis becomes chronic hypertension • Outcomes usually good. However, if severely elevated BP, outcomes similar to PEC • Requires enhanced surveillance • May be a predictor of chronic hypertension in the future
Chronic hypertension	• Hypertension prior to conception or before 20 weeks GA

Chronic hypertension with superimposed preeclampsia	• Women with chronic hypertension who develop proteinuria after 20 weeks GA
	• Women with chronic hypertension and proteinuria before 20 weeks GA who then
	 • Experience sudden increase in hypertension or require more antihypertensive medications
	 • Experience other signs or symptoms:
	  • Abnormal elevation in liver enzymes
	  • Platelets decrease to <100 000/µL
	  • Right upper quadrant pain
	  • Severe headaches
	  • Visual disturbances
	  • Pulmonary edema
	  • Renal insufficiency (creatinine doubles or increases to ≥1.1 in absence of other renal disease)
	  • Significantly increased protein excretion

Preeclampsia and Eclampsia	**Preeclampsia** • Usually occurs after 20 weeks GA, most often near term • New-onset hypertension / proteinuria (classic definition) • Some women present without proteinuria (but with other systemic signs of disease such as thrombocytopenia, impaired liver function, renal insufficiency, pulmonary edema, or symptoms) **Eclampsia** • New-onset grand mal seizures with PEC • Can be before, during, or after labor • Often preceded by headaches and hyperreflexia; but not always

Data from ACOG Task Force on Hypertension in Pregnancy, *Hypertension in Pregnancy*, 2013.

Terminology
• PEC *without* severe features: No longer termed "mild" because even in the absence of severe disease, morbidity and mortality are significantly increased. See Table 1-22
• PEC *with* severe features: Diagnosed if ANY of the criteria in Table 1-23 are present
• *HELLP syndrome:* A specific constellation of laboratory findings; often considered a PEC subtype
  • *H*emolysis, *E*levated *L*iver enzymes, *L*ow *P*latelet count
  • **Differential diagnosis:** Acute fatty liver of pregnancy, gastroenteritis, hepatitis, appendicitis, gallbladder disease, ITP, TTP, lupus flare, antiphospholipid syndrome, hemolytic-uremic syndrome
  • *If platelets very low (<50 000), may administer dexamethasone 10 mg IV every 12 hours until platelets are over 100 000. However, this has not been proven to improve outcome*

Diagnostic Criteria for PEC (Table 1-22)

TABLE 1-22 DIAGNOSTIC CRITERIA FOR PREECLAMPSIA

Blood Pressure	• ≥140 mm Hg systolic or ≥90 mm Hg diastolic on two occasions at least 4 hours apart after 20 weeks GA in a woman with previously normal BP • If severely elevated (≥160 mm Hg systolic or ≥110 mm Hg diastolic), diagnosis can be confirmed without waiting 4 hours so antihypertensive medications may be administered

and

Proteinuria	• ≥300 mg per 24 hour urine collection *OR* • Urine protein/creatinine ratio ≥0.3 • Dipstick reading of 1+ (only if no other test available)

Or in the absence of proteinuria, new-onset hypertension with the new onset of any of

Thrombocytopenia	• Platelet count <100 000/μL
Renal insufficiency	• Serum creatinine ≥1.1 mg/dL or a doubling of the baseline
Impaired liver function	• Elevated liver enzymes to twice normal
Pulmonary edema	
Cerebral/Visual symptoms	

Diagnostic Criteria for PEC with Severe Features (Table 1-23)

TABLE 1-23 PRECLAMPSIA WITH SEVERE FEATURES*

- Systolic BP of ≥160 mm Hg, or diastolic BP ≥110 mm Hg on two occasions at least 4 hours apart while on bed rest (unless antihypertensive therapy have been administered within 4 hours of first reading)
- Thrombocytopenia (platelets <100 000/μL)
- Impaired liver function (elevated liver enzymes (twice normal) or severe right upper quadrant/ epigastric pain without alternative diagnosis
- Renal insufficiency (serum creatinine >1.1 mg/dL or a doubling of baseline with no other renal disease)
- Pulmonary edema
- New-onset cerebral or visual disturbances
- *Since there is not a strong relationship between urine protein and pregnancy outcome in PEC, proteinuria over 5 g has been eliminated from the criteria for severe PEC*

* Presence of ANY of these findings meets criteria for severe.
Data from ACOG Task Force on Hypertension in Pregnancy, *Hypertension in Pregnancy*, 2013.

Risk Factors for PEC

• Primiparity	• Family history of PEC
• Previous PEC	• Pregestational or gestational diabetes
• Chronic hypertension or chronic renal disease	• Obesity
• History of thrombophilia	• Systemic lupus erythematosus
• Multifetal pregnancy	• Advanced maternal age (>40 years)
	• In vitro pregnancy

Prevention of PEC

- Women with a history of early-onset PEC with delivery at < 34-0/7 weeks or PEC in more than one prior pregnancy are advised to *initiate daily low-dose aspirin (60–80 mg)* beginning in the late first trimester. (Typical low-dose aspirin in United States is 81mg).

Prediagnostic Findings Warranting Increased Surveillance

- Maternal: New headaches, visual disturbances, right upper quadrant or epigastric pain, edema, rapid weight gain, new-onset proteinuria after 20 weeks GA, elevations in BP > 15 mmHg diastolic or 30 mmHg systolic
- Fetal: IUGR

Management of Gestational Hypertension, PEC, and HELLP

- *Initial Evaluation*
  - Labs: CBC, creatinine, liver enzymes, 24-hour urine or protein/creatinine ratio
  - Maternal: Evaluate for symptoms
  - Fetal: Ultrasound for estimated fetal weight and AFI; NST, BPP if NST nonreactive
- If GA is ≥37-0/7 weeks, DELIVER.
- If GA is ≥34-0/7 weeks and severe features are present, DELIVER.
- If GA is < 34-0/7 weeks, and PEC with severe features, see Table 1-24
- If GA is < 37-0/7 weeks, and PEC without severe features:
- Consider antenatal steroids if <34-0/7 weeks
- May manage as in- or out-patient
- Maternal evaluation twice weekly
- Fetal evaluation
  - If gestational hypertension, consider weekly NST
  - If PEC, consider twice weekly NST
- *Bed Rest:* For gestational hypertension or PEC without severe features, strict bed rest should not be prescribed

TABLE 1-24   MANAGEMENT OF PEC WITH SEVERE FEATURES AT LESS THAN 34 WEEKS GA

Initial Management:

- Observe in Labor and Delivery for 24-48 hours
- Administer antental corticosteroids
- Administer magnesium sulfate for seizure prophylaxis
- Administer antihypertensive medications as needed
- Monitor maternal symptoms and lab tests
- Assess fetus with ultrasound, FHR monitoring

IF any of the following are present, deliver once patient is stable:

- Eclampsia
- Pulmonary edema
- Disseminated intravascular coagulation
- Uncontrollable hypertension
- Nonviable / Previable fetus
- Abnormal fetal testing
- Placental abruption

If any of the following are present, deliver 48 hours after first corticosteroid administration:

- ≥33-5/7 weeks
- Persistent symptoms
- HELLP / partial HELLP
- IUGR (<5th percentile)
- Severe oligohydramnios
- Reversed end-diastolic flow in Umbilical artery Doppler studies
- Labor/PPROM
- Significant renal dysfunction

To continue expectant management:

- Facility must have adequate resources for maternal/fetal intensive care
- Patient remains inpatient
- Frequent maternal and fetal monitoring is performed (See Table 1-25)
- Oral antihypertensive therapy may be needed

Indications for Delivery:

- 34-0/7 weeks GA
- Delivery may be indicated prior to 34-0/7 weeks for either maternal or fetal indications
  - Maternal indications include:
    - Recurrent severe hypertension or symptoms of PEC
    - Renal insufficiency (doubling of creatinine or greater than ≥1.1 mg/dl)
    - Persistent thrombocytopenia or HELLP
    - Pulmonary edema
    - Eclampsia
    - Suspected placental abruption
  - Fetal indications include:
    - Severe IUGR (<5th percentile)
    - Persistent oligohydramnios
    - BPP of ≤4/10 on 2 occasions less than 6 hours apart
    - Abnormal umbilical artery Dopplers (reversed end-diastolic flow)
    - NST with recurrent variables or late decelerations

Data from ACOG Task Force on Hypertension in Pregnancy, *Hypertension in Pregnancy*, 2013.

TABLE 1-25 MONITORING DURING EXPECTANT MANAGEMENT IN PEC WITH SEVERE FEATURES

Maternal and Fetal Monitoring	
Maternal Assessment	**Fetal Assessment**
• Vital signs, strict ins and outs, symptoms monitored every 8 hours • Labs: CBC, including platelets, liver enzymes, creatinine daily. Can check every other day if stable	• NST daily • BPP twice weekly • Serial fetal growth every 2 (per ACOG) weeks and umbilical artery Doppler studies every 2 weeks if IUGR is suspected

Data from ACOG Task Force on Hypertension in Pregnancy, *Hypertension in Pregnancy*, 2013.

Seizure Prophylaxis
• Recommended in PEC with severe features

Magnesium Sulfate

• IV: 4 (or 6) g IV bolus, then 2 g/h
• IM: May be given IM into upper outer quadrant of buttocks
  • Loading dose: 5 g in each buttock
  • Maintenance dose: 3 g in alternating buttocks every 4 hours
• *Therapeutic levels: 4–7 mEq/L (4.8–8.4 mg/dL)*

• If CD, continue magnesium administration intra-operatively
• *Magnesium Toxicity* (Table 1-26)
  • *Treatment of Magnesium Toxicity*
    • Discontinue magnesium. Check blood level; treat based on clinical signs
    • Maintain airway/oxygenation. Mechanical ventilation may be needed
    • Administer: Calcium gluconate 1 g IV over at least 3 minutes
    • Diuretic agents (furosemide, mannitol) may be administered
• Can use Phenytoin (*Dilantin*) or Fosphenytoin if unable to use magnesium

TABLE 1-26 SIGNS OF MAGNESIUM TOXICITY

	Serum Magnesium		
	mmol/L	**mEq/L**	**mg/dL**
Loss of patellar reflexes	3.5–5	7–10	8.5–12
Respiratory depression	5–6.5	10–13	12–16
Altered cardiac conduction	>7.5	>15	>18
Cardiac arrest	>12.5	>25	>30

Antihypertensive Therapy
• *Antihypertensive Therapy:* Not recommended if systolic BP <160 or diastolic BP <110
• Antihypertensive Agents for Urgent Blood Pressure Control in Pregnancy (Table 1-27)
• Common Oral Antihypertensive Agents in Pregnancy (Table 1-28)

TABLE 1-27 ANTIHYPERTENSIVE AGENTS FOR URGENT BLOOD PRESSURE CONTROL IN PREGNANCY

Drug	Dose and Route	Concerns and Comments
Labetalol	10–20 mg IV, then 20–80 mg every 20–30 minutes, maximum of 300 mg total dose For infusion: 1–2 mg/min IV	• Considered first-line agent • Tachycardia less common; fewer adverse effects • Contraindicated in patients with asthma, heart disease, or congestive heart failure
Hydralazine	5 mg IV or IM, then 5–10 mg every 20–40 minutes For infusion: 0.5–10.0 mg/h	• Higher or frequent dosage associated with maternal hypotension, headaches, and fetal distress—may be more common than other agents
Nifedipine	10–20 mg orally, repeat in 30 minutes if needed; then 10–20 mg every 2–6 hours	• Theoretical concern about combination of nifedipine and magnesium resulting in hypotension and neuromuscular blockade (both calcium channel antagonists). Thus, monitor carefully

TABLE 1-28 COMMON ORAL ANTIHYPERTENSIVE AGENTS IN PREGNANCY

Drug	Dose and Route	Concerns and Comments
Labetalol	200–2400 mg/day orally in two to three divided doses	• Well tolerated • Potential bronchoconstrictive effects • Avoid in patients with asthma and congestive heart failure
Nifedipine	30–120 mg/day orally of a slow-release preparation	• Do not use sublingual form
Methyldopa	0.5–3 g/day orally in two to three divided doses	• Childhood safety data up to 7 years of age • May not be as effective in control of severe hypertension
Thiazide diuretics	Depends on agent	• Second-line agent

Route of Delivery
• Should be determined by fetal GA, presentation, cervical status, and maternal–fetal condition
• With IOL, *likelihood of CD* increases with decreasing GA
  • <28 weeks 93–97%
  • 28–32 weeks 53–65%
  • 32–34 weeks 31–38%

Management of Chronic Hypertension
• Baseline Labs/Evaluation
  • Serum creatinine, electrolytes, liver enzymes
  • Platelet count, uric acid
  • Urine protein (consider 24-hour collection if dipstick is 1+ or higher; spot protein/creatinine ratio)
  • ECG or echocardiogram if severe hypertension for more than 4 years
  • Screen for presence of secondary hypertension (resistant hypertension, hypokalemia, palpitations, age <35 years)
• Antihypertensive Therapy
  • Recommended if persistent hypertension with systolic BP of ≥160 mm Hg or diastolic ≥105 mm Hg
  • Maintain BP between 120/80 and 160/105
  • BP goals are lower if evidence of end-organ damage (chronic renal disease or cardiac disease)—systolic BP <140 mm Hg and diastolic <90 mm Hg

Other Information
- If diagnosed with gestational hypertension, PEC, or superimposed PEC, BP should be monitored in the hospital for at least 72 hours postpartum (or equivalent outpatient surveillance be performed) and again 7–10 days after delivery. Earlier follow-up is needed if patient experiences any symptoms
- For women who present in the postpartum period with new-onset hypertension associated with headaches or blurred vision or PEC with severe hypertension, administration of magnesium sulfate is suggested
- For women with persistent postpartum hypertension, systolic BP of ≥150 or diastolic BP ≥100 on at least two occasions at least 4–6 hours apart, antihypertensive therapy is suggested. Persistent BP of 160/100 or higher should be treated within 1 hour

DIABETES IN PREGNANCY

Pregestational Diabetes Mellitus (DM)

Classification

Type 1	Type 2
• Insulin sensitive	• Insulin resistant
• History of severe hypoglycemia or diabetic ketoacidosis (DKA)	• Onset at any age except early childhood
	• Usually insulin-requiring in pregnancy
• Risk of hypoglycemia or DKA in pregnancy	• Risk of hyperosmolar coma
• Insulin dependent	

Fetal Malformations
- Increase with increasing HbA1C in first trimester
  - HbA1C less than 6.0–6.5 is desired

HbA1C (%)	Risk of Malformation (%)
<6	2–3 (same as general population)
7–8.9	5–10
9–10.9	10–20
≥11	>20

- Types of Malformations: Cardiovascular, renal, neural tube defects. Double outlet right ventricle, truncus arteriosus, and caudal regression syndrome seen with higher frequency than expected. Sacral agenesis/caudal regression syndrome is almost pathognomonic (500-fold increase)

Workup for Pregestational DM or Gestational Diabetes Mellitus (GDM) Diagnosed at < 20 weeks GA
- Labs: HbA1C; TFTs (40% with Type 1 diabetes have thyroid disorders)
- Ophthalmology consult; consider ECG
- 24-hour urine for total protein and creatinine clearance (need serum creatinine) for baseline (or spot protein/creatinine ratio)
- Ultrasounds: Dating, anatomy at 18–20 weeks; fetal growth at 28–30 and 36 weeks
- Fetal echocardiogram around 22 weeks GA

Gestational Diabetes (GDM)
- Definition: Carbohydrate intolerance leading to hyperglycemia with onset or first recognition during pregnancy
- Types
  - Class A1 = Diet-controlled
  - Class A2 = Requires medication
- Occurs in 6–7% of pregnancies (1–14% depending on population and diagnostic test used)
- 20–50% develop overt diabetes in the next 5–10 years; 33–50% will have recurrent GDM
- Meta-analysis: If diagnosed with GDM, there is a 7.4-fold risk for developing Type 2 DM
- Treatment of mild GDM as compared with usual care resulted in reduced rates of PEC, gestational hypertension, and reduced risks of fetal overgrowth, shoulder dystocia, CD

Screening and Diagnosis of GDM
- If early pregnancy, can diagnose overt diabetes if
  - Fasting plasma glucose ≥126 mg/dL, or
  - HbA1C ≥6.5%, or
  - Random plasma glucose ≥200 mg/dL (with confirmation test)
- If GDM is diagnosed <20 weeks GA, counsel/manage as Type 2 pregestational DM
- Currently, a two-step approach is recommended
  - *Screen with 50-g glucose challenge test (GCT)*
    - Screen at 24–28 weeks
    - May be done in fasted or fed state (more sensitive in fasting state)
    - Threshold for diagnosis varies from 130 to 140 mg/dL
      - Sensitivities and specificities vary by study. Lower cutoff is slightly more sensitive; however, more women will have false-positive tests
      - Because there is no clear evidence supporting a cutoff, ACOG recommends providers choose a consistent cutoff (130, 135, or 140). If screen is positive (at chosen cutoff), proceed with 3-hour glucose tolerance test (GTT)
  - *Diagnostic test: 3-hour GTT (100 g)*
    - Ideally, fast for 8 hours after 3-day carbohydrate-rich diet (>150 g/day)
    - Diagnostic criteria for GDM (Table 1-29)

TABLE 1-29 DIAGNOSIS OF GDM BASED ON 3-HOUR GTT

	Diagnosis of GDM from 3-hour GTT	
	Carpenter and Coustan*	National Diabetes Data Group
Fasting	<95	<105
1 hour	<180	<190
2 hours	<155	<165
3 hours	<140	<145

*Used at Johns Hopkins.
Values mg/dl. Two abnormal values needed for diagnosis of GDM.

- **Perform early GCT at first prenatal visit if high-risk for GDM**
  - Personal history of GDM, BMI ≥30, prior infant weighing over 4000 g, strong family history, prior diagnosis of polycystic ovary syndrome (PCOS)
  - If normal glucose screen, repeat screen at 24–28 weeks
  - If GCT is abnormal, do 3-hour GTT
  - If GTT is normal, repeat GTT at 24–28 weeks

Management of Pregestational DM and GDM

- Nutrition consult, carbohydrate-controlled diet with three meals and three snacks
- Home glucose monitoring can this be 4–5 times per day [fasting, 1 or 2 hours postprandial ± bedtime (QHS)]
- Poorly controlled pregestational DM: Fasting, premeals, and QHS D-sticks until control improves. Then change to fasting and postprandial. Can test up to eight times per day (fasting, premeal, postmeal, QHS)
- If in hospital for poor control or infection: Fasting, premeal, postmeal, QHS
- Type 1 diabetics, especially if on insulin pump, may test 7–10 times per day—this regimen should be continued when hospitalized
- Insulin regimen for hospitalized patients
  - Adjust on daily basis as needed
  - Use correctional boluses (Novolog or Humalog) premeal or QHS, as needed
  - Avoid postmeal correctional boluses unless blood glucose is over 180 mg/dL

Goal Blood Glucose Levels for Adequate Control

Fasting	60–90 (or 95) mg/dL
Premeal	60–100 mg/dL
1 hour postprandial	<140 mg/dL
2 hours postprandial	<120 mg/dL
Bedtime	<120 mg/dL
2:00–6:00 AM	60–120 mg/dL

Important Points

- Avoid hospitalization for diabetic control; patient will eat better and be more active at home. Control in the hospital has little to do with control in real life
- For cough, avoid regular Robitussin (sugar syrup vehicle). Use sugar-free Robitussin or Tessalon Perles
- Terbutaline and steroids may cause hyperglycemia (sometimes severe) in diabetics
- Treatment of hypoglycemia: Patient on insulin should have glucagon 1 mg IM and someone trained in its administration. Carry glycemic food at all times
- *IN GENERAL*
  - 10-g carbohydrate increases blood glucose 30 mg/dL
  - 1 unit rapid acting insulin decreases blood glucose 30 mg/dL
- Recommendations for Antenatal Testing and Delivery Timing (Table 1-30)
- Consider CD to prevent brachial plexus injury when the EFW is over 4500 g

TABLE 1-30 RECOMMENDATIONS FOR ANTENATAL TESTING AND DELIVERY IN DIABETES

	Antenatal Testing	Delivery
GDM-A1	Not at increased risk for fetal demise prior to 40 weeks GA. No antepartum testing is required beyond that recommended for normal pregnancy	Usual obstetric indications There are no evidence-based recommendations.
Pregestational and GDM-A2	Twice weekly NSTs ± BPP starting at 32–34 weeks (28 weeks if other complications: nephropathy, IUGR)	Deliver between 39 and 40 weeks

Pharmacologic Management of Diabetes

Oral Hypoglycemics: Acceptable alternative to insulin when diet fails

- Glyburide
  - Second generation sulfonylurea: Stimulates functional beta cells in pancreatic islets, increasing insulin release
  - *Starting dose:* Usually 2.5 mg at bedtime or 2.5 mg twice daily
  - *Max dose* is 20 mg/day; lowest available dose is 1.25 mg
  - Side effects: Hypoglycemia, nausea, heartburn, allergic skin reactions
  - Likely won't be effective in GDM if fastings are over 110 mg/dL
- Metformin (*Glucophage*): Shown to be safe in pregnancy
  - Biguanide: Decreases hepatic glucose production and intestinal glucose absorption; increases peripheral glucose uptake and utilization by improving insulin sensitivity
  - *Dose:* 500 mg once or twice daily, maximum of 2500 mg/day
  - Side effects: Diarrhea, flatulence, indigestion, nausea/vomiting
  - GERD is a relative contraindication
  - *Lactic acidosis:* Rare metabolic complication due to accumulation; fatal in about 50%. Temporarily stop medication prior to any IV contrast or surgery

Insulin

- Dosing Guidelines (Table 1-31)
- Total daily dose is divided into **thirds**; two-thirds in morning and one-third in evening
  - **Morning** dose (before breakfast)
  - Two-thirds dose as NPH insulin
    - One-third dose as a rapid acting insulin (Humalog or Novolog)

TABLE 1-31 INSULIN DOSING GUIDELINES

Gestational Age (weeks)	Total Calculated Daily Insulin Needed
1–18	0.7 U/kg actual body weight
18–26	0.8 U/kg actual body weight
26–36	0.9 U/kg actual body weight
36–40	1.0 U/kg actual body weight

Usually do not start more than 60 U insulin/day.

- **Evening** dose typically divided into predinner and bedtime
  - One-half as rapid acting (Humalog or Novalog) → Pre-dinner
  - One-half as NPH at bedtime. Sometimes given with pre-dinner for patient convenience, but best given at bedtime
- *If persistent fasting hyperglycemia with normal postprandial values, may start bedtime NPH insulin alone*
- Insulin requirements may decrease after 35 weeks, especially if pregestational. If this occurs, assess fetal well-being as it could be the result of placental insufficiency

Insulin Pump

- *To Start*
  - Start with 80% of total daily insulin dose. About half of insulin is used in basal rate
  - Uses rapid-acting insulin analog (Humalog or Novolog)
- *Basal Rates*
  - Can be changed every hour. Usually 0.5–1.5 units/h in Type 1; higher in Type 2
  - Usual basal rates: Start with 3–4 basal rates in pregnancy (1 when not pregnant)
    - MN–4 AM; 4 AM–8 AM; 8 AM–4 PM; 4 PM–MN
- *Boluses*
  - Premeals: Based on carbohydrate counting (usually 1:10 in pregnancy; 1:15 nonpregnancy)
  - Correction Factor (CF)
    - Based on patient's sensitivity to exogenous insulin
    - Rule: 1800/total insulin dose
    - Usually 25–30 in pregnancy (40–60 in nonpregnant)
    - For every "CF mg/dL" over target blood sugar, add 1 unit of insulin
      - *Example: If CF is 30, goal 120, current glucose 180, then add 2 units insulin*
- *Managing Insulin Pump on Labor and Delivery*
  - **Don't turn off pump** and start insulin drip. USE PUMP!
  - Average their basal rates and use as a single rate during labor or CD
  - If hyperglycemic, may bolus with pump or give IV insulin, depending on urgency
- *Post-delivery*
  - Decrease basal rate by 50–70%. Individualize bolus rates

Diabetic Management During Labor

- For IOL, have patient take NPH the evening before; hold AM insulin
- Discontinue Metformin the night before scheduled CD or at time of admission
- If not on a pump, start insulin drip
  - **Insulin Drip:** 100 units regular insulin in 100 mL NS (1 unit per mL)
- Hourly D-sticks in active labor
  - **Goal glucose = 70–110 mg/dL**
  - *Type 1 diabetics* need baseline insulin if glucose >60 mg/dL (at least 0.5 units/h)

Postpartum Care

- Pregestational DM
  - Postdelivery: Decrease pre-delivery insulin regimen by at least half OR use pre-pregnancy regimen
  - D-sticks: Fasting, premeal, and bedtime
- GDM
  - Discontinue oral hypoglycemic medications or insulin
  - 6–12 weeks postpartum: *2-hour 75-g GTT.* Patient must be fasted. See Table 1-32 for diagnostic criteria for DM, impaired fasting glucose, and impaired glucose tolerance

TABLE 1-32 DIAGNOSTIC CRITERIA FOR DIABETES MELLITUS, IMPAIRED FASTING GLUCOSE, IMPAIRED GLUCOSE TOLERANCE

Test	Diabetes	Impaired Fasting Glucose	Impaired Glucose Tolerance
Fasting plasma glucose	Fasting plasma glucose is ≥126 mg/dl	Fasting plasma glucose is 100–125 mg/dl	NA
2-hour 75-g GTT	Fasting plasma glucose is ≥126 mg/dl OR 2-hour plasma glucose is ≥200 mg/dl	Fasting plasma glucose is 100–125 mg/dl	2-hour plasma glucose is 140–199 mg/dl

Diabetic Ketoacidosis (DKA) (see algorithm in Table 1-33)

- Can occur in 5–10% of pregestational Type 1 diabetics
- Symptoms include abdominal pain, nausea and vomiting, and altered sensorium
- Fetal mortality up to 10%

DKA Diagnostic Criteria
- Blood glucose >200 mg/dL
- Plasma bicarbonate <15 mEq/L
- Moderate ketonuria
- Arterial pH usually <7.3; elevated anion gap

Initial Management
- Continuous fetal monitoring if ≥24 weeks GA until resolution of DKA
- DO NOT DELIVER for nonreassuring fetal status unless ominous; in utero resuscitation much better for perinatal outcome
- Start IV fluids: One liter normal saline for 1 hour, then reevaluate
- Keep patient NPO
- Insert Foley catheter if patient cannot spontaneously void
- Obtain baseline ECG
- Labs

Critical Care Labs	Other Labs
· Arterial blood gas (ABG)	· Complete blood count
· Bicarbonate	· Chloride
· Sodium and potassium	· Urine culture
· Whole blood glucose	
· Creatinine	

- Correct serum sodium for hyperglycemia (for each 100 mg/dL glucose, add 1.6 mEq to sodium)
- Continue monitoring on L&D for at least 4 hours

TABLE 1-33 PROTOCOL RECOMMENDED BY THE AMERICAN COLLEGE OF OBSTETRICIANS AND GYNECOLOGISTS (2012) FOR MANAGEMENT OF DIABETIC KETOACIDOSIS DURING PREGNANCY

Laboratory assessment
Obtain arterial blood gases to document degree of acidosis present; measure glucose, ketones, and electrolyte levels at 1- to 2-hour intervals
Insulin
Low-dose, intravenous Loading dose: 0.2–0.4 U/kg Maintenance: 2–10 U/hr
Fluids
Isotonic sodium chloride Total replacement in first 12 hours of 4–6 L 1 L in first hour 500–1000 mL/hr for 2–4 hours 250 mL/hr until 80% replaced
Glucose
Begin 5-percent dextrose in normal saline when glucose plasma level reaches 250 mg/dL (14 mmol/L)
Potassium
If initially normal or reduced, an infusion rate up to 15–20 mEq/hr may be required; if elevated, wait until levels decrease into the normal range, then add to intravenous solution in a concentration of 20–30 mEq/L
Bicarbonate
Add one ampule (44 mEq) to 1 L of 0.45 normal saline if pH is <7.1

HIV AND PREGNANCY

Quick Points for L&D

- Check *ultrasensitive* HIV RNA copy number (viral load; VL) and CD4 count on admission if not done recently (within 4–5 weeks if VL <20; 2 weeks if >20) *AND* you anticipate patient will NOT deliver soon
- As of 2014: Zidovudine (generic name; also referred to as Retrovir, ZDV, AZT) should be administered to women with **HIV RNA >1000 copies/mL** (or unknown HIV RNA near delivery), but it is *not* required in women on antiretroviral therapy (ART) who have HIV RNA ≤1000 copies/mL near time of delivery
- Artificially rupture membranes *only* if not making adequate cervical dilation and delivery is anticipated soon
- Avoid invasive monitoring or operative vaginal delivery, unless obstetric indication
- If spontaneous ROM occurs early in labor, consider oxytocin to decrease the interval to delivery
- **Avoid methergine** if on Protease Inhibitors or Efavirenz—exaggerated vasoconstriction
- If rapid HIV test is positive in patient of unknown HIV status who presents in labor, start IV ZDV without waiting for results of confirmatory test. Follow up on confirmatory test

Transmission

- See Table 1-34 for Risk of Transmission Rates
- To reduce transmission risk
  - **Landmark Study (ACTG 076):** Zidovudine (antepartum, intrapartum, and to neonate) decreased risk of perinatal transmission from 25.5% to 8.3% (67.5% reduction). Although zidovudine alone has substantially reduced the risk for perinatal transmission, ART *monotherapy* is now considered *suboptimal* for treatment of HIV infection and combination drug regimens are considered the standard of care both for treatment of HIV infection and for prevention of perinatal transmission
- Antiretroviral (ARV) drugs reduce perinatal transmission by several mechanisms. Risk of transmission is decreased even when VL <1000 copies/mL. Combined antepartum, intrapartum, and infant ARV prophylaxis is recommended to prevent transmission
- All HIV-infected women should be counseled about and administered ARV drugs during pregnancy for prevention of perinatal transmission, regardless of their HIV RNA levels or CD4 T-lymphocyte count. Although risk of perinatal transmission in women with undetectable HIV RNA levels is extremely low, transmission has been reported even in women with very low or undetectable levels of maternal HIV RNA on ART
- http://AIDSinfo.nih.gov is a useful up-to-date Web site for further information

TABLE 1-34 RISK OF TRANSMISSION

No antiretroviral treatment during pregnancy	25–30%
ZDV only (intrapartum + neonatal)	10%
ZDV only (ante and intrapartum + neonatal)	8.3%
Antiretroviral therapy (ART)	<2%
ART and undetectable viral load	<1%

Data from Public Health Service task Force Recommendations, November 2007; Connor et al. Reduction of maternal-infant transmission of human immunodefiiency virus type 1 with zidovudine treatment. Pediatric AIDS clinical trials Group Protocol 076 Study Group. *NEJM.* 1994;331:1173–1180; Wade et al. Abbreviated regimens of zidovudine prophylaxis and perinatal transmission of the human immunodefiiency virus. *NEJM.* 1998;339:1409–1414.

Recommendations—Antepartum

- Obtain baseline labs: HIV RNA, CD4 cell count, CBC, renal and liver function testing
- Genotypic ARV drug-resistance studies should be performed before starting an ARV drug regimen if HIV RNA level is above threshold (>500 copies/mL)
- Perform repeat ARV drug resistance testing and assess adherence to guide changes in ARV drugs in women who do not achieve virologic suppression on regimen
- When HIV is diagnosed later in pregnancy, combination ART should be initiated promptly without waiting for results of resistance testing
- Screen for Hepatitis A, B, and C and TB
- Vaccinate for pneumococcus (if CD4 >200 cells/μL), Hepatitis A and B, and influenza
- Administer Tdap vaccine per recommendations
- Assess need for prophylaxis against opportunistic infections, such as mycobacterium avium complex (MAC) and pneumocystis pneumonia (PCP)

Antiretroviral Therapy
- ARV drugs are used to: (1) treat patient and (2) reduce vertical transmission
- *When to start antiretrovirals?*
  - Decision to start regimen in the first trimester or delay until 12 weeks depends on CD4 count, HIV RNA levels, and maternal conditions (nausea/vomiting). Earlier initiation of ARV regimen may be more effective in reducing transmission, but benefits must be weighed against potential fetal effects of first trimester drug exposure and risks of noncompliance if hyperemesis is present
  - In general, if patient is on ART and presents for care during the first trimester, they should continue ART during pregnancy, assuming it is tolerated and effective
  - If patient is AIDS-defined, start ARV regimen ASAP
- *Antiretroviral Medications*
  - Combined ART regimen should contain at least three agents
    - A dual nucleoside reverse transcriptase inhibitor (NRTI) backbone
    - A non-nucleoside reverse transcriptase inhibitor (NNRTI) *or*
    - One or more protease inhibitors (PI)
  - There is a possible small increased risk of preterm birth if receiving PI-based combination ARV regimens; however, given the clear benefits of such regimens for both a woman's health and prevention of mother-to-child transmission, PIs should not be withheld for this reason

Monitoring During Pregnancy
- CD4 count: Initial visit and at least every 3 months
- HIV-RNA levels
  - Initial visit
  - 2–4 weeks after initiating or changing ARV regimen
  - Monthly until levels are undetectable, then at least every 3 months
  - At 34–36 weeks for decision on mode of delivery
  - If concern regarding adherence or resistance, then more frequent monitoring

Recommendations—Intrapartum

- As of 2014: Zidovudine (ZDV/AZT) should be administered to women with **HIV RNA ≥1000 copies/mL** (or unknown HIV RNA near delivery), but it is *not* required in women on combination ARV who have HIV RNA ≤1000 copies/mL consistently during late pregnancy and near delivery and no concerns regarding adherence

> - *Zidovudine* loading dose: *2 mg/kg* IV over 1 hour, then
> - Continuous infusion of *1 mg/kg/h* until delivery

- Continue ART during labor. If oral ZDV is part of ART regimen and HIV RNA is >1000 copies/mL, the oral ZDV component of regimen should be stopped while receiving IV ZDV. When CD is planned, oral medications can be continued preoperatively with sips of water
- AVOID, unless clear obstetric indications (potential increased risk of transmission)
  - Artificial rupture of membranes (AROM)
  - Routine use of fetal scalp electrode
  - Operative delivery with forceps or vacuum and/or episiotomy
- **Ruptured Membranes**
  - Risk of transmission higher if ROM over 4 hours (double risk; likely higher with longer duration). Unknown if risk applies if undetectable HIV RNA or on ART
  - Recent study: In women on combination ART with HIV-RNA <1000, there were no cases of perinatal transmission with up to 25 hours of ROM. HIV RNA >10000 copies/mL was the only independent risk factor for transmission
  - When ROM occurs before 37 weeks, decisions about timing of delivery should be based on best obstetrical practices. Steroids should be given, if appropriate, because no data exist to suggest these recommendations need to be altered for HIV-infected women. When the decision is made to deliver, route of delivery should be according to obstetrical indications
- **Cesarean Delivery**
  - Recommended when HIV RNA is >1000 copies/mL or unknown near time of delivery (whether or not patient is receiving ART) to decrease transmission
    - Schedule at *38 weeks* if HIV RNA >1000 copies/mL
    - Schedule at *39 weeks* if HIV RNA <1000 and CD is for obstetrical reasons
  - IV ZDV should be started **3 hours** before scheduled CD and run until cord clamp
  - Data are insufficient to evaluate benefit of CD in patients on ART with HIV RNA <1000 copies/mL. Given low rate of transmission, unlikely that CD confers added benefit
  - Administer routine perioperative antibiotic prophylaxis
  - HIV-infected women have increased post-op complications, mostly infectious
  - If HIV-infected patient scheduled for CD presents in labor or with ROM
    - UNCLEAR if CD after ROM or labor provides benefit in reducing transmission

- Management must be individualized based on duration of rupture, progress of labor, HIV RNA, current ART, and other clinical factors
- If cervical dilation is minimal and long labor anticipated, begin ZDV loading dose and proceed expeditiously with CD to decrease duration of ROM and avoid vaginal delivery in patients who meet criteria for CD (>1000 copies/mL) OR begin oxytocin to expedite delivery
- If labor is progressing rapidly, women should be allowed to deliver vaginally
- When an unscheduled CD is indicated and HIV RNA ≥1000 copies/mL, consider shortening interval between starting IV ZDV and delivery. Some experts recommend giving 1-hour loading dose and then proceeding with delivery

Recommendations—Postpartum

- **Methergine use:** *Avoid* in patients on PI if possible (exaggerated vasoconstriction). Only use if no alternative—lowest dose, for shortest duration
- Continue or stop ART after delivery?
  - Consult with HIV provider
- Breast-feeding is *not* recommended for HIV-infected women in the United States
- Drug interactions have been documented between oral contraceptives and many ARV drugs. See up-to-date perinatal HIV guidelines for details

Miscellaneous

- *Amniocentesis:* In women on effective combined ART, no perinatal transmissions have been reported after amniocentesis, but a small risk cannot be ruled out. If amniocentesis is indicated, it should be done only after initiation of an effective ART regimen, and if possible, when HIV RNA levels are undetectable
- *Chorionic Villus Sampling (CVS):* Some experts consider CVS and cordocentesis too risky to offer to HIV-infected women and recommend limiting invasive procedures to amniocentesis (but data are limited)
- **Consideration can also be given to noninvasive testing using cell-free fetal DNA to reduce the need for invasive procedures**

ASTHMA

- Asthma complicates 4–8% of pregnancies
- Wheezing, dyspnea, nonproductive cough
- Risks of severe, poorly controlled asthma in pregnancy: Prematurity, IUGR, CD, PEC

Pulmonary Physiology During Pregnancy

- Relative hyperventilation
- Increased minute ventilation
- Increased tidal volume
- Stable respiratory rate, stable forced expiratory volume in the first second (FEV1)
- Decreased functional residual capacity (FRC)
- Decreased inspiratory capacity (IC)
- Decreased IC + Decreased FRC = Decreased in total lung capacity (TLC)

Acute Asthma Management

- History and physical (include triggers, history of prior hospitalizations, intubations or steroid use, current and prior medication, baseline peak flow)
- Document peak flow and O_2 saturation
- Consider chest x-ray, ABG, and respiratory virus panel based on clinical evaluation and response to initial treatments
- Appropriate evaluation of fetal status depending on GA
- Continue to monitor response to medical treatment with patient's symptoms, oxygenation status, and peak flows
- Supplemental oxygen and IV hydration; optimize asthma regimen when time for discharge

Medications

- Medication considerations should be similar to treating the nonpregnant patient
  - *Beta 2 agonist:* Albuterol metered dose inhaler (MDI) or nebulizer (every 20 minutes for three doses and then every 1–4 hours as needed for ongoing treatment)
  - *Ipratropium nebulizer* (often given simultaneously with Beta 2-Agonist)
  - *Systemic steroids:* Consider if nonresponsive to initial nebulizer treatments or on chronic oral steroids
    - Severe exacerbations: 60–80 mg IV methylprednisolone
    - Oral prednisone: 40–80 mg orally in single or divided dose
  - Adjunct therapies
    - Magnesium sulfate 2 g IV over 20 minutes
    - Terbutaline 0.25 mg every 20 minutes × 3 doses

Classification of Asthma Severity and Control in Pregnant Patients (Table 1-35)

TABLE 1-35   CLASSIFICATION OF ASTHMA SEVERITY AND CONTROL IN PREGNANT PATIENTS

Asthma Severity	Symptom Frequency	Nighttime Awakening	Interference with Normal Activity	FEV$_1$ or Peak Flow
Intermittent (well controlled)	≤2 days/week	≤ Twice per month	None	≥80%
Mild persistent (not well controlled)	≥2 days/week, but not daily	> Twice per month	Minor limitation	≥80%
Moderate persistent (not well controlled)	Daily symptoms	>Once per week	Some limitation	>60–<80%
Severe persistent (very poorly controlled)	Throughout the day	Frequent	Extremely limited	≤60%

Step Therapy Medical Management of Asthma During Pregnancy (Table 1-36)

TABLE 1-36   STEP THERAPY MEDICAL MANAGEMENT OF ASTHMA DURING PREGNANCY

Mild intermittent	No daily medications Albuterol* as needed
Mild persistent	Low-dose inhaled glucocorticoid†
Moderate persistent	Medium-dose inhaled glucocorticoid† OR Low-dose inhaled glucocorticoid† plus long-acting beta agonist‡ OR Medium-dose inhaled glucocorticoid† plus long-acting beta agonist‡
Severe persistent	High-dose inhaled glucocorticoid† plus long-acting beta agonist‡

*Albuterol is preferred inhaled short-acting beta 2-agonist in pregnancy.
†Budesonide is preferred inhaled corticosteroid in pregnancy.
   Low-dose: 200–600 µg/day
   Medium-dose: 600–1200 µg/day
   High-dose: >1200 µg/day
‡Salmeterol is preferred long-acting inhaled beta 2-agonist in pregnancy.
Data from NAEPP Expert Panel Report. Managing Asthma During Pregnancy: Recommendations for Pharmacologic Treatment–Update 2004. US Department HHS, Bethesda, MD. NIH Publication No. 04-5246, March 2004.

THROMBOPHILIA AND PREGNANCY

- Pregnancy is considered a hypercoagulable state
- Venous thromboembolism (VTE) complicates about 1 in 1600 births and is a leading cause of maternal morbidity in the United States

Thrombophilias

High-Risk Inherited Thrombophilias

- Antithrombin deficiency
- Factor V Leiden homozygous
- Prothrombin G20210A homozygous
- Double heterozygous for prothrombin G20210A and Factor V Leiden

Low-Risk Inherited Thrombophilias

- Factor V Leiden heterozygous
- Prothrombin G20210A heterozygous
- Protein C deficiency
- Protein S deficiency

MTHFR (methylenetetrahydrofolate reductase) Mutations

- Homozygosity is most common cause of hyperhomocysteinemia
- MTHFR mutations themselves do not appear to increase risk for VTE

- Elevated homocysteine levels are a weak risk factor for VTE and intervention studies with vitamin B supplementation in nonpregnant patients show no reduction in VTE
- Thus, per ACOG → insufficient evidence to support measuring MTHFR or fasting homocysteine levels in the evaluation of a thrombophilic etiology for VTE

Screening

- IS CONTROVERSIAL!
- Routine screening for thrombophilias is not recommended in all pregnant women
  Do Screen if
  - Personal history of VTE that was associated with a nonrecurrent risk factor (fracture, surgery, immobilization)
  - First degree relative with a history of a high-risk thrombophilia or VTE before age 50 in the absence of other risk factors
  HISTORICALLY, a thrombophilia workup has also been recommended if
  - VTE during pregnancy (workup after delivery)
  - Previous unexplained fetal death in utero (FDIU) at 20 weeks or greater*¶
  - Severe early (before 34 weeks) PEC or HELLP*
  - Severe IUGR*
  - History of placental abruption*
  *ACOG no longer recommends screening in these situations as there is insufficient evidence that antepartum prophylaxis with LMWH/UFH prevents recurrence.
  ¶Screening for antiphospholipid antibodies may be appropriate.

Thrombophilia Workup

- *Recommended by ACOG*

• Factor V Leiden mutation • Protein C activity • Antithrombin deficiency	• Prothrombin gene mutation G20210A • Protein S activity

- Other tests often ordered (not recommended by ACOG)
  - Plasminogen Activator Inhibitor-1 (PAI-1 mutation 4G/4G; if not available, plasma PAI-1 activity)
  - MTHFR mutation screen and/or fasting plasma homocysteine levels
  - Antiphospholipid Syndrome (APS) workup may be appropriate for women with repeated fetal losses (see section on APS)

Thromboprophylaxis Regimens in Pregnancy (Table 1-37)

TABLE 1-37 THROMBOPROPHYLAXIS REGIMENS IN PREGNANCY

Prophylactic Dose

Low Molecular Weight Heparin *(LMWH)*
- Enoxaparin 40 mg SC once daily
- Enoxaparin 30 mg SC twice daily*
- Dalteparin 5000 units SC once daily
- Tinzaparin 4500 units SC once daily

Unfractionated Heparin *(UFH)*
- UFH 5000 units SC every 12 hours (minidose)
- UFH 5000–10 000 units SC every 12 hours
  - First trimester: UFH 5000–7500 units SC every 12 hours
  - Second trimester: UFH 7500–10 000 units SC every 12 hours
  - Third trimester: UFH 10 000 units SC every 12 hours (unless aPTT is elevated)

Intermediate Dose

LMWH
- Enoxaparin 40 mg SC every 12 hours
- Dalteparin 5000 units SC every 12 hours

UFH
- UFH SC every 12 hours
  - *Target an anti-Xa UFH level of 0.1–0.3 units/mL 6 hours after injection*

TABLE 1-37 THROMBOPROPHYLAXIS REGIMENS IN PREGNANCY (*Continued*)

Therapeutic (or "Weight-Adjusted" or "Full Treatment") Dose

LMWH

- Enoxaparin 1 mg/kg SC every 12 hours
- Enoxaparin 1.5 mg/kg SC every 24 hours[†] [Not per ACOG]
- Dalteparin 200 units/kg SC every 24 hours
- Dalteparin 100 units/kg SC every 12 hours
- Tinzaparin 175 units/kg SC every 24 hours
    - *Target an anti-Xa LMWH level of 0.6–1.0 units/mL for twice daily regimen (slightly higher for once daily regimen) 4 hours after injection*

UFH

- UFH 10 000 units or more SC every 12 hours
    - *Target an anti-Xa UFH level of 0.35–0.7 units/mL or therapeutic range aPTT (ratio of 1.5–2.5) 6 hours after injection*

Postpartum Anticoagulation (for 4–6 weeks)

- Prophylactic LMWH/UFH for 4–6 weeks *OR*
- Warfarin with target INR of 2.0–3.0 with initial UFH/LMWH overlap until INR ≥2.0 for 2 days

*Some experts recommend twice daily dosing in certain circumstances (ie, antiphospholipid antibodies in SLE) secondary to pharmacokinetic properties of LMWH in pregnancy; however, comparison data are lacking. Additionally, women at the extremes of weight may require different dosing.
[†]Chunilal SD, Bates SM. Venous thromboembolism in pregnancy: Diagnosis, management and prevention. *Thromb Haemost.* 2009;101:428–438.
Data from Bates SB, Greer IA, Middlekorp S et al. VTE, thrombophilia, Antithrombotic therapy, and pregnancy. Antithrombotic Therapy and Prevention of Thrombosis, 9th ed: American College of Chest Physicians Evidence-Based Clinical Practice Guidelines. *Chest.* 2012;141(2 Suppl):e691S–736S; ACOG. Thromboembolism in pregnancy. Practice Bulletin No. 138, September 2013, reaffirmed 2014.

Recommended Approach to Pregnant Patients at Risk for VTE

- See Table 1-38 for recommendations in selected clinical scenarios
- Please see ACOG Practice Bulletins and CHEST guidelines for updated information

TABLE 1-38 RECOMMENDED THROMBOPROPHYLAXIS APPROACH IN SELECT CLINICAL SCENARIOS

Clinical Scenario	Antepartum / Postpartum *
Low-risk thrombophilia, no prior VTE	Antepartum: Surveillance Postpartum: Surveillance or prophylactic LMWH/UFH if additional risk factors **
Prior VTE associated with a transient risk factor (immobility, surgery) that is no longer present; no thrombophilia.	Antepartum: Surveillance Postpartum: Prophylactic LMWH/UFH
Prior single episode of VTE without an associated risk factor; no thrombophilia; not on long-term anticoagulation.	Antepartum: Prophylactic LMWH/UFH Postpartum: Prophylactic LMWH/UFH
Prior single episode of VTE that was pregnancy or estrogen-related; no thrombophilia.	Antepartum: Prophylactic LMWH/UFH Postpartum: Prophylactic LMWH/UFH
High risk thrombophilia without prior VTE	Antepartum: Surveillance or prophylactic LMWH/UFH Postpartum: Prophylactic LMWH/UFH
Low risk thrombophilia with a single episode of VTE; not on long-term anticoagulation	Antepartum: Surveillance or prophylactic or intermediate-dose LMWH/UFH Postpartum: Prophylactic LMWH/UFH or intermediate dose LMWH/UFH
High risk thrombophilia with single prior VTE or an affected first degree relative; not on long-term anticoagulation	Antepartum: Prophylactic, intermediate- or adjusted-dose LMWH/UFH Postpartum: Therapy should be at least as high as antepartum

*Typically for 6 weeks postpartum.
**First degree relative with VTE before age 50; obesity, prolonged immobilization, surgery, etc.
Data from ACOG inherited thrombophilias in pregnancy. Practice Bulletin no. 138, September 2013.

Anticoagulation in Pregnancy
- Regional anesthesia considerations
  - Consider transitioning patient on LMWH to subcutaneous UFH around 36 weeks (or sooner if delivery seems imminent) due to shorter half-life than LMWH. Alternative is to stop therapeutic anticoagulation and induce labor within 24 hours
  - **Heparin**
    - Prophylactic: No restrictions
    - Therapeutic: Must have normal coagulation lab studies
  - **LMWH**
    - Prophylactic: Last dose 12 hours prior to administration of regional anesthesia
    - Therapeutic: Last dose 24 hours before administration of regional anesthesia
- Do not restart anticoagulation until 2 hours after catheter removal
- Postpartum
  - May start anticoagulation **4–6 hours** after vaginal delivery and **6–12 hours** after CD
  - Warfarin: Initial dose should be 5 mg for 2 days, then adjust according to INR. Maintain on therapeutic doses of UFH/LMWH for 5 days and until INR is therapeutic (2–3) for 2 consecutive days
  - UFH/LMWH/Warfarin are all compatible with breast feeding

ANTIPHOSPHOLIPID SYNDROME (APS)

- Autoimmune disorder defined by presence of clinical features and specified levels of circulating antiphospholipid antibodies (Table 1-39)
- 1–5% of healthy individuals have antiphospholipid antibodies, usually due to IgM antibodies at low titers (influenced by increasing age, chronic disease, infections, malignancies, and certain drugs). Persistent positivity is rare

TABLE 1-39 SYDNEY CLASSIFICATION CRITERIA FOR APS

Clinical Criteria (one or more present)

- Vascular thrombosis: One or more objectively confirmed episodes of arterial, venous, or small vessel thrombosis occurring in any tissue or organ
- Pregnancy morbidity
  - One or more unexplained deaths of a morphologically normal fetus at or beyond 10 weeks GA, or
  - One or more premature births of a morphologically normal neonate before 34 weeks GA because of eclampsia/PEC, placental insufficiency, or
  - Three or more unexplained consecutive spontaneous abortions before 10 weeks GA

Lab Criteria (one or more, present on two or more occasions at least 12 weeks apart)

- Lupus anticoagulant, detected according to the guidelines of the International Society on Thrombosis and Haemostasis. [Several different tests are used to confirm the presence of a lupus anticoagulant and may include PTT, PT, dilute Russell viper venom screen (dRVVT), or kaolin clotting time]
- Anticardiolipin antibody of IgG and/or IgM isotype, present in medium or high titer (greater than 40 GPL or MPL, or greater than the 99th percentile), measured by a standardized ELISA
- Anti-β_2-glycoprotein-1 antibody of IgG and/or IgM isotype, present in titer greater than the 99th percentile, measured by a standardized ELISA

Pregnancy Management
- If APS and no history of thrombosis, should receive prophylactic anticoagulation and low-dose aspirin during pregnancy and postpartum period
- If APS and previous thrombosis, should receive full anticoagulation antepartum and postpartum
- Consider serial growth scans (risk of IUGR) and antenatal testing

INTRAHEPATIC CHOLESTASIS OF PREGNANCY

- Pruritis with elevated serum bile acids
- *Prevalence*: Varies widely; geographic variations. Highest rates in Chile, Bolivia, and Scandinavia. In the United States, between 0.001% and 0.32%; 5.6% in Latina population in Los Angeles
- *Etiology*: Multifactorial. Genetic, hormonal, environmental factors may play a role
- Usually develops in third trimester, occasionally late second trimester (80% after 30 weeks)
- Increased risk with multiple gestation
- Pruritis
  - No rash; excoriations from scratching may be present
  - Primarily on palms and soles; extending to legs and abdomen. Worse at night

- Precedes lab abnormalities by a mean of 3 weeks
- Usually relieved within 48 hours of delivery
- Jaundice occurs in approximately 10–25% of patients, 1–4 weeks after the pruritus
- Recurs in 50–70% of subsequent pregnancies

Labs

- *Bile Acids*
  - Order *Total* and *Fractionated Bile Acids*
  - Fasting is preferred BUT THIS IS NOT A REQUIREMENT
  - *Diagnosis:*
    - Total bile acids: **10–14 µmol/L**
    - Fractionated bile acids: Chenodeoxycholic acid, deoxycholic acid, cholic acid Cholic acid raised more than chenodeoxcholic acid (increased ratio may be most sensitive indicator, but no diagnostic cutoff)
- May see mildly elevated direct bilirubin (20% of women) and alkaline phosphatase
- Transaminase levels are normal to moderately elevated in up to 60% (may be delayed, so assess serially); normalize by 2–8 weeks postpartum
- Consider screening for Hepatitis C (higher cholestasis incidence in these patients)
- Typically normalize within 4 weeks of delivery

Complications

- Linked to increased perinatal morbidity and mortality (preterm delivery, meconium, intrapartum FHR abnormalities, FDIU)
- Appear to **correlate with total bile acids, especially if over 40 µmol/L**

Treatment

- Antihistamines and topical emollients (hydroxyzine)
- **Ursodeoxycholic acid** (*Ursodiol*) increases bile flow and is highly effective in controlling pruritus and lab abnormalities. *May* decrease fetal risks
  - Doses range from 8 to 15 mg/kg/day divided twice to three times daily
  - Common starting dose is 300 mg twice daily. Can increase to 600 mg twice a day if pruritis persists after 1 week of treatment
- **Cholestyramine** (8–18 g/day, divided two to four times daily); effective if mild to moderate. NOT first line therapy

Antepartum Fetal Testing

- Recommended; no evidence-based guidelines on type, duration, frequency
- May not be predictive of poor fetal outcome
- Reasonable to start twice weekly NSTs upon diagnosis

Delivery

- No evidence-based recommendation
- Typical management: Delivery between 37 and 38 weeks. Consider obstetrical history, lab values, etc when determining timing
- Some advocate amniocentesis at 36 weeks to detect meconium followed by delivery if present

ACUTE FATTY LIVER OF PREGNANCY

- A medical and obstetric emergency
- Most common cause of acute liver failure in pregnancy
- Microvesicular fatty infiltration of hepatocytes
- One in 7000 to 1 in 20000 deliveries; typically late in pregnancy
- More common in multiple gestations
- *Symptoms:* Nausea or vomiting (in 75%), abdominal pain, malaise, anorexia, and jaundice. Approximately half of patients have signs suggestive of PEC. May be difficult to differentiate from HELLP syndrome
- Possible *laboratory abnormalities*

• Hemoconcentration	• **Hypoglycemia**
• Mild to moderate thrombocytopenia	• WBC elevated higher than expected
• Hypofibrinogenemia	• Elevated LDH
• Elevated creatinine	• Elevated bilirubin
• Elevated liver enzymes	• Elevated uric acid
• Prolonged clotting times	• Ammonia level

- Liver biopsy is diagnostic, but not always practical
- *Treatment:* Supportive care, maternal stabilization (ie, reverse DIC), delivery of fetus
- Substantial morbidity may occur (hepatic encephalopathy, severe coagulopathy, renal failure). Maternal mortality may range from 4% to 7%
- Hepatic function typically normalizes within a week of delivery
- Association with inherited defects in mitochondrial beta-oxidation of fatty acids, *long-chain 3-hydroxyacyl CoA dehydrogenase deficiency (LCHAD);* therefore, pediatrics should be notified to evaluate infant

THYROID AND PREGNANCY

- Universal screening not recommended before pregnancy or at first prenatal visit
- Consider screening if high risk

• Over 30 years of age	• Presence of type 1 diabetes or other autoimmune disorder
• Family history	
• Goiter	• Infertility
• Known presence of thyroid antibodies	• History of miscarriage or preterm delivery
• Signs/symptoms of thyroid dysfunction	• Prior head/neck irradiation or thyroid surgery

Thyroid—Changes in Pregnancy (Figure 1-29)

- Increase in size of thyroid gland (10–15%)
- Estrogen-mediated increase in thyroid binding globulin (TBG) twofold to threefold
- Production of thyroxine (T4) and tri-iodothyronine (T3) increases by 50%
- Transient decrease in thyrotropin (or TSH) weeks 8–14
- Reduction in iodide (increased clearance)
- Maternal T3, T4 cross placenta; TSH does not
- Reference range for TSH is lower during pregnancy than in nonpregnant state
- **TSH is the most accurate indicator of thyroid status in pregnancy** (Table 1-40)
- Consider growth ultrasounds in women with thyroid disorders

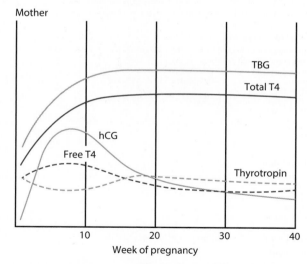

Figure 1-29 Maternal changes during pregnancy. (Used with permission from Cunningham F, et al. Chapter 4. Maternal Physiology. In: Cunningham F, et al., eds. *Williams Obstetrics*, 24th ed. New York, NY: McGraw-Hill; 2013.)

Fetal Thyroid

- Early first trimester, fetus depends on maternal thyroid
- After 10–12 weeks, fetus begins concentrating iodine and synthesizing thyroid hormone

TABLE 1-40 TRIMESTER-SPECIFIC TSH RANGES

Trimester	TSH (mIU/L)
First	0.1–2.5
Second	0.2–3.0
Third	0.3–3.0

Data from the American Thyroid Association taskforce on thyroid disease during pregnancy and postpartum.
Guidelines of the American Thyroid Association for the diagnosis and management of thyroid disease during pregnancy and postpartum. *Thyroid*. 2011;10:1081–1125.

Thyroid Antibodies

- Thyroid peroxidase (TPO) antibody
  - Suggests autoimmune cause of thyroid disease
    - Hashimoto's thyroiditis; Graves' disease
  - Is a relationship with pregnancy loss
- Thyroglobulin antibody (TgAb)
  - Thyroid cancer; Hashimoto's thyroiditis
- TSH receptor antibody (TRAb)
  - Graves' disease
  - Composed of
    - Thyroid stimulating immunoglobulins (TSI)
    - Thyrotropin binding inhibitory immunoglobulins (TBII)
  - Order if symptoms of hyperthyroidism
  - Used to monitor effectiveness of antithyroid therapy

Hypothyroidism

- *Most common cause:* Hashimoto's thyroiditis. Many with TPO antibodies
- *Signs/Symptoms:* Fatigue, sensitivity to cold, constipation, dry skin, unexplained weight gain, thinning hair, slow heart rate, depression
- *Risks if untreated*
  - Premature birth, low birth weight, neonatal RDS, gestational hypertension
  - Significant childhood IQ reduction, affects cognitive development

Treatment

- **Levothyroxine** is the treatment of choice
  - If newly pregnant and hypothyroid, increase dose 25–30% by 4–6 weeks gestation
    - Can increase daily dose OR
    - Have patient take two extra pills per week (9 versus 7 pills)
  - Typical starting dosage is 100–150 µg/day. Adjust as follows:
    - If TSH 5–10 mIU/mL: Need 25–50 µg/day increment
    - If TSH 10–20: Need 50–75 µg/day
    - If TSH >20 Need 75–100 µg/day increment
- Ferrous sulfate can interfere with absorption—stagger by at least 4 hours
- Monitor **TSH** levels every 4 weeks in the first half of pregnancy, then every 4–6 weeks
- After delivery, reduce dosing to pre-pregnancy levels; check TSH 6 weeks postpartum

Hyperthyroidism

- *Signs/Symptoms:* Heat intolerance, fatigue, anxiety, diaphoresis, tachycardia. May have goiter, exophthalmos
- *Diagnosis*
  - TSH: Low or undetectable
  - Free T4: Elevated
  - Free T3: Elevated
  - TSI present in Graves' disease; mimics TSH and stimulates thyroid cells

Types of Hyperthyroidism

- *Transient hyperthyroidism (gestational thyrotoxicosis)*
  - Associated with elevated β-hCG (multiple gestation, molar pregnancy)
  - Limited to the first half of pregnancy
  - Elevated free T4 and suppressed or undetectable TSH, in the absence of thyroid autoimmunity
  - Associated with hyperemesis gravidarum
    - *Measure TSH and free T4 in women with hyperemesis gravidarum (5% weight loss, dehydration, ketonuria) and clinical features of hyperthyroidism. Free T3 is elevated less frequently*
  - *No treatment needed*: Free T4 levels normalize as β-hCG falls

- *Graves' disease—most common cause (80–85%)*
  - Autoimmune disease with antibodies that activate TSH receptors
  - Treatment:
    - Monitor **free T4** levels every 2–4 weeks and adjust dosing as needed to maintain **free T4** in the upper limits of normal with the lowest dosing possible. Then, monitor every 4–6 weeks

Medications for Hyperthyroidism
- Thionamides: Propylthiouracil (PTU) or methimazole (MMI)
  - Agranulocytosis is most serious side effect of both
  - PTU and MMI are considered equally efficacious
  - Use clinical judgment in choosing therapy
  - If switch from PTU to MMI, check TFTs in 2 weeks
  - *10 mg MMI = 100–150 mg PTU*
    - **Propylthiouracil**
      - Recommended in first trimester
      - Starting dose: 50–100 mg every 8 hours
      - Risk of hepatotoxicity. Monitor LFTs
    - **Methimazole**
      - Typically switch to MMI after first trimester
      - Typical starting dose: 5–15 mg/day
      - Rare complications include *aplasia cutis* and "MMI embryopathy" (choanal/esophageal atresia; dysmorphic facies)
      - May be better if compliance is an issue
  - **Beta Blocker:** (for symptoms)
    - **Propranolol** 20–40 mg every 6–8 hours. Often stopped in 2–6 weeks

Complications
- PEC (most common)
- Fetus/Neonate: May develop thyrotoxicosis or hypothyroidism
- If poorly controlled, associated with increased miscarriage, PTL, IUGR/low birth weight; FDIU
- Overtreatment of mother can lead to iatrogenic fetal hypothyroidism

Thyroid Storm (medical emergency–severe, acute exacerbation)

- Often is an inciting event (infection, labor, delivery, surgery)
- Signs and symptoms
  - Fever
  - Tachycardia out of proportion to fever
  - CNS: Agitation, confusion, delirium, coma
  - GI: Vomiting, diarrhea
  - Heart failure
- Treatment
  - Stabilize patient (airway, circulation)
  - Administer PTU 600–800 mg orally, then 150–200 mg every 4–6 hours (MMI is an option if unable to take PTU)
  - 1–2 hours later, administer one of the following:
    - Potassium iodide, 2–5 drops orally every 8 hours
    - Sodium iodide, 0.5–1.0 g IV every 8 hours
    - Lugol's solution (8 drops every 6 hours)
    - Lithium carbonate, 300 mg orally every 6 hours
  - Dexamethasone 2 mg IV or IM every 6 hours for four doses (or hydrocortisone 100 mg IV every 8 hours)
  - Propranolol 20–80 mg orally every 4–6 hours or 1–2 mg IV every 5 minutes for a total of 6 mg, then 1–10 mg IV every 4 hours
  - Phenobarbital 30–60 mg orally every 6–8 hours as needed (restlessness)

SYSTEMIC LUPUS ERYTHEMATOSUS (SLE) IN PREGNANCY

- Active SLE at time of conception is strongest predictor or adverse outcome
- Exacerbation or "flares": Variable. Rates between 25% and 65%
  - Majority of flares mild to moderate
- In general, pregnancy outcome is better if
  - Lupus activity has been quiescent for at least 6 months before conception
  - There is no active renal involvement or history of lupus nephritis
  - There is no baseline hypertension
  - Superimposed PEC does not develop
  - There is no evidence of antiphospholipid antibody activity

- Hydroxychloroquine has not been discontinued
- SLE patients have increased risk of
  - Pregnancy loss
  - Preterm delivery
  - IUGR
  - PEC: Complicates 16–30% of SLE pregnancies (3–5 fold higher risk)

Neonatal Lupus Syndrome

- Passively acquired from maternal antibodies, anti-SSA (Ro) and anti-SSB (La)
- Rash, hematological and hepatic abnormalities
- Resolves by 6–8 months of life

Fetal Congenital Heart Block (CHB)

- Permanent damage to conduction system
- High fetal mortality (15–30%)
- Increased risk if anti-Ro or anti-La antibodies present. Affects about 2% of children born to primigravid women with anti-Ro antibodies (increases to 16–20% in subsequent pregnancies)
- Most often develops between 18 and 24 weeks
- If **anti-Ro** and/or anti-La antibodies, may increase fetal surveillance. No consensus on type or frequency of monitoring. At JHH, we monitor with weekly M-mode echocardiography starting at 16 weeks until delivery.
- Dexamethasone 4 mg daily has been used if evidence of CHB

Prenatal Care

- Initial Labs: Complement (C3, C4, CH50), anti-DS DNA, anti-cardiolipin antibodies, lupus anticoagulant (Russell viper venom time), anti-Ro, anti-La, 24-hour urine for protein, calcium, creatinine clearance, spot protein/creatinine
- Prenatal visits: Every 2 weeks after 20 weeks; weekly after 28 weeks
  - Fetal echo if nti-Ro or La positive
- Growth scans every 3–4 weeks
- Antenatal testing beginning at 26–28 weeks (NST and/or BPP), depending on status
- Difficult to differentiate "flare" from PEC
  - To evaluate for flare: C3, C4, CH50, anti-DS DNA
  - Disease flare: Complement (C3 and C4) decreases (increases in normal pregnancies and PEC), anti-DS DNA titer increases, responds to steroids

Other Points

- If antiphospholipid antibodies
  - Increased risk of pregnancy morbidity and loss
  - Present in about 25–50% of women with SLE; however, not all meet criteria for APS
  - Increase risk of PEC, IUGR, preterm delivery
  - Low-dose aspirin is recommended
  - **IF APS**, then low-dose aspirin plus prophylactic heparin is recommended (if LMWH, requires twice-daily administration—typically 30 mg twice daily)

Common Medications

- Steroids: Methylprednisolone/prednisone. Short courses used during disease flares
  - If long-term use, should receive stress dose steroids at delivery
- Hydroxychloroquine (*Plaquenil*)
  - Should be continued in all SLE pregnancies
- Antihypertensives
- Azathioprine (immunosuppressant)

ANEMIA

- Definition by CDC
  - Hemoglobin less than 11.0 g/dL in first and third trimester
  - Hemoglobin less than 10.5 in second trimester
- MCV
  - If microcytic (MCV <80 fL), iron studies and hemoglobin electrophoresis are indicated. A decreased serum ferritin (parallels iron storage) is most sensitive indicator of iron deficiency. Levels under 10–15 µg/L confirm iron-deficiency anemia
  - If macrocytic (MCV >100 fL), check folate and B12
  - CDC and ACOG currently recommend daily iron (30 mg elemental) for prophylaxis. If anemic, 60–120 mg of daily elemental iron is recommended. See Table 1-41 for various preparations

TABLE 1-41 IRON PREPARATIONS AND ELEMENTAL IRON CONTENT

Iron Preparation	Elemental Iron
Oral	
Ferrous fumarate 325 mg	106 mg
Ferrous sulfate 325 mg	65 mg
Ferrous gluconate 325 mg	34–38 mg
IV	
Iron dextran*	50 mg/mL
Ferric gluconate	12.5 mg/mL
Iron sucrose	20 mg/mL

*Anaphylaxis in 1%. Fewer reactions in other preparations.

SICKLE CELL DISEASE (SCD)

- *Complications*
  - Miscarriage, IUGR stillbirth, PEC, premature birth
  - Increased risk of infections (urinary-pyelonephritis, pulmonary-pneumonia); possibly more painful crises
  - Risk of acute chest syndrome
    - New infiltrate with fever, respiratory symptoms
    - Approximately 15% require ventilator support; 3% mortality rate
  - 25–50% are alloimmunized because of transfusion history
- *Prenatal Care Recommendations*
  - **Vaccines:** Haemophilus influenza type b; meningococcal; pneumococcal
  - Check hemoglobin electrophoresis of father of baby
  - Obtain spot urine protein/creatinine ratio for baseline
  - Consider echocardiogram to screen for pulmonary hypertension
  - Check urine culture every trimester
  - Provide DVT prophylaxis when hospitalized
- *Medications*
  - Increased folic acid advised. No consensus. Per ACOG: 4 mg/day
  - Consider low-dose aspirin after first trimester (for high risk of PEC)
  - Prophylactic penicillin may be continued during pregnancy
  - Iron supplements should *only be prescribed if iron deficient*. Check ferritin levels
- *Fetal Surveillance*
  - Consider antenatal testing starting at 32 weeks
  - Consider growth scan in third trimester, more frequently if needed depending on disease severity

MULTIPLE GESTATION

Types of Twins

- **Dizygotic twins**
  - Result from fertilization of two separate ova ("fraternal")
  - Two-third of spontaneous twin pregnancies
  - 93% of ART twin pregnancies
  - Dichorionic-diamniotic (placentas may be fused or separate)
- **Monozygotic twins**
  - Result from a single fertilized ovum that divides ("identical")
  - One-third of all spontaneous twin pregnancies
  - Timing of division determines placentation and amnionicity
  - May be dichorionic-diamniotic (15–25%), monochorionic-diamniotic (75%), monochorionic-monoamniotic (1–2%), or conjoined

Morbidity and Mortality in Multiple Gestation

- The average delivery time for twins and triplets is 35.3 and 31.9 weeks, respectively
- The average birth weight for twins is 2336 grams, tripets is 1660 grams.

Complications with Multiples

- Preterm Labor: Over half of twins deliver preterm
- Gestational Diabetes
  - 3–6% of twin pregnancies; 22–39% of triplet pregnancies

- Hypertension/PEC
  - Hypertensive complications: Twins 12.7%, triplets 20%
  - Incidence of PEC 2.6 fold higher in twins
  - If PEC, likely occurs earlier and is more severe
- Increased incidence of hyperemesis, anemia, hemorrhage, CD, postpartum depression, acute fatty liver, VTE

Miscellaneous

- Fetal fibronectin: Can be used in multiple gestation
- Prophylactic cerclage: Not shown to prolong gestation or improve outcome in multiple gestation
- Progesterone: Not effective in twins for reducing preterm delivery

Chorionicity

- Clinically important due to significant differences in perinatal morbidity and mortality between monochorionic and dichorionic placentation
- Best if determined in first trimester (10–14 weeks)
- *Monochorionic*
  - Single placenta; thin dividing membrane. Septum forms a "T" as it meets the base. Absence of chorion in septum makes septum thin (only two layers) or hard to see—can give false impression of monochorionic-monoamniotic twins
  - Ultrasound example of monochorionic diamniotic twins shown in Figure 1-30
- *Dichorionic*
  - Twin Peak Sign (or Lambda) in dichorionic twins. Thick dividing chorion
  - Ultrasound example of dichorionic twins shown in Figure 1-31

Monochorionic Twins—Risks

- Perinatal loss and handicap rate up to three to five times higher than dichorionic
- Increased risk of congenital heart defects (almost ninefold; risk 4–5%, normal is 0.5%)
- Fetal demise in one twin: 40–50% risk of death/neurologic handicap for surviving co-twin
- Selective IUGR due to unequal placental sharing
- Twin reversed arterial perfusion (TRAP) sequence: Sudden changes in blood flow affects development; one baby may die, the surviving baby continues to send blood to dead co-twin (about 1% of monochorionic twins)
- Twin anemia polycythemia sequence (TAPS) complicates 3–5% of monochorionic twins; discordance in hemoglobin levels in absence of amniotic fluid abnormalities
- **Twin-twin transfusion syndrome (TTTS)**: Complicates up to 10–15% of monochorionic twins

Management of Multiple Gestations

- ALL Twins: Obtain early ultrasound to determine chorionicity. Best by 10–14 weeks
- *Dichorionic*
  - 18–20 weeks: Anatomy ultrasound
  - Growth: Evaluate every 3–4 weeks
  - 36 weeks: Consider antenatal testing (earlier if indicated)
- *Monochorionic*
  - Consider primary risk stratification (evaluate for early discordance) between 11-14 weeks
  - 16 weeks: Begin ultrasound for TTTS checks every 2 weeks
  - 18–20 weeks: Anatomy ultrasound
  - 22 weeks: Fetal echocardiograms
  - Growth: Evaluate every 2–4 weeks
  - 32–34 weeks: Consider antenatal testing (earlier if indicated)
- *Monoamniotic*
  - Same as monochorionic
  - Admission for increased fetal surveillance at 26–28 weeks
- Iron supplementation
  - Iron deficiency 2.4–4 times higher than singleton pregnancy
  - Take 60–120 mg elemental iron daily (ferrous sulfate 325 mg has 65 mg elemental iron)
  - Folic acid 1 mg daily minimum

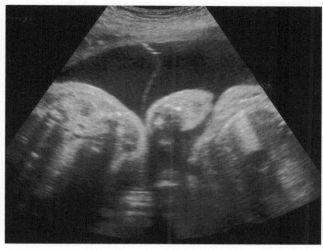

A

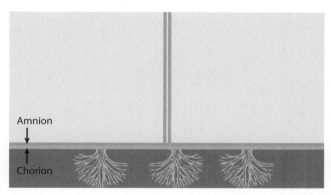

B

Figure 1-30 Monochorionic-diamniotic. (Used with permission from Cunningham F, Leveno KJ, Bloom SL, et al. Chapter 45. Multifetal pregnancy. In: Cunningham F, Leveno KJ, Bloom SL, et al., eds. *Williams Obstetrics*. 24th ed. New York, NY: McGraw-Hill; 2013.)

Delivery Timing

Monochorionic-Monoamniotic	
• No complications	32-0/7–34-0/7
Monochorionic-Diamniotic	
• No complications	34-0/7–37-6/7
• Isolated IUGR	32-0/7–34-6/7
Dichorionic-Diamniotic	
• No complications	38-0/7–38-6/7
• Isolated IUGR	36-0/7–37-6/7
• IUGR with abnormal Dopplers, hypertension, etc	32-0/7–34-6/7

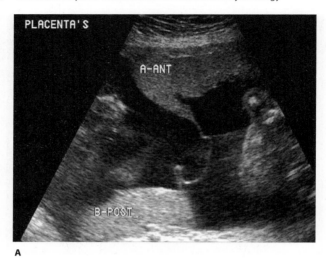

Figure 1-31 Dichorionic-diamniotic. (Used with permission from Cunningham F, et al. Chapter 45. Multifetal pregnancy. In: Cunningham F, et al., eds. *Williams Obstetrics*, 24th ed. New York, NY: McGraw-Hill; 2013)

NAUSEA AND VOMITING OF PREGNANCY

- *Hyperemesis Gravidarum*: Clinical diagnosis. Severe vomiting with weight loss (usually >5% pre-pregnancy weight), ketonuria, electrolyte disturbances
- Thiamine supplementation (100 mg intravenously daily for 2–3 days) is recommended for women who have vomited for more than 3 weeks to prevent Wernicke's Encephalopathy
- *Dietary changes*
  - Eat small, frequent meals; eat bland foods; avoid spicy and fatty foods
  - Avoid strong odorous foods
  - Take prenatal vitamin at night with a snack and not in AM on empty stomach
  - Avoid supplements with iron until symptoms resolve
- *Complementary/Alternative Treatments*
  - Herbal supplements (ginger 250 mg orally four times per day)
  - P6 acupuncture or acupressure wristbands (Seabands) apply continuous pressure on the P6 (or Nei-Kuan) point on each wrist using a plastic stud
- Pharmacologic Therapy for Nausea and Vomiting of Pregnancy (Tables 1-42 and 1-43).

TABLE 1-42 MEDICATIONS FOR NAUSEA AND VOMITING OF PREGNANCY

Medication	Dosage
First-line oral medications	
Pyridoxine (Vitamin B$_6$)	25 mg orally three times daily as single agent
Pyridoxine + Doxylamine *(Diclegis)* *Take on empty stomach. Do not crush*	10/10 mg; Max is 4 tabs per day. Start with 2 tabs at bedtime. If symptoms persist, take 2 tabs at bedtime the next night and then 1 tab the next morning and 2 the next night. If symptoms still not controlled, take one tab the next morning, one tab mid-afternoon, and 2 tabs at bedtime. *Doxylamine is also available in over-the-counter sleeping pills (Unisom; 25 mg)*
If persistent N/V add antihistamine	
Diphenhydramine *(Benadryl)*	25–50 mg orally/IV every 4–6 hours
Meclizine *(Antivert)*	25 mg orally every 4–6 hours
If persistent	
Promethazine *(Phenergan)* Prochlorperazine *(Compazine)* Metoclopramide *(Reglan)*	12.5–25 mg orally/PR/IM/IV every 4–6 hours 5–10 mg orally every 6–8 hours 5–10 mg IV every 6–8 hours Orally: 30 minutes before meals and at bedtime
Ondansetron *(Zofran)* Zofran ODT *(oral dissolving tab)*	4–8 mg orally/IV every 8 hours 4–8 mg orally every 8 hours
May also consider	
Dimenhydrinate *(Dramamine)* Methylprednisolone *(Medrol)*	50–100 mg orally every 4–6 hours See taper in Table 1-48

TABLE 1-43 STEROID TAPER FOR NAUSEA AND VOMITING OF PREGNANCY

Methylprednisolone Taper Orally/IV (mg)			
Day	**AM**	**Midday**	**Bedtime**
1	16	16	16
2	16	16	16
3	16	16	16
4	16	8	16
5	16	8	8
6	8	8	8
7	8	4	8
8	8	4	4
9	8	4	
10	8	4	
11	8		
12	8		
13	4		
14	4		

Used with permission from Safari HR, Fassett MJ, Souter ic, et al. the efficy of methylprednisolone in the treatment of hyperemesis gravidarum: A randomized, double-blind, controlled study. *Am J Obstet Gynecol.* 1998;179:921–924.

PRENATAL CLINIC

- Timing of various laboratories and tests (Table 1-44)
- Frequency of clinic visits (general guideline)
  - 0–28 weeks every 4 weeks
  - 28–32 weeks every 3 weeks
  - 32–36 weeks every 2 weeks
  - 36 weeks to delivery every week
- *Weight Gain Recommendations* (Table 1-45)
- **Poor weight gain/excessive weight gain/size greater than or less than dates**
  - Nutrition consult
  - Fundal height (FH) and weight checks
  - GA by fundal exam
    - 6–8 weeks = orange size
    - 8–10 weeks = grapefruit size (top normal nonpregnant size)
    - 12 weeks = at the pubic symphysis
    - 16 weeks = halfway between pubic symphysis and umbilicus
    - 20 weeks = at the umbilicus
    - >20 weeks FH in cm = GA
  - Schedule fetal growth ultrasound if FH differs more than 2 weeks from GA for two or more visits or if difference is more than 3 weeks

TABLE 1-44 PRENATAL CARE—TIMING OF VARIOUS INTERVENTIONS

11–13-6/7 weeks	Offer first trimester screening
16–18 weeks	Offer Quad screen if first trimester screening not done (window: 15-0/7 to 22-6/7 weeks) or maternal serum AFP alone if first trimester screening done
18–20 weeks	Anatomy ultrasound
27–36 weeks	Administer Tdap vaccine (tetanus, diphtheria, pertussis)
	Administer to women during *every* pregnancy
	May give at any time in pregnancy, but weeks *27–36 is optimal*
	Transplacental transfer of maternal antibodies from mother to infant provides some protection to infants in early life
	Encourage vaccine for family members
28 weeks	Repeat labs and glucose screen. RhoGAM if Rh negative
36 weeks	GBS, GC/CT cultures

TABLE 1-45 RECOMMENDED WEIGHT GAIN DURING PREGNANCY

Category	Pre-pregnancy BMI	Weight Gain (lbs)	Guidelines for Twins (lbs)
Underweight	<18.5	28–40	
Normal weight	18.5–24.9	25–35	37–54
Overweight	25.0–29.9	15–25	31–50
Obese (all classes)	≥30	11–20	25–42

Data from The Institute of Medicine. Weight gain during pregnancy: Reexamining the guidelines, 2009. http://www.nap.edu/openbook.php?record_id=12584&page=R5.

Special Considerations

Rh negative—Unsensitized
- RhoGAM at 28 weeks and within 72 hours after delivery (if infant is Rh positive)
- Also give RhoGAM for vaginal bleeding, abdominal trauma, amniocentesis or CVS

Advanced Maternal Age (≥35 years of age at delivery)
Offer genetic counseling

History of UTIs
- Pregnant patients are at increased risk for UTI/pyelonephritis
  - Progesterone causes decreased ureteral peristalsis
  - Intermittent glucosuria provides medium for bacteria to grow
  - Compression of the ureters by the gravid uterus
- If a patient has **two** UTIs or one episode of pyelonephritis during pregnancy, start suppression antibiotics (typically Macrobid 100 mg daily) for entire pregnancy
- Both symptomatic *and* asymptomatic UTIs in pregnancy should be treated for 7–10 days and a test of cure should be obtained after treatment

Syphilis in Pregnancy—Treatment Recommendations
- Primary, secondary, or early latent syphilis (acquired within last 1 year)
  - **Benzathine PCN G** 2.4 million units IM × 1 dose
- *Late Latent Syphilis or Latent Syphilis of Unknown Duration*
  - **Benzathine penicillin G** 7.2 million units total, administered as three doses of 2.4 million units IM each at 1-week intervals
- **Penicillin Allergy:** No alternatives to penicillin have been proved effective for treatment of syphilis during pregnancy. Pregnant women with a penicillin allergy should be **desensitized** and treated with penicillin. Skin testing may be helpful

Hepatitis B
- Nomenclature in Table 1-46
- Transmission is primarily parenteral, sexual, or vertical
- Many infections are asymptomatic
- Neonatal transmission is more frequently associated with third trimester maternal infection than with maternal chronic carrier
- Breastfeeding is not contraindicated
- Neonates should receive
  - Hepatitis B immunoglobulin (HBIG)
  - Hepatitis B vaccine

TABLE 1-46 HEPATITIS B NOMENCLATURE

HBsAg	Hepatitis B surface antigen	Marker of infectivity. Indicates either acute or chronic HBV infection
Anti-HBs *or* HBsAb	Antibody to Hep B surface antigen	Marker of immunity. Immune response to HBV infection or vaccination, or presence of passively acquired antibody
Anti-HBc *or* HBcAb	Antibody to hepatitis B core antigen	Marker of acute, chronic, or resolved infection. NOT a marker of vaccine-induced immunity
IgM anti-HBc		Indicates acute infection (<6 months)
IgG anti-HBc		Indicates past or current infection. If it and HBsAg are both (+) (in absence of IgM anti-HBc), then it is chronic infection
HBeAg	Hepatitis B "e" antigen	Marker of high degree of infectivity; correlates with a high level of HBV replication
Anti-HBe	Antibody to hepatitis B "e" antigen	May be present in an infected or immune person. In persons with chronic HBV, indicates low viral titer and low infectivity
HBV-DNA		Marker of viral replication, correlated well with infectivity. Used to monitor treatment of patients

ANEUPLOIDY SCREENING

Maternal Age-Related Aneuploidy Risk (Table 1-47)

Screening Tests
- Numerous tests (and combinations of tests) are available
- See Table 1-48 for detection rates

TABLE 1-47 MATERNAL AGE AND ANEUPLOIDY RISK

Age	Down Syndrome		Any Aneuploidy	
	Mid-trimester	Term	Mid-trimester	Term
35	1/250	1/385	1/132	1/204
36	1/192	1/303	1/105	1/167
37	1/149	1/227	1/83	1/130
38	1/115	1/175	1/65	1/103
39	1/89	1/137	1/53	1/81
40	1/69	1/106	1/40	1/63
41	1/53	1/81	1/31	1/50
42	1/41	1/64	1/25	1/39
43	1/31	1/50	1/19	1/30
44	1/25	1/38	1/15	1/24
45	1/19	1/30	1/12	1/19

Used with permission from Cunningham F, Leveno KJ, Bloom SL, et al. Chapter 14. Prenatal diagnosis. In: Cunningham F, Leveno KJ, Bloom SL, et al., eds. *Williams Obstetrics*. 24th ed. New York, NY: McGraw-Hill; 2013.

TABLE 1-48 SCREENING TEST DETECTION RATES

Screening Test	Detection Rate
First Trimester Screen	
• Nuchal Translucency measurement	64–70
• Nuchal Translucency, maternal serum (PAPP-A, and free or total β-hCG)	79–87 85–90[†]
• Nuchal Translucency, maternal serum, and nasal bone*	95
Second Trimester	
• Quad screen (MS-AFP, hCG, unconjugated estriol, inhibin A)	74
First Plus Second Trimester	
• Integrated (first trimester screen and Quad test). Results withheld until Quad completed.	94–96
• Stepwise sequential (first trimester screen and Quad test) • If positive first trimester result, diagnostic test offered • If negative, Quad screen offered. Results withheld until Quad test completed	95
• Contingent sequential • If positive first trimester result, diagnostic test offered • If negative, no further testing • If intermediate, Quad screen offered. Results withheld until Quad test completed	88–94
Circulating cell-free fetal DNA (Non-Invasive Prenatal Testing)	>98

*PerkinElmer Labs/NTD
[†]*Fetal Medicine Foundation*
Numbers vary in different studies, populations.
Data from Cunningham F, et al. Chapter 14. Prenatal Diagnosis. In: Cunningham F, et al., eds. *Williams Obstetrics*, 24th ed. New York, NY: McGraw-Hill; 2013; ACOG: Screening for fetal chromosomal abnormalities. Practice Bulletin No. 77, January 2007.

First Trimester Screen

- 11-0/7–13-6/7 weeks
- Nuchal Translucency (NT): CRL has to be within 45–84 mm to use NT
- Linked with congenital heart defects when >99th percentile
- Maternal Age, NT, maternal serum markers [β-hCG, pregnancy associated plasma protein-A (PAPP-A)]. NT is dependent on GA
- Nasal bone (NB) may be incorporated (increases detection rate of Down syndrome). Absent NB correlates with Down syndrome. One study showed absent NB in 65–70% of fetuses with DS, but only 1% of normal fetuses. Not a good independent marker

Second Trimester Screen

- **Quad Screen:** 15-0/7–22-6/7 weeks. Provides risk for DS, open neural tube defects (NTD), trisomy 18
- **MS-AFP:** If elevated, increased risk of NTD or abdominal wall defects

Other Screening Tests

- **Circulating cell-free fetal DNA (*Non-Invasive Prenatal Testing*; NIPT)**
  - Trisomy 21, 18, 13
  - May be collected after 10 weeks GA and up until a couple of hours after delivery
  - Not recommended in multiple gestations

Invasive Testing

- **CVS:** Usually performed at 10–13 weeks. CVS not recommended before 10 weeks. Unsensitized Rh negative women require RhoGAM after CVS
- **Amniocentesis:** Usually performed after 16 weeks. Unsensitized Rh negative women require RhoGAM

Ultrasound

- See Table 1-49 for ultrasonographic markers of aneuploidy and their follow-up

TABLE 1-49 ISOLATED SECOND-TRIMESTER ULTRASONOGRAPHIC MARKERS FOR DOWN SYNDROME

Ultrasound Marker	Likelihood Ratio	Other Considerations; Follow-up
Choroid plexus cyst	–	Linked to Trisomy 18 (not Down syndrome) No need for follow-up if isolated and no increased risk for Trisomy 18
Echogenic cardiac focus	1.4–1.8	None; not linked with congenital heart defects (fetal echo not warranted)
Renal pyelectasis	1.5–1.6	Mild renal pyelectasis (≥4 mm) is often a transient physiologic state. Follow-up at 32 weeks. If measures ≥7 mm at 32 weeks, postnatal follow-up is suggested
Short humerus length	2.5–5.8	Consider third-trimester growth ultrasound
Short femur length	1.2–2.2	Consider third-trimester growth ultrasound
Nuchal thickening (≥6 mm at 15–20 weeks)	11–18.6	Genetic counseling; 40–50% sensitivity and >99% specificity for Down syndrome
Echogenetic bowel	5.5–6.7	Genetic counseling; also associated with IUGR, congenital infection (eg, CMV), intraamniotic bleeding, cystic fibrosis, GI obstruction. Follow up with 32-week ultrasound to evaluate growth and bowel
Absent/hypoplastic nasal bone	As high as 83	Genetic counseling

Data from Cunningham F, et al. Chapter 14. Prenatal Diagnosis. In: Cunningham F, et al., eds. *Williams Obstetrics*, 24th ed. New York, NY: McGraw-Hill; 2013; ACOG: Screening for fetal chromosomal abnormalities. Practice Bulletin No. 77, January 2007.

ANTEPARTUM FETAL SURVEILLANCE

- Antepartum fetal surveillance tests have high false-positive rates and low positive predictive values
- Usually initiate testing at 32 weeks. If very high-risk pregnancy, may initiate at an earlier GA if delivery would be considered for perinatal benefit (ie, 26–28 weeks)
- Optimal frequency of testing is unknown. Should be individualized. NST, BPP, and modified BPP are typically repeated weekly; but in certain high-risk conditions, such as post term pregnancy, type 1 diabetes, IUGR or gestational hypertension, twice-weekly is performed
- Any significant deterioration in the maternal medical status requires fetal reevaluation, as does any acute diminution in fetal activity, regardless of the amount of time that has elapsed since the last test
- Negative predictive value of NST is 99.8%; for CST, BPP, and modified BPP it is 99.9%
- See Table 1-50 for testing indications

TABLE 1-50 INDICATIONS FOR ANTENATAL FETAL SURVEILLANCE*

Hypertension (chronic, gestational)	Late-term or post term pregnancy
Diabetes (pregestational, gestational requiring medications)	Isoimmunization
	Morbid obesity
Systemic Lupus Erythematosis	Advanced maternal age
Sickle cell disease or other hemoglobinopathy	Assisted reproductive technologies
Poorly controlled thyroid disease	Decreased fetal movement
Maternal cyanotic heart disease	Oligohydramnios/polyhydramnios
Maternal thrombophilia or antiphospholipid syndrome	Multiple pregnancy (no specific guidelines available)
Renal disease	Prior fetal demise
Poorly controlled thyroid disease	IUGR

*Plus any condition that is thought to be associated with increased perinatal morbidity/mortality.
Data from ACOG: Antepartum fetal surveillance. Practice Bulletin No. 145, July 2014; Liston R, Sawchuck D, Young D. Fetal health surveillance: antepartum and intrapartum consensus guideline. Society of Obstetrics and Gynaecologists of Canada, British Columbia Perinatal Health Program. *J Obstet Gynaecol Can.* 2007;29:S3–56.

Testing Techniques

- **Kick Counts**
  - Numerous protocols appear to be acceptable
    - Patient lies on her side and counts distinct fetal movements. Perception of 10 distinct movements in a period of up to 2 hours is considered reassuring. Once 10 movements have been perceived, the count may be discontinued
    - Count fetal movements for 1 hour three times per week. Reassuring if count equals or exceeds previously established baseline
- **NST**
  - Reactive NST: Two or more FHR accelerations of at least 15 bpm above the baseline and last 15 seconds from baseline to baseline within a 20-minute period
  - Nonreactive NST: Lacks sufficient FHR accelerations over 40 minutes
  - Before 32 weeks, accelerations are defined as 10 bpm or more for 10 seconds
  - Should be conducted for at least 20 minutes
  - Vibroacoustic stimulation may elicit FHR accelerations (may reduce testing time and is valid)
- **Contraction Stress Test (CST)**
  - FHR response to uterine contractions. Premise is that fetal oxygenation is transiently worsened by contractions
  - Three contractions lasting at least 40 seconds in a 10-minute period. May use oxytocin or nipple stimulation to induce contractions
  - Interpretation
    - Negative: No late or significant variable decelerations
    - Positive: Late decelerations following 50% or more of contractions
    - Equivocal-suspicious: Intermittent late decelerations or significant variable decelerations
    - Unsatisfactory: Fewer than three contractions in 10 minutes
- **Biophysical Profile (BPP)** (Table 1-51)
  - May be used as early as 26–28 weeks
  - Correlates well with fetal acid–base status
  - Earliest manifestations of fetal acidosis: Nonreactive NST and loss of fetal breathing
  - Antenatal corticosteroid administration may decrease score if done within 48 hours—usually fetal breathing and NST, but also movement. Returns to normal by 48–96 hours

TABLE 1-51 BIOPHYSICAL PROFILE

	Normal (Score = 2)	Abnormal (Score = 0)
NST	Reactive	Nonreactive
Fetal breathing	≥1 episode of breathing lasting ≥30 seconds within 30 minutes	Absent or no episode of breathing meeting criteria
Fetal movement	≥3 discrete body or limb movements within 30 minutes	Less than 3 movements
Fetal tone	≥1 episode of extension of an extremity with return to flexion or opening or closing of hand	No extension/flexion movements
Amniotic fluid volume	A single deepest vertical pocket of more than 2 cm	Fluid pocket ≤2 cm

Management Based on BPP
- BPP = 8 or 10 is normal
  - BPP = 6 is considered equivocal
    - If ≥37-0/7 weeks, further evaluation and consider delivery
    - If <37-0/7 weeks, repeat BPP in 24 hours. In the interim, maternal corticosteroid administration should be considered for pregnancies < 34 weeks. Repeat equivocal scores should result either in delivery or continued intensive surveillance
  - BPP = 4 is abnormal
    - Usually indicates that delivery is warranted, although if <32-0/7 weeks, management should be individualized and extended monitoring may be appropriate
  - BPP <4
    - Should generally result in delivery

Oligohydramnios
- Has been defined as
  - Single deepest vertical pocket of ≤ 2 cm *or*
  - AFI of ≤ 5 cm
  - Percentile should NOT be used in management decisions
  - *Data support using deepest vertical pocket of ≤ 2 cm to diagnose oligohydramnios*
- Regardless of BPP score, oligohydramnios requires further evaluation
- Modified BPP
  - Combines the NST (a short-term indicator of fetal acid–base status) *AND* amniotic fluid assessment (an indicator of long-term placental function)
  - Normal if reactive NST and amniotic fluid volume >2 cm in deepest pocket
- Umbilical Artery Doppler Velocimetry
  - Umbilical arterial Doppler waveforms reflect the status of placental circulation. In the umbilical artery, end-diastolic flow (EDF) may be normal, reduced, absent, or reversed, reflecting progressive increases in placental resistance
  - Betamethasone administration may be associated with a transient return of EDF

MEDICATIONS IN PREGNANCY

Antidiarrheals

Diphenoxylate/atropine (*Lomotil*) 2 tabs orally four times daily
Loperamide (*Imodium*) start with 4 mg, then 2 mg after each loose stool (max 16 mg/day)
Note: Pepto Bismol is *not* usually recommended as may contain aspirin

Antiemetics

- See section on Nausea and Vomiting of Pregnancy

Antihistamines/Decongestants

Diphenhydramine (*Benadryl*) (usual doses)
Pseudoephedrine (*Sudafed*) 30 mg four times daily. Caution if hypertension
Loratadine (*Claritin*) 10 mg orally daily

Constipation

Docusate sodium (*Colace*) 100 mg orally daily or twice daily (stool softener)
Polyethylene glycol (*MiraLax*) 17 g (diluted in 8 ounces water, juice) orally once daily
Magnesium citrate 1 bottle divided daily or twice daily (laxative; for severe constipation)
Milk of Magnesia 15 mL orally every 6 hours as needed

Cough Syrup

Robitussin (Plain or DM) 1 tsp every 4 hours as needed
Benzonatate (*Tessalon Perles*) 100 mg orally two to three times daily (use in diabetics)

Ear Infection

Amoxicillin 500–875 orally twice daily for 7–10 days;
Amoxicillin/clavulanate (*Augmentin*) 875/125 mg orally twice daily for 10–14 days (if recurrent or diabetic)
Cefuroxime 500 mg orally twice daily for 7–14 days

Gastroesophageal Reflux/Gastritis

Ranitidine (*Zantac*) 150 mg orally twice daily or 300 mg at night
Famotidine (*Pepcid*) 20 mg orally twice daily
Calcium carbonate (*Maalox*) 30 cc orally every 6 hours as needed
Pantoprazole (*Protonix*) 40 mg orally once daily; **Prevacid** 30 mg once daily; other PPIs

Headaches/Migraines

Acetaminophen (*Tylenol*) 650 mg orally every 6–8 hours as needed
Metoclopramide (*Reglan*) 10 mg IM every 3–4 hours as needed

Recalcitrant Headaches: Can Try Neuro "Cocktail"
Metoclopramide (*Reglan*) 10 mg IV (may repeat every 20 minutes × 3 doses, giving benadryl 25 mg with first and third doses) + **methylprednisolone** (*Solumedrol*) 100 mg IV ± **ketorolac** (*Toradol*) 30–60 mg IM/IV (consider GA)
Can also add **magnesium sulfate** 2 g IV

Headache Prevention
Propranolol 40 mg XR orally once daily
Cyclobenzaprine (*Flexeril*) 5–10 mg orally three times daily
Can consider sumatriptan (*Imitrex*) (in case-specific circumstances)

HSV in Pregnancy (Table 1-52)

TABLE 1-52 TREATMENT OF HSV IN PREGNANCY

Indication	Acyclovir	Valacyclovir
Primary or first-episode infection	400 mg orally three times for 7–10 days	1 g orally twice daily for 7–10 days
Symptomatic recurrence	400 mg orally three times for 5 days	500 mg orally twice daily for 3 days
	OR	*OR*
	800 mg orally twice daily for 5 days	1 g orally every day for 5 days
Daily suppression* (from 36 weeks to delivery)	400 mg orally three times	500 mg orally twice daily

*Earlier if preterm labor.

Urinary Tract Infection

Amoxicillin 500–875 mg orally twice daily for 7–10 days
Nitrofurantoin (*Macrobid*) 100 mg orally twice daily for 7–10 days
Cephalexin (*Keflex*) 500 mg orally twice daily for 7–10 days
TMP-SMX DS (*Bactrim*) orally twice daily 7–10 days (avoid in first trimester and near delivery if possible for theoretical risks of NTD in first trimester and kernicterus near term)

Pyelonephritis (hospitalize until 24 hours afebrile and asymptomatic)

- **Ceftriaxone** 1 g IV every 24 hours *OR*
- **Ampicillin** 2 g IV every 6 hours *PLUS*
  Gentamicin (8 hour dosing if pregnant); 2 mg/kg load, then 1.5 mg/kg every 8 h *OR*
- **Cefazolin** (*Ancef*) 1 g IV every 6–8 hours
- *THEN:* Oral antibiotics to complete 14 days of treatment (per sensitivities)
- UTI suppression - after diagnosis of pyelonephritis (or 2 UTIs in pregnancy) until delivery
  - **Nitrofurantoin** (*Macrobid*) 100 mg once daily *OR*
  - **Ampicillin** 500 mg once daily *OR*
  - **Cephalexin** (*Keflex*) 500 mg once daily

Stress-Dose Steroids

Administer stress-dose steroids when patient is in active labor (about 8 cm) or before CD to patients on chronic steroids. This includes patients who took more than 5 mg/day prednisone or its equivalent (methylprednisolone 4 mg; hydrocortisone 20 mg) for over 3 weeks

- Moderate surgical stress
  - 50 mg hydrocortisone IV before procedure (or in active labor) *THEN*
  - 25 mg hydrocortisone IV every 8 hours for 24 hours
  - Resume usual dose thereafter
- Major surgical stress
  - Take usual AM steroid dose
  - 100 mg IV hydrocortisone before procedure (or in active labor) *THEN*
  - 50 mg IV hydrocortisone every 8 hours for 24 hours
  - Resume usual dose thereafter

Mastitis

- Mastitis typically presents as a hard, red, tender, swollen area of one breast. Patient complains of fever, myalgia, chills, malaise, and flu-like symptoms
- Most lactation-related breast infections are caused by *Staphylococcus aureus*. Other pathogens include *S. pyogenes* (Group A or B), *E. coli*, bacteroides species, corynebacterium species, and coagulase negative staph
- Ultrasound is the most effective method of differentiating mastitis from a breast abscess

Treatment

- Anti-inflammatory agents (eg, ibuprofen); cold compresses or ice packs reduce swelling and pain
- Encourage continued milk drainage, either by breast feeding or pumping
- Antibiotics for 10–14 days
  - **Dicloxacillin** 500 mg orally every 6 hours
  - **Cephalexin** (*Keflex*) 500 mg orally every 6 hours
  - **Amoxicillin-clavulanate** (*Augmentin*) 875/125 mg orally every 12 hours
  - **Clindamycin** 300 mg orally every 6 hours

If high risk for MRSA treat with one of the following

- Trimethoprim-sulfamethoxazole (*Bactrim DS*) 1 tab every 12 hours
- Clindamycin 300 mg orally every 6 hours
- Linezolid 600 mg orally every 12 hours

DIAGNOSTIC IMAGING AND PREGNANCY

- **Gray (Gy):** SI unit of energy for the absorbed dose of radiation. One *gray* is the absorption of 1 joule of radiation energy by 1 kg of matter. *1 Gy = 100 rad*
- **RAD:** Radiation Absorbed Dose. A unit which measures radiation in terms of the absorbed dose
- *Exposure to less than 5 rad has* not *been associated with an increase in fetal anomalies or pregnancy loss*
- Ultrasonography and MRI are not associated with known adverse fetal effects
- See Table 1-53 for selected imaging methods used in obstetrics and estimated fetal exposure

TABLE 1-53 ESTIMATED FETAL EXPOSURE FROM SOME COMMON RADIOLOGIC PROCEDURES

Procedure	Fetal Exposure
Chest x-ray (2 views)	0.02–0.07 mrad
Abdominal film (single view)	100 mrad
Intravenous pyelography	≥1 rad[a]
Hip film (single view)	7–20 mrad
Barium enema or small bowel series	2–4 rad
CT scan of head or chest	<1 rad
CT scan of abdomen and lumbar spine	3.5 rad
CT pelvimetry	250 mrad

[a]Exposure depends on the number of films.
CT, computed tomography.
Adapted from Cunningham F, et al. Chapter 46. General Considerations and Maternal Evaluation. In: Cunningham F, et al., eds. *Williams Obstetrics*, Twenty-Fourth Edition. New York, NY: McGraw-Hill; 2013.

Gynecology

GYN SURGERY: PREOPERATIVE CONSIDERATIONS

Antibiotic Prophylaxis for Gynecologic Procedures

• Antimicrobial Prophylactic Regimens by Procedure (Table 2-1)

Key Points to Remember

• Antibiotics must be given within 1 hour prior to skin incision. Anesthesia induction is a convenient time
• Give *repeat dose* of antibiotic if
  • Long procedure (over one to two times antibiotics half-life; *ex: re-dose cefazolin at 3 hours*)
  • EBL over 1500 cc
• Neither treatment for several days before a procedure nor subsequent doses after procedure are indicated for prophylaxis
• Prophylactic antibiotics are recommended for induced abortion/dilation and curettage (D&C) *even if negative* gonorrhea/chlamydia (GC/CT) testing

TABLE 2-1 ANTIMICROBIAL PROPHYLACTIC REGIMENS BY PROCEDURE

Procedure	Antibiotic	Dose
• Hysterectomy • Urogynecology procedures, including those involving mesh	Cefazolin[1] (preferred) *If PCN allergic:* Clindamycin[2] *plus* Gentamicin[3] (preferred for PCN allergic) OR Metronidazole[2] *plus* Gentamicin[3] (alternative for PCN allergic)	Weight <120 kg: 2 g IV Weight ≥120 kg: 3 g IV 600 mg IV 5 mg/kg IV[4] 500 mg IV 5 mg/kg IV[4]

• Laparoscopy
  Diagnostic/Operative
  Tubal sterilization
	None	

• Laparotomy	None	

• Hysteroscopy
  Diagnostic/Operative
  Endometrial ablation
  Essure
	None	

• Hysterosalpingogram or chromotubation	Doxycycline[5]	100 mg orally twice daily for 5 days
• IUD insertion	None	
• Endometrial biopsy	None	
• Induced abortion/D&C	Doxycycline	100 mg orally 1 hour before procedure and 200 mg orally after the procedure
	Metronidazole	500 mg orally twice daily for 5 days
• Urodynamics	None	

[1]Acceptable alternatives: Cefotetan, cefoxitin, cefuroxime, ampicillin-sulbactam.
[2]Antimicrobial agents of choice if history of immediate hypersensitivity to penicillin (PCN). Combination of drugs recommended to broaden coverage.
[3]Quinolones (cipro-, levo-, moxi-floxacin) or aztreonam (1 g IV) can be alternatives to gentamicin.
[4]Gentamicin is recommended as a single dose preoperatively based on actual body weight (ABW) unless ABW is >20% above ideal body weight (IBW); in this case, calculate weight for dose by IBW + 0.4 (ABW-IBW).
[5]If history of PID or dilated fallopian tubes. No prophylaxis is indicated for a study without dilated tubes.
Data from ACOG Practice Bulletin No. 104, May 2009, Reaffirmed 2011; Bratzler DW, Dellinger EP, Olsen KM, et al. Clinical practice guidelines for antimicrobial prophylaxis in surgery. *Am J Health-Syst Pharm.* 2013;70:195–283.

Endocarditis Prophylaxis

- Cardiac conditions associated with the highest risk of adverse outcomes from endocarditis that require antibiotic prophylaxis are shown in Table 2-2. Suggested antibiotics are listed in Table 2-3

TABLE 2-2   CARDIAC CONDITIONS REQUIRING ENDOCARDITIS PROPHYLAXIS

- Prosthetic cardiac valve or prosthetic material used for cardiac valve repair
- Previous infective endocarditis
- Congenital heart disease (CHD)*
- Unrepaired cyanotic CHD, including palliative shunts and conduits
  - Completely repaired CHD with prosthetic material or device, whether placed by surgery or by catheter intervention, during the first 6 months after the procedure†
  - Repaired CHD with residual defects at the site or adjacent to the site of a prosthetic patch or prosthetic device (which inhibit endothelialization)
- Cardiac transplantation recipients who develop cardiac valvulopathy

*Except for conditions listed above, prophylaxis is not recommended for any other form of CHD.
†Prophylaxis is reasonable because endothelialization of prosthetic material occurs within 6 months after the procedure.
Used with permission from Wilson W, et al. Prevention of Infective Endocarditis: Guidelines From the American Heart Association. Circulation. 2007; 116: 1736–1754.

TABLE 2-3   ANTIBIOTIC PROPHYLAXIS FOR INFECTIVE ENDOCARDITIS

Treatment	Antibiotic	Regimen
IV Therapy	Ampicillin	2 g IV
	or	
	Cefazolin or ceftriaxone*	1 g IV
Allergic to penicillin or ampicillin*,†	Cefazolin or ceftriaxone	1 g IV
	or	
	Clindamycin	600 mg IV
Oral	Amoxicillin	2 g

*Cephalosporins should not be used in patients with a significant sensitivity to penicillins.
†These regimens don't cover enterococcus. If enterococcus is a concern, use Vancomycin.
Preferable to administer 30–60 minutes before procedure.
Used with permission from Wilson W, et al. Prevention of Infective Endocarditis: Guidelines From the American Heart Association. Circulation. 2007;116:1736–1754.

Venous Thromboembolism (VTE) Prophylaxis

- Risk factors for VTE include, but are not limited to, surgery, immobility, trauma, cancer, previous VTE, estrogen-containing medications, obesity, inherited or acquired thrombophilia, pregnancy and the postpartum period, erythropoiesis-stimulating agents, nephrotic syndrome, myeloproliferative disorders, and central venous catheterization
- Prevalence of VTE in patients that undergo major gynecologic surgery is 15–40%
- Risk of VTE and subsequent prophylaxis recommendations depend on
  - Patient's age and associated risk factors
  - Type and duration of procedure
- VTE prophylaxis
  - Recommended according to risk classification (Table 2-4)

TABLE 2-4   RISK CLASSIFICATION AND VTE PROPHYLAXIS IN PATIENTS UNDERGOING SURGERY

Level of Risk	Definition	Successful Prevention Strategies
Low	Surgery lasting less than 30 minutes in patients younger than 40 with no additional risk factors	No specific prophylaxis; early and "aggressive" mobilization
Moderate	Surgery lasting less than 30 minutes in patients with additional risk factors	Low-dose UFH (5000 units every 12 hours), LMWH (2500 units dalteparin or 40 mg enoxaprin daily), graduated compression stockings, or SCDs
	Surgery lasting less than 30 minutes in patients aged 40–60 with no additional risk factors	
	Major surgery in patients under age 40 with no additional risk factors	

TABLE 2-4 RISK CLASSIFICATION AND VTE PROPHYLAXIS IN PATIENTS UNDERGOING SURGERY (*Continued*)

Level of Risk	Definition	Successful Prevention Strategies
High	Surgery lasting less than 30 minutes in patients older than 60 or with additional risk factors Major surgery in patients over 40 or with additional risk factors	Low-dose UFH (5000 units every 8 hours), LMWH (5000 units dalteparin or 40 mg LMWH daily), or SCDs
Highest	Major surgery in patients over 60 plus prior VTE, cancer, or molecular hypercoagulable state	Low-dose UFH (5000 units every 8 hours), LMWH (5000 units dalteparin or 40 mg enoxaparin daily), or SCDs/graduated compression stockings + low-dose UFH or LMWH. Consider continuing prophylaxis for 2–4 weeks after discharge

UFH, unfractionated heparin; LMWH, low molecular weight heparin; SCDs, sequential compression devices.
Data from Geerts et al. Prevention of venous thromboembolism: the Seventh ACOG conference on Antithrombotic and thrombolytic therapy. Chest. 2004;126(suppl):338S–400S.

Per ACOG
- Consider preoperative administration of 5000 units UFH within 2 hours preoperatively followed by postoperative administration every 8 (high risk) to 12 hours (moderate risk) until discharge. Alternative: LMWH (*lovenox* 40 mg) 12 hours preoperatively followed by once daily postoperative administration until discharge (moderate and high risk)
- Dual prophylaxis with UFH and graduated compression stockings/SCDs is recommended for patients with the highest risk of VTE

Data from ACOG. Prevention of deep vein thrombosis and pulmonary embolism. Practice Bulletin No. 84, August 2007, reaffirmed 2013.

LAPAROTOMY

Common Abdominal Incisions in Gynecologic Surgery

- *Midline vertical:* Start 3–4 cm above pubic **symphysis** and extend superiorly in midline; provides excellent exposure and ability to extend superiorly to xyphoid; less bleeding
- *Pfannenstiel:* Horizontal incision 3–4 cm above pubic symphysis; keeping incision within lateral rectus border and curving incision cephalad will help to avoid ilioinguinal/iliohypogastric nerve injuries (see Table 2-5). Cosmetic, however, more bleeding, and less exposure
- *Maylard:* Wide horizontal skin incision (anterior inferior iliac spine (ASIS) to ASIS), dissection of rectus sheath, followed by transection of rectus muscles and possible suture ligation of inferior epigastric vessels. Cut ends of muscle are transfixed to the rectus sheath to prevent retraction and permit closure at end of case. Provides exposure
- *Cherney:* Horizontal skin/fascial incision; tendons of rectus and pyrimidalis are transected 1–2 cm above their attachment to the pubic symphysis and are reapproximated at end of case. Provides exposure

Complications of Gynecologic Surgery

- *Intestinal injury (less than 1% risk)*
  - Repair with suture line perpendicular to long axis of bowel to prevent narrowing of bowel lumen
- *Urologic injury (approximately 1% risk)*
  - Increased risk when surgery indicated for malignancy or prolapse
  - Small bladder injury (<1 cm) in the dome of the bladder may be treated with Foley for 7–10 days or repaired
  - Larger bladder injury (≥1 cm) requires repair; two layer closure
  - Ureteral injury may not be apparent until 1–5 days after surgery (urinoma or ascites develops)
  - Cystoscopy can be helpful to assess for bladder defects and ureteral function
  - See Figure 2-1—Path of Ureter
- *Fistula formation:* Relatively rare; may be urologic or gastrointestinal
- *Fascial dehiscence*
  - Can occur early or late, average 4–14 days postoperatively
  - Risk factors: Chronic pulmonary disease, post-op cough, ascites, malignancy, obesity, wound infection, poor nutrition, history of radiation

- • Diagnosis: "Popping" sensation, copious serosanguinous discharge from wound, bulge at incision; may be partial or complete opening of fascia
  - • Treatment: Surgical emergency; moist dressing over wound and go to OR; 10% mortality
  - • Prevention: Proper fascial closure without tension and delayed absorbing suture; postoperative teaching and precautions
- • *Evisceration:* Dehiscence with protrusion of abdominal contents out of incision
- • *Wound infection* (cellulitis, abscess); hematoma/seroma
- • *Wound hematoma/seroma*
- • *Incisional hernia*
- • *VTE*
- • *Nerve injury:* Risk can be reduced by knowledge of anatomy, careful positioning of patient and retractors (in open surgery) (Table 2-5)

Path of the ureter: 15 cm in abdomen, 15 cm in pelvis

Renal pelvis
↓
Over psoas muscle
↓
Crosses pelvic brim over bifurcation of iliac vessels
↓
Courses through ovarian fossa medial to vessels
↓
Dives medial and anterior in median leaf of broad ligament
↓
Courses under the uterine artery, 2 cm away from the internal os of the cervix ("water under the bridge")
↓
Travels on anterolateral surface of the cervix to insert posteriorly into the trigone of the bladder

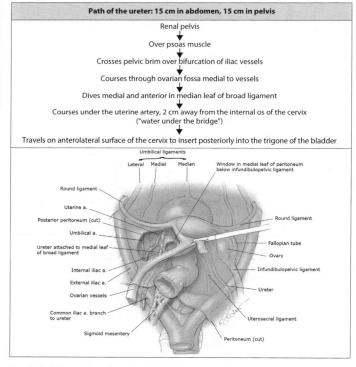

Figure 2-1 Path of ureter. (Used with permission from Hoffman BL, et al. Chapter 38. Anatomy. In: Hoffman BL, et al., eds. *Williams Gynecology*, 2nd ed. New York, NY: McGraw-Hill; 2012.)

TABLE 2-5 NERVE INJURIES WITH GYNECOLOGIC SURGERY

Nerve	Common Cause of Injury	Deficit
Femoral (L2-4)	Pressure from deep retractors (self-sustaining retractors, increased risk with wide incision—Pfannenstiel/Maylard) Excessive hip flexion (candy canes) Inguinal dissection	*Sensory:* Anterior/medial thigh, leg, foot *Motor:* Decreased hip flexion, knee extension, knee deep tendon reflexes

TABLE 2-5 NERVE INJURIES WITH GYNECOLOGIC SURGERY (*Continued*)

Nerve	Common Cause of Injury	Deficit
Lateral femoral cutaneous (L2-3)	Pressure from deep retractors (self-sustaining retractors, increased risk with wide incision—Pfannenstiel/Maylard) Excessive hip flexion (candy canes)	*Sensory only:* Lateral thigh
Genitofemoral (L1-2)	Pelvic side wall dissection	*Sensory only:* Mons, labia, and upper thigh
Obturator (L2-4)	Retroperitoneal dissection, lymphadenectomy paravaginal repair	*Sensory:* Medial thigh *Motor:* Decreased thigh adduction
Common peroneal (L4-5, S1-2)	Compression from Yellofin stirrups on lateral knee	*Sensory:* Lateral calf and dorsal foot *Motor:* Loss of dorsiflexion of the foot ("foot drop")
Ilioinguinal (L1) (3 cm medial/3 cm inferior to ASIS) Iliohypogastric (L1) (2 cm medial/1 cm inferior to ASIS)	Lateral port placement Pfannenstiel incision, especially if extended beyond the border of oblique muscles Can also be incorporated into fascial repair resulting in nerve entrapment syndrome	*Sensory:* Mons, labia, and inner thigh Pain may extend from surgical incision laterally into the inguinal and suprapubic regions. May radiate to lower abdomen
Pudendal (S2-4) (through Alcock's canal)	Sacrospinus ligament suspension, pelvic reconstruction	Damage/entrapment causes vulvar pain; pain radiates down posterior leg or perineum; bowel and bladder may be affected
Phrenic nerve (C3–5)	Diaphragmatic resection near esophageal hiatus	Diaphragm muscle dysfunction; impaired work and efficiency of breathing; difficulty weaning from ventilator

Suture Selection

Suture Types (Table 2-6)
- Absorbable (monocryl, vicryl, chromic, PDS) versus nonabsorbable (nylon, gortex, silk, fiberware, ethibond, prolene, steel)
- Braided (silk, vicryl, ethibond) versus nonbraided/monofilament (monocryl, PDS, ethilon/nylon)
  - Nonbraided may cause less tissue reactivity/tearing; knots more likely to loosen

Suture Size
- More zeroes, the smaller the diameter (eg, 4-0 or 0000 is larger than 5-0 or 00000)
- Then sizes are 0, #1, #2, etc (larger the number, larger the diameter)
- Typically, 0 is for fascia

Needle Types
- Tapered: Used on tissue that is more easily pierced (eg, bowel, fascia, muscle)
  - TP or CTX—fascia
  - CT or CT1—suprafascial deep tissue layers
  - CT2—uterus
  - SH—bowel
  - CV or BV—vessel and nerve repair
- Cutting: Used on skin and other tough tissue
  - GS—fascia or soft tissue
  - FSLX—large skin closure when tension present
  - FSL—for sewing drains to skin or skin closure needing higher tension closure
  - FS2 or PS2—skin closure

TABLE 2-6 SUTURES

Suture Type	Material	Natural/Synthetic	Construction	Available Sizes	Strength Retention Profile	Absorption Time	Common Uses in Gyn
Plain gut	Beef serosa or sheep submucosa	Natural	Monofilament	3 to 7-0	7–10 days	70 days	Tubal
Chromic	Beef serosa or sheep submucosa	Natural	Monofilament	3 to 7-0	21–28 days	90 days	Tubal, hysterotomy, peritoneum
Vicryl	Polyglactin 910	Synthetic	Braided	3 to 8-0	75% at 14 days 50% at 21 days 25% at 28 days	56–70 days	Hysterotomy, fascia, peritoneum, subcutaneous, skin, B-Lynch
Monocryl	Poliglecaprone 25	Synthetic	Monofilament	2 to 6-0	50–60% at 7 days 20–30% at 14 days	91–119 days	Skin
PDS	Polydioxanone	Synthetic	Monofilament	2 to 9-0	70% at 2 weeks 50% at 4 weeks 25% at 6 weeks	180–210 days	Fascia, B-Lynch
Silk	Silk	Natural	Braided	5 to 9-0	About 1 year	n/a	Bowel, interrupted skin, securing drains to skin
Nylon	Nylon 6	Synthetic	Ethilon (monofilament) Nurolon (braided)	2 to 11-0 1 to 6-0	20% loss/year	n/a	Interrupted skin
Mersilene	Polyester/Dacron	Synthetic	Braided	5 to 6-0	Indefinite	n/a	Cerclage
Prolene	Polypropylene	Synthetic	Monofilament	2 to 10-0	Indefinite	n/a	Cerclage
Biosyn	Polyester	Synthetic	Monofilament	1 to 6-0	21 days	90–110 days	Skin
Maxon	Polyglyconate	Synthetic	Monofilament	1 to 5-0	42 days	180 days	Fascia
Polysorb	Glycolide/lactide copolymer	Synthetic	Braided	2 to 8-0	21 days	56–70 days	Vaginal cuff, hysterotomy, fascia
Absorbable V-Loc	Polyglyconate	Synthetic	Monofilament barbed	0 to 4-0	14–21 days	90–110 days	Vaginal cuff

HYSTEROSCOPY

Types of Hysteroscopes

- Diagnostic
  - Flexible (2.8–5.0 mm in diameter)
  - Rigid (1.0–5.0 mm in diameter; 12 degrees, 30 degrees most common)
- Operative (8.0–10.0 mm in diameter)
  - Electrosurgical resectoscopes: Monopolar, bipolar (Versapoint)
  - Hysteroscopic morcellators (Smith & Nephew TRUCLEAR™, Hologic MyoSure®)
  - Operative sheath with instruments inserted through channels

Preoperative/Intraoperative Considerations

- Optimal timing is during follicular phase of menstrual cycle
- If performing operative (not diagnostic) hysteroscopy such as myomectomy, essure, or ablation, consider preoperative *Depo-Provera* several weeks ahead of time to thin endometrial lining and aid visualization
- Consider use of misoprostol (eg, 200 or 400 μg orally or vaginally) for cervical ripening if cervical stenosis is anticipated (evidence-based only for premenopausal women)
- Distension of uterine cavity typically requires 60–70 mm Hg
- Keeping intrauterine pressure less than mean arterial pressure (MAP) will decrease fluid intravasation
- If using monopolar energy, patient must be grounded

Contraindications

- Pregnancy; active genital tract infections; active herpetic infection

Media: Table 2-7

TABLE 2-7 HYSTEROSCOPY MEDIA

Type	Use	Management	Complications
Carbon dioxide gas	Diagnostic only	Limit flow to less than 100 mL/min Intrauterine pressure less than 100 mm Hg	Gas embolization
Electrolyte-poor fluid (1.5% glycine, 3% sorbitol, 5% mannitol*)	Primarily operative with monopolar resectoscope	Fluid deficit = 750 cc signals need to complete case[†] Fluid deficit = 1500 cc → stop case, check electrolytes, manage complications	Hyponatremia[‡] Hyperammonemia Decreased serum osmolality Seizures Cerebral edema, death
Electrolyte-containing fluid (normal saline)	Diagnostic and operative Compatible with bipolar scope, MyoSure®, and TRUCLEAR™	Fluid deficit = 1500 cc signals need to complete case Fluid deficit = 2500 cc → stop case, check electrolytes, manage complications	Fluid overload resulting in pulmonary edema, congestive heart failure

*Mannitol acts as a diuretic and therefore does decrease serum osmolality
[†]In patients with cardiovascular or renal compromise, consider stopping immediately
[‡]If signs or symptoms of hyponatremia (confusion, headache, nausea/vomiting, weakness, hypertension): Compensatory mechanism results in free water, cerebral edema, increased intracranial pressure, central pontine myolysis.

Complications (Primarily with Operative Hysteroscopy)

- Hemorrhage 2.4%, uterine perforation 1.5%, cervical laceration 1–11%
- Air embolism: Decrease risk by avoiding Trendelenburg position, prime tubing, limiting CO_2 flow; treatment if air embolism is suspected is left lateral decubitus position, head tilted down 5 degrees, aspiration of air from right ventricle
- Fluid overload: Check electrolytes, consider furosemide *(Lasix)* 20–40 mg IV; if Na is less than 125 mEq/L, stop procedure

LAPAROSCOPY

Selecting Patients for Laparoscopy

- Prior abdominal surgery: Greater than 20% risk of adhesions of omentum and/or bowel to the anterior abdominal wall. Consider left upper quadrant (LUQ) entry
- Pulmonary disease: Hypercarbia and decreased ventilation associated with laparoscopy may be problematic for patients with pulmonary disease

Setting up the OR

- Antibiotics: Not needed unless doing hysterectomy or dealing with infected tubes
- Bowel prep: Does not decrease incidence of complications, but useful if bowel resection required, so consider if complicated case. No longer standard practice prior to routine gynecologic surgery
- Have nasogastric (NG) tube orogastric (OG) tube placed for decompression (especially with LUQ entry)
- *Positioning*
  - Consider placing the patient on a "bean bag," gel, or foam pad to limit sliding while in deep Trendelenburg
  - Lithotomy: Thigh should be slightly flexed, no more than 90 degrees from the plane of the abdomen. Avoid hyperextension to reduce chance of nerve injury
  - Buttocks slightly over table edge (allows for uterine manipulation); sacrum should be completely supported by table to reduce chance of back strain
  - Tuck both or one arm(s) with padding; arms should be supported in a neutral position with hand against thigh to avoid ulnar nerve injury
  - The patient should be flat (not in Trendelenburg) for umbilical trocar placement to minimize chance of injury to aorta/iliacs

Uterine Manipulation

- A variety of uterine manipulators are available. Several examples are shown in Figure 2-2

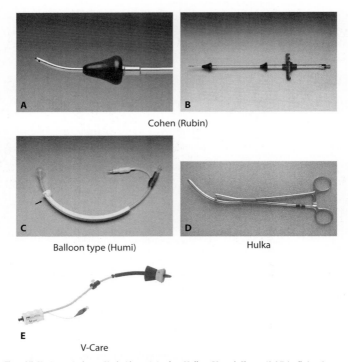

Figure 2-2 Uterine manipulators. (Used with permission from Hoffman BL, et al. Chapter 42. Minimally invasive surgery. In: Hoffman BL, et al., eds.*Williams Gynecology*, 2nd ed. New York, NY: McGraw-Hill; 2012.)

Options for Creating Pneumoperitoneum

- Use Veress needle: Two "pops"—first, the fascia; second, the peritoneum; DO NOT wiggle needle side to side after entry—can enlarge an inadvertent injury
- Direct visual entry using trocar with transparent tip (Xcel®, Visiport™, Optiview®)
- Open laparoscopy and place Hassan trocar, then insufflate
- Insufflate to 12–15 mm Hg. (Can start with 20 mm Hg and decrease to 12–15 mm Hg)

Confirming Access to Peritoneal Cavity

- Plunger on syringe attached to Veress is withdrawn to make sure no blood (indicating a vessel injury) or brown/green content (bowel injury) appear
- Hanging drop test: Drop of normal saline is sucked into abdominal cavity (negative pressure)
- Low intra-abdominal pressure (ideally below 7 mm Hg)

Trocar Placement

- *Umbilicus:* Distance between skin and peritoneal cavity is shorter at umbilicus than any another site—there is no fat or muscle between skin and peritoneum
  - In average weight patients, insert Veress toward hollow of sacrum
  - In obese patients (BMI ≥30), use a more vertical approach
  - See Figure 2-3
- *LUQ entry at Palmer's point:* Left hypochondrium, two fingerbreadths below the left costal margin in the midclavicular line
- *Secondary trocars*
  - In midline, 3 cm above pubic symphysis
  - Laterally, approximately 8 cm from the midline and 8 cm above pubic symphysis to avoid inferior epigastric vessels (inferior epigastrics are approximately 5 cm from midline and 3 cm above symphysis; on laparoscopic view, are medial to lateral insertion of round ligament and just lateral to the obliterated umbilical vessels.). See Figure 2-4 for location of anterior abdominal wall blood vessels

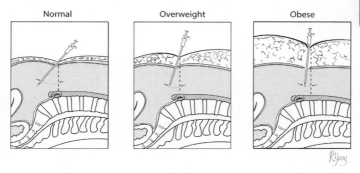

Figure 2-3 Trocar placement in laparoscopy. (Used with permission from Hoffman BL, et al. Chapter 42. Minimally invasive surgery. In: Hoffman BL, et al., eds. *Williams Gynecology*, 2nd ed. New York, NY: McGraw-Hill; 2012.)

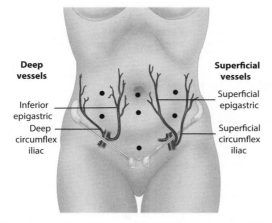

Figure 2-4 Location of anterior abdominal wall vessels. (Used with permission from Cain J, et al. Chapter 41. Gynecology. In: Brunicardi F, et al., eds. *Schwartz's Principles of Surgery*, 9th ed. New York, NY: McGraw-Hill; 2010.)

Energy Sources

- *Monopolar:* Risk of injury to adjacent structures if instrument touches them
- *Bipolar:* Offers a greater margin of safety. Damage is limited by thermal spread (approximately 22 mm) rather than by electrical current; cutting ability is reduced
- *Laser:* Offers a precise, rapid, and accurate method of thermally destroying the tissue, although hemostatic effects are less and the cost is more
- *Advanced bipolar sealing devices:* Enseal, plasma kinetic dissection forceps (Gyrus), and LigaSure™ use pressure and pulsed current to seal vessels with minimal lateral thermal spread
- *Harmonic scalpel:* Blade vibrates at 55.5 mHz to break hydrogen bonds in tissue, resulting in cutting or coaptation of vessels

Principles of Electrosurgery

- Dissection of tissue using high-energy alternating currents
  - Cut mode: Low voltage, continuous current; deeper tissue penetration, less lateral spread
  - Coagulation mode: High voltage, interrupted current; superficial tissue penetration, more lateral spread
- Monopolar (example: *Bovie*)
  - Instrument contains a single active electrode
  - Path of energy: Generator → active electrode → tissue → dispersed through the body to the return electrode (ie, grounding pad) → generator
- Bipolar (example: *Kleppinger*)
  - Instrument contains active and return electrodes
  - Path of energy: Generator → active electrode → tissue → return electrode → generator and the intervening tissue is dessicated

Complications of Laparoscopy

- *Retroperitoneal vessel injury (aorta/iliacs):* (risk approximately 0.1–1%)
  - Treatment: Make midline vertical incision, transfuse blood products, call vascular surgeon, ask anesthesiologist to place central line
- *Abdominal wall vessel injury:* (risk approximately 0.2–2%)
  - Inferior epigastric (from external iliac), superficial epigastric (from femoral)
  - Avoid injury: Transilluminate to see superficial epigastric; look intraperitoneally beneath the peritoneum between the insertion of the round ligament at the inguinal canal and the obliterated umbilical artery to see the inferior epigastric
  - Treatment: Coagulate the vessel with electrosurgery from another port site, or place a Foley catheter through the trocar and inflate the balloon or place a transabdominal suture
- *Intestinal injury:* (risk approximately 0.1–0.4%)
  - May not be recognized at time of surgery. Usually manifests 24–48 hours post-op: fevers, leukocytosis, nausea/vomiting, distension, abdominal pain
- *Incisional hernia:* (risk approximately 0.2–5%)
  - May decrease risk by visualizing closure of the fascia for port sites larger than 10–12 mm
- *Gas embolism:* (risk approximately 0.001–0.6%)
  - Uncommon; may be caused by inadvertent placement of Veress in vessel
  - Signs: Decreased end-tidal carbon dioxide, decreased oxygen saturation, a loud mill-wheel murmur, severe hypotension, and possible cardiac arrest
  - Treatment: Stop insufflation, remove the needle, place the patient in the left lateral decubitus position, administer 100% oxygen, place a central line for aspiration of the gas from the right side of the heart and from the pulmonary vasculature

POSTOPERATIVE PAIN MANAGEMENT

Important Points

- Half-life of opioids is approximately 3 hours (takes approximately 15 hours to achieve steady state)
- Acetaminophen + oxycodone (*Percocet/Tylox*): acetaminophen limits dose-maximum 4000 mg in 24 hours
  - *Tylox* contains 5 mg oxycodone + 500 mg acetaminophen
  - *Percocet* contains 5 mg oxycodone + 325 mg acetaminophen
- If need more narcotic
  - Oxycodone: 5–20 mg every 3–4 hours (often given without acetaminophen to avoid toxicity)
  - Hydromorphone *(Dilaudid)* 1–4 mg every 3–4 hours
- To switch to morphine sulfate controlled release (*MS Contin*), take last 24 hours cumulative dose of morphine and give one-half of that as *MS Contin* every 12 hours or one-third every 8 hours
- Morphine sulfate immediate release (MSIR): 30–60 mg orally every 3–4 hours
- See Table 2-8 for equivalent analgesic dosing for various narcotic medications

TABLE 2-8 EQUIVALENT NARCOTIC DOSING**

Medication	Time to Effect	Duration of Action	Route	Equivalent Analgesic Dose
Codeine	30–60 mins	3–6 hours	Orally	200 mg
Fentanyl	Almost immediate	30–60 mins	IM/IV	0.1 mg (= 100 µg)
Hydrocodone	10–20 mins	4–8 hours	Orally	20–30 mg
Hydromorphone	5 mins (IV)	2–4 hours IV/IM	IV	1.5 mg
	15–30 mins (orally)	3–6 hours orally	Orally	7.5 mg
Morphine	20 mins IM; 5 mins IV	1–2 hours IV; 3–4 hours IM	IM/IV	10 mg
	30–60 mins (orally)	3–6 hours orally	Orally	30 mg*
Oxycodone	10–15 mins	3–6 hours	Orally	15–30 mg (20 mg)

For example 1.5 mg hydromorphone IV = 20 mg oxycodone orally = 10 mg morphine IV = 0.1 mg fentanyl.
*60 mg if chronic use
**Many variables affect these numbers use as guideline only.

COMMON POSTOPERATIVE COMPLICATIONS

Low Urine Output

• *Definition:* Less than 0.5 cc/kg/hour, or less than 30 cc/hour for 60 kg woman
• *Differential Diagnosis*
  • Prerenal: Dehydration, hemorrhage
  • Renal: Acute tubular necrosis (ATN), acute interstitial nephritis
  • Postrenal: Obstruction, retention
• *Physical Exam*
  • Vital signs (orthostatics, fever, tachycardia), ins/outs (I/Os), heart, lungs, abdomen, extremities
  • Is Foley catheter working? Unkink! Flush! Replace!
• *Labs:* If cause is obvious, go to management. Otherwise consider
  • CBC to check hematocrit if concerned about bleeding or patient is orthostatic
  • Send urine for specific gravity, sodium (less than 20 mEq/L generally indicative of hypovolemia), and creatinine (to calculate fractional excretion of sodium (FENa); see below)
  • Need basic metabolic panel labs if doing FENa (for serum Na and Cr)
    • Findings suggestive of
      • *Prerenal*: Urine specific gravity (>1.025), BUN/Cr >20, urine Na <20 mEq/L, FENa <1%
      • *Renal*: Normal to low specific gravity, BUN/Cr <20, urine Na >40 mEq/L, FENa >2%

FENa: Measures percentage of filtered Na excreted in urine*

$$FENa(\%) = \frac{Urine\ Na \times Plasma\ Cr}{Plasma\ Na \times Urine\ Cr} \times 100$$

<1%: Pre-renal
>2%: Intrinsic Renal (eg, ATN)

*Difficult to interpret if patient is on diuretic!

• *Management*
  • Strict I/O's (monitor with Foley)
  • **Prerenal:** If patient is obviously dry with no signs of acute blood loss, give IV fluid bolus and follow urine output. The healthy patient should tolerate a fluid challenge of 10 mL/kg of NS or LR run over 20–30 minutes; fluid resuscitate, rule out bleeding (hematoma), rule out sepsis. Consider CT scan if concerned about bleeding
  • **Renal:** Stop nephrotoxic medications (ketorolac, ibuprofen, gentamicin)
    • **ATN:** May be caused by sepsis, shock, toxins (radio-contrast dye, amino-glycosides). Presence of large amounts of tubular epithelial cells and epithelial cell (granular) casts pathognomonic for ATN (ischemic damage)
  • **Postrenal:** Place/flush Foley, rule out ureteral obstruction (renal sono)/injury. If evidence of pulmonary edema, diurese (ie, *Lasix*, follow K+)

Postoperative Fever

- *Definition*
  - ≥38.0°C (100.4°F) on two occasions at least 4–6 hours apart and *more than* 24 hours after surgical procedure. EXCLUDES fever during first 24 hours post-op
  - ≥39.0°C (102.2°F) recorded on any occasion in post-op period
- *Causes*
  - 20% due to infection; 80% due to noninfectious causes
    - Noninfectious: Atelectasis, hypersensitivity reactions to medications, pyrogenic reaction to tissue trauma, hematoma formation
    - Infectious: Aspiration pneumonia, wound infection, abscess formation
  - Most early post-op fevers are caused by inflammatory stimulus and resolve spontaneously
  - Increased risk of post-op fever with operative time over 2 hours and intraoperative transfusion
  - Think about the **5 Ws**: Wind (atelectasis), water (UTI), wound (infection/hematoma), walk (superficial/deep vein thrombophlebitis), wonder drugs (drug-induced fever)
  - See Figure 2-5 for timing of fever onset with various complications
- *Evaluation*
  - Careful history and exam guides which lab tests, IF ANY, are indicated
  - Study of post-op GYN patients
    - Urine culture positive in only 9% of patients cultured and less than 2% of febrile patients
    - Chest x-ray with significant findings in 1.5% of febrile patients
    - Blood cultures—none were positive
  - *In the first 48 hours*
    - Nonseptic causes most common. Atelectasis causes up to 90%
    - Diagnostic studies performed have a very low yield
    - Evaluate: History, vital signs, urine output, physical exam: pharynx; lungs, back for costovertebral angle (CVA) tenderness, incision, extremities (DVT, thrombophlebitis), drains, IV sites
    - Keep in mind: In post-hysterectomy patients, vaginal cuff cellulitis/hematoma/abscess may be a fever source
  - *After the first 48 hours*
    - Most common sites of infection in post-op laparotomy patient are pulmonary system, wounds, and urinary tract
    - *"Fever Workup"* (if indicated)
      - Consider CBC with differential, basic metabolic panel, chest x-ray, urinalysis with culture
      - Blood cultures two times (if fever ≥39°C, or HIV-infected, or Oncology patient, patient with central line)—realize they have very low yield in the majority of instances
      - Sputum culture if respiratory symptoms; wound culture
      - If exam warrants, consider pelvic ultrasound, CT scan, lower extremity Dopplers, etc

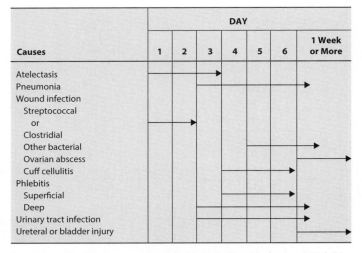

	DAY						
Causes	1	2	3	4	5	6	1 Week or More
Atelectasis							
Pneumonia							
Wound infection							
Streptococcal							
or							
Clostridial							
Other bacterial							
Ovarian abscess							
Cuff cellulitis							
Phlebitis							
Superficial							
Deep							
Urinary tract infection							
Ureteral or bladder injury							

Figure 2-5 Onset of fever for various postoperative complications. (Used with permission from Lentz GM, Lobo RA, Gershenson DM, et al. *Comprehensive Gynecology*, 6th ed. 2012.)

- Consider drug fever
  - May take several days or weeks to develop
  - Fever is usually constant, not spiking
  - Generally improves
- **Be more aggressive if persistent fever, immunosuppressed (Oncology patients), frail/unstable patients, unusual signs/symptoms**
- *Treatment:* Depends on the suspected source

Gynecologic Infections

Cuff cellulitis

- Infection of surgical margin in upper vagina
- Signs/symptoms: Can begin late hospital course or after discharge: Lower abdominal pain, back pain, fever, vaginal discharge
- Diagnosis: Erythema of cuff on vaginal exam
- Management: Broad spectrum coverage (amoxicillin/clavulanate (*Augmentin*), levofloxacin/metronidazole, etc)

Pelvic Abscess/Cuff Abscess/Infected Cuff Hematoma

- Tender, fluctuant mass near vaginal cuff, possible purulent drainage
- Signs/symptoms: Pain, fever, drainage
- Diagnosis: Pelvic exam findings, imaging (CT scan or pelvic ultrasound)
- Management: Culture for aerobic/anaerobic pathogens; consider drainage, broad spectrum IV coverage (ertapenem, piperacillin/tazobactam (*Zosyn*)/vancomycin, etc)

Septic Pelvic Thrombophlebitis

- Complicates 0.1–0.5% of gynecological surgical procedures
- Signs/symptoms: Often occurs 2–4 days post-op; fever, tachycardia, GI distress, unilateral abdominal pain
- Diagnosis: May be confirmed by CT scan or MRI—but, can be missed by imaging. Diagnosis of exclusion when fevers do not respond to appropriate antibiotic treatment in absence of abscess or infected hematoma
- Management: Some suggest extended antibiotic coverage; others anticoagulate with UFH or LMWH; however, optimal duration of anticoagulation has not been identified

Wound Infection

- Signs/symptoms: Erythema, warmth, swelling, tenderness
- Diagnosis: Exam findings; consider imaging if high-grade fever or drainage
- Management
  - Cellulitis/no drainable fluid collection: Oral cephalosporin, clindamycin or trimethoprim/sulfamethoxazole (*Bactrim DS*) for 7–10 days
  - Drainable fluid collection: Open incision; clean/pack. Wound care consult as needed; IV versus oral antibiotics depending on clinical presentation

Necrotizing Fasciitis

- Severe complication from synergistic bacterial infection of fascia, subcutaneous tissue, and skin. More common in diabetics, immunocompromised
- Signs/Symptoms: Pain out of proportion to exam, clinical signs of sepsis, viscous, cloudy, malodorous drainage. Wound edges may be purple or necrotic. May see bullae of skin; crepitus in subcutaneous tissue
- Diagnosis: Exam; consider CT scan to confirm/determine extent
- Management: Prompt and extensive resection of involved tissue. Broad IV coverage (*Zosyn*/vancomycin/clindamycin)

- *Oncology patients often have more complicated infections and you should have a low threshold for work up, including imaging*

ABNORMAL UTERINE BLEEDING

See Figure 2-6.

Definitions

- Normal menses: Generally menses every 21–35 days, lasting 2–7 days
- Abnormal uterine bleeding (AUB):
  - Cycle less than 21 days or more than 35 days, bleeding more than 8–10 days
  - Menstrual blood loss over 80 mL/cycle OR subjectively heavy menses; some sources suggest soaking through more than six tampons or pads in a day is abnormal
  - Intermenstrual bleeding

Diagnostic Workup

- History
  - Previous menstrual bleeding patterns versus current pattern
  - Underlying endocrine conditions

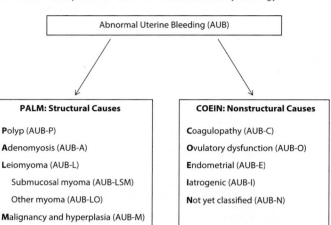

Figure 2-6 Abnormal uterine bleeding. Basic PALM–COEN classification system for the causes of abnormal uterine bleeding in nonpregnant women of reproductive age. This system, approved by the International Federation of Gynecology and Obstetrics, uses the term AUB paired with descriptive terms that describe associated bleeding patterns (HMB or IMB), or a qualifying letter (or letters), or both to indicate its etiology(ies). (Data from ACOG. Diagnosis of abnormal uterine bleeding in reproductive-aged women. Practice Bulletin No. 128, July 2012; also see ACOG Committee Opinion No. 557. Management of acute abnormal uterine bleeding in nonpregnant reproductive-aged women. *Obstet Gynecol.* 2013;121:891–896).

- Screen for bleeding disorder (present in up to 20% women with heavy menses)
- Medications (ie, anticoagulants, hormones), herbal remedies
- Physical Exam
  - Height, weight, BMI (obesity associated with anovulation)
  - Clinical signs of androgen excess (hirsutism, acne) or insulin resistance (acanthosis nigricans)
  - Thyroid enlargement/nodularity
  - Findings suggestive of prolactinoma: Visual field defect, nipple discharge
  - Pelvic exam: Look for cervical/vaginal lesions and pelvic mass or tenderness, and assess uterine size
- Labs (consider based on clinical presentation)
  - β-hCG, CBC, TSH, prolactin, pap, GC/CT, wet mount
  - Suspect PCOS: FSH, LH, estradiol, DHEA-S, free and total testosterone
  - Suspect coagulopathy: CBC with platelets, PT/PTT, including tests for von Willebrand disease (VWD) (vWF—ristocetin cofactor activity, vWF antigen, and factor VIII activity)
- Endometrial biopsy for
  - Women with AUB 45 years of age or older
  - Women under 45 years old with risk factors for hyperplasia such as unopposed estrogen exposure (obesity/PCOS), failed medical management, persistent AUB
  - Pipelle samples 5–15% of cavity, but sensitivity for diagnosis of cancer/hyperplasia is approximately 80–90%
- Imaging
  - Pelvic ultrasound (most helpful immediately after menses)
  - Consider hysteroscopy, sonohysterogram, MRI if additional info needed

Differential Diagnosis

- **Uterus:** Pregnancy, anovulation, polyps, fibroids, endometrial hyperplasia, cancer, adenomyosis, endometritis, retained products of conception
- **Cervix:** Cervicitis, polyps, cervical intraepithelial neoplasia (CIN), cancer, cervical endometriosis, trauma
- **Vagina:** Vaginitis, benign growths, vaginal intraepithelial neoplasia (VAIN), cancer, atrophy, trauma
- **Vulva:** Cysts, dermatitis, herpes simplex virus (HSV), vulval intraepithelial neoplasia (VIN), cancer, trauma
- **Ovary:** Granulosa cell tumors
- **Fallopian tubes:** Malignancy can result in abnormal bleeding
- **Outside the genital tract:** Urethritis, bladder cancer, UTI, inflammatory bowel disease, hemorrhoids, colon cancer

- **Systemic disease:** Thyroid disease, hyperprolactinemia, liver disease, renal disease, hormone releasing tumors, coagulopathies (ie, VWD), Crohn's disease, Behçet's disease, Cushing's disease, etc
- **Drugs:** Hormonal contraception, paraGard® IUD, hormone therapy, anticoagulation, Tamoxifen, steroids, chemotherapy, antipsychotics
- Age-specific considerations
  - Children: Rectal or urethral prolapse, trauma, foreign body
  - Adolescents: Anovulation, coagulopathy
  - Reproductive-aged women: Pregnancy!
  - Perimenopausal: Anovulation
  - Postmenopausal: 30–90% from atrophy
- Consider abuse and sexually transmitted infections (STIs) in differential for ALL ages

Treatment

- Based on the cause. See Table 2-9 for general management guidelines

Structural causes

- Endometrial polyps
  - Generally benign; remove for therapeutic purposes or if postmenopausal and bleeding
    - Postmenopausal, no bleeding, risk of hyperplasia/carcinoma about 1.5% (up to 3%)
    - Postmenopausal, with bleeding, risk of hyperplasia/carcinoma 4–5% (up to 11%)
  - Hysteroscopy to identify and resect
- Uterine leiomyoma
  - Benign growths, present in up to approximately 80% of women
  - Submucosal, intramural, or subserosal
    - Management based on size and location of leiomyoma
    - Medical management
      GnRH agonists: Approximately 30–60% reduction in size in 3 months; may cause initial increase in bleeding followed by amenorrhea
      Options listed in Table 2-9 may help to control associated bleeding
    - Surgical management: Uterine artery embolization, myomectomy, hysterectomy
- Adenomyosis
  - Endometrium invades underlying stroma; common and present in 20–30% hysterectomy specimens
  - Medical management: Continuous oral contraceptive pills (OCPs), *Depo-Provera*, high-dose progestins, Mirena® IUD, GnRH agonists
  - Surgical management: Uterine artery embolization, hysterectomy

Suspected coagulopathy

- Von Willebrand disease
- Affects 1% general population; only 1% of those are symptomatic
- Work with hematologist for management; desmopressin acetate typically used for prevention of bleeding/flares
- Menstrual control: Hormonal options versus nonhormonal (tranexamic acid)
- Avoid NSAIDs/ASA (medications that interfere with platelet function)

Ovulatory dysfunction

- Treat underlying cause if able (hyperprolactinemia, hypothyroidism, etc)
- Hormonal management to regulate cycles/control bleeding/decrease risk of hyperplasia

Management of Acute Heavy Bleeding

- Determine stability of patient
  - Orthostatics
  - Hematocrit/hemoglobin compared to baseline if available
  - Consider age, medical co-morbidities, and blood dyscrasias

Management of Unstable Patient (orthostatic and/or dropping hemoglobin)

- Two large bore IVs, IV fluids, type and cross, strict vitals and I/Os
- Can consider uterine tamponade with packing or Foley balloon
- **Estrogen 25 mg IV** every 4 hours (up to 24 hours)
  - Can consider if patient stabilizes with IV hydration, etc
  - Need to consider medical contraindications to estrogen (VTE/stroke risk, etc)
  - May cause nausea, prescribe antiemetic
  - Once bleeding is controlled with high-dose estrogen, transition to oral regimen
- Uterine curettage (in operating room)
- Uterine Artery Embolization
- Hysterectomy

TABLE 2-9 MANAGEMENT OF HEAVY MENSTRUAL BLEEDING

Med	Dose	Nonsurgical		Contraindications
		Advantages	Disadvantages	
Progestin-releasing IUD (Mirena*)	20 µg levonorgestrel per day	Effective, simple, provides contraception, decreases blood loss 74–97% after 1 year of use Approximately ½ of patients amenorrheic at 2 years	Irregular bleeding, especially in first 3–6 months	Uterine anomalies, high STI risk (relative contraindication)
NSAIDs	Days 1–5 or end of menses Naproxen 500 mg every 12 hours Ibuprofen 600 mg daily Mefenamic acid 500 mg every 8 hours	Simple, inexpensive, relieves dysmenorrhea, reduces blood loss 20–50%	GI upset	Gastritis, peptic ulcer disease
Progestins	Norethindrone 5 mg three times daily on days 15–26 Medroxyprog acetate (Provera) 10 mg on days 15–26 Norethindrone 0.35 mg daily (Micronor) Medroxyprog esterone (Depo Provera) 150 mg IM every 3 months	Cyclical methods: Inexpensive 87% decrease in mean blood loss, induces regular withdrawal bleed Depo-Provera: Approximately 55% amenorrheic at 1 year	Oral progestins: Frequent pill taking, headache, breast pain, acne, nausea, breakthrough bleeding Depo-Provera: Weight gain, mood changes, irregular bleeding	Undiagnosed bleeding
Antifibrinolytics	Tranexamic acid 1300 mg three times daily on days 1–5	Effective, simple 47% decrease in mean blood loss	Nausea, leg cramps, diarrhea	Risk factors for VTE
Combined OCPs	Ethinyl estradiol + progestin	Simple, inexpensive, contraception 43% decrease in mean blood loss	Daily pill taking, nausea, breast pain, breakthrough bleeding	Risk factors for VTE, MI
Danazol	50–100 mg daily; up to 400–800 mg/day	Effective, but side effects; over 50% decrease in mean blood loss	Irreversible androgenic side effects, expensive	Risk factors for VTE, MI, liver disease
GnRH Therapy	Leuprolide 11.25 mg IM every 3 months	Decrease size of leiomyomas	Menopausal symptoms; treatment usually limited to 6–12 months	

TABLE 2-9 MANAGEMENT OF HEAVY MENSTRUAL BLEEDING (*Continued*)

| Procedure | Surgical | |
	Advantages	Disadvantages/Comments
Endometrial ablation	Minimally invasive	May require second ablation or subsequent hysterectomy. Need pathologic diagnosis before ablation! Contraindicated if desire future fertility. Does not provide contraception
D&C	Quick, provides tissue specimen	Usually not curative, only temporary relief
Myomectomy	Preserves uterus, less extensive	Fibroids may recur; if get pregnant, risk abnormal placentation, uterine rupture
Uterine artery embolization	Minimally invasive, quick	Fibroids may recur, possible treatment failure, may require subsequent surgical management, implications for future pregnancy not completely known
Hysterectomy	Definitive treatment	Invasive procedure, major surgery, risks for complications

Management of Stable Patient

- No orthostatic hypotension hemoglobin over 10 g/dL, hospitalization not required
- **OCP taper (use MONOPHASIC pill containing at least 30 μg ethinyl estradiol.)**
  - A variety of tapers exist; one example is:
    - 4 pills for 4 days (every 6 hours)
    - 3 pills for 3 days (every 8 hours)
    - 2 pills for 2 days (every 12 hours)
    - 1 pill daily thereafter
  - Provide antiemetics!
- **High-dose Progestins** (5–10 day course)
  - Megestrol acetate (*Megace*) 10–80 mg orally daily or every 12 hours
  - Medroxyprogesterone acetate (*Provera*) 10–20 mg orally daily or every 12 hours
  - Norethindrone (*Aygestin*) 5 mg daily or every 12 hours
  - May cause nausea, headache, and in high doses may increase blood pressure
- **Tranexamic acid** (*Lysteda*) (5-day course)
  - Antifibrinolytic, acts within 2–3 hours
  - 1-1.5 g orally every 6–8 hours
  - May cause nausea, dizziness, diarrhea
  - Caution in patients at risk for VTE
- **GnRH agonist** (*Depo Lupron*)
  - Consider if other modalities have failed or are contraindicated; typically used following initial treatment of acute bleeding rather than as first line
- **Endometrial ablation**
  - Consider if medical management has failed or is contraindicated

PELVIC PAIN

- *Incidence:* 15% women will experience sometime in their life; indication for 15–40% of laparoscopies and 12% of hysterectomies in the United States
- *Differential diagnosis:* Table 2-10

TABLE 2-10 DIFFERENTIAL DIAGNOSIS OF PELVIC PAIN

Differential Diagnosis of Pelvic Pain	
Gynecologic	**Musculoskeletal**
Uterine	• Abdominal wall myofascial pain
• Adenomyosis	• Chronic coccygeal pain
• Dysmenorrhea/Ovulatory pain	• Compression of lumbar vertebrae
• Cervical stenosis	• Degenerative joint disease
• Chronic endometritis	• Disc herniation/rupture
• Polyps/Leiomyomata	• Hernias: Ventral, inguinal, femoral, Spigelian
• IUD	• Low back pain
• Genital prolapse	• Muscle strain/sprain
• Malignancy	• Malignancy of spinal cord/sacral nerve
Outside of the uterus	• Iliohypogastric, ilioinguinal, or genitofemoral neuralgia
• Adhesive disease	• Levator ani spasm
• Adnexal masses	• Piriformis syndrome
• Salpingitis	• Rectus tendon strain
• Endometriosis	• Spondylosis
• Chronic ectopic pregnancy	• Poor posture
• Malignancy	
• Ovarian remnant syndrome	
• Pelvic congestion syndrome, pelvic varicosities	
• Peritoneal inclusion cysts	
• Acute or chronic pelvic inflammatory disease (PID)	
• Tuberculous salpingitis	

TABLE 2-10 DIFFERENTIAL DIAGNOSIS OF PELVIC PAIN (*Continued*)

Differential Diagnosis of Pelvic Pain	
Urologic	**Gastrointestinal**
• Malignancy	• Malignancy
• Acute or recurrent cystitis/urethritis	• Colitis
• Chronic UTI	• Constipation
• Interstitial cystitis; radiation cystitis	• Chronic/Intermittent bowel obstruction
• Nephro/urolithiasis	• Diverticular disease
• Detrusor dyssynergia (bladder contractions)	• Hernias
• Urethral diverticulum or caruncle	• Inflammatory or irritable bowel disease
Iatrogenic	**Other**
• Post-endometrial ablation	• Abdominal migraine or epilepsy
• Post-Essure/Post-tubal ligation	• Abuse/Depression/Bipolar disorders
• Post-mesh pain	• Shingles
• Postsurgical neuropathy/adhesions/cutaneous nerve entrapment	• Familial Mediterranean fever
• Post-delivery neuropathy/pelvic floor weakness/ episiotomy pain	• Porphyria
	• Sleep disturbances
	• Somatic referral

Used with permission from Howard F. chronic pelvic pain. *Obstet Gynecol.* 2003;101:594–611..

- *History*
  - Comprehensive medical, surgical, gynecologic, obstetric, family, social history
  - Specific pain questions: Age and timing of onset, exacerbating factors, prior treatments, position changes that have improved pain; providers seen
- *Physical:* HEENT, heart, lungs, breasts, abdomen, back, extremities, pelvic exam

ENDOMETRIOSIS

- *Incidence:* 6–10% premenopausal women, increased prevalence in women with infertility or a family history of endometriosis
- *Common presentation:* Pelvic pain or infertility
  - Ask specifically about bowel/bladder-related symptoms as endometriosis may infiltrate either
- *Diagnosis:* Biopsy of suspicious lesions at the time of laparoscopy confirming presence of endometrial glands and stroma
  - Lesion appearance: Red, white, clear, or black powder-burn (classic)
- *Classification:* ASRM classification used to record operative findings, but does not correlate with severity of symptoms or infertility
  - Common implant locations: Uterosacral and broad ligaments, ovaries, posterior cul-de-sac
  - Non-gyn organs to evaluate: Bowel/appendix, bladder, diaphragm, umbilicus, thorax, inguinal canal
- *Management*
  - Suspected endometriosis can be treated without definitive diagnosis; trial of continuous OCPs, NSAIDs; consider 3-month trial of GnRH agonist if initial regimen fails
  - **Medical**
    - Common first line: Continuous OCPs, NSAIDs, *Depo-Provera*
    - Alternatives: Mirena® IUD, etonogestrel implant (*Nexplanon*), oral progestins, GnRH agonist, danazol
    - GnRH agonist: May cause vasomotor symptoms and bone loss with prolonged use; hormonal *add back* therapy may alleviate these effects
      - Norethindrone 5 mg daily ± conjugated estrogen 0.625 mg daily
      - Also recommend calcium supplementation 1000 mg daily
      - GnRH agonist use FDA approved for approximately 12 months
    - Aromatase inhibitors: Possible utility in resistant cases, evidence lacking thus far
  - **Surgical**
    - Surgical management may improve fertility rates in infertile couples
    - Ablation of lesions: Laser vaporization, electrosurgical fulguration
    - Resection of lesions
    - Presacral neurectomy: May decrease midline pain, but may cause bowel/bladder dysfunction
    - Hysterectomy plus/minus bilateral salpingo-oophorectomy (BSO)
      - Women who retain ovaries at the time of hysterectomy may have an increased risk of recurrent symptoms (approximately 60%) and re-operation (approximately 30%)
      - Hormone therapy following BSO has not been shown to increase risk of recurrent disease

ECTOPIC PREGNANCY

- Accounts for about 6% of all pregnancy-related deaths
- Risk of recurrence: 8–15% if one previous ectopic (risk increased with salpingostomy); over 25% if two or more
- Heterotopic pregnancy (occurrence of intrauterine and extrauterine pregnancy): Varying reports; approximately 1:3900 pregnancies overall to 1 in 100 assisted reproductive technology (ART) pregnancies
- Interstitial pregnancies (some use the term "cornual"; some say they are not the same!). Tubal segment traversing muscular wall of uterus. Higher morbidity/mortality because interstitial portion of tube dilates more freely and painlessly than rest of the tube. Later clinical presentation and potential for massive hemorrhage. Diagnosis suggested when what appears to be an intrauterine pregnancy (IUP) is visualized high in fundus, not surrounded in all planes by 5 mm of myometrium. See Figure 2-7
- Ectopic and IUD: Ectopic pregnancy unlikely in IUD users due to efficacy of IUD. But, if pregnancy occurs, 1/2 Mirena® users and 1/16 ParaGard® users will have ectopic pregnancies
- Ectopic and bilateral tubal ligation (BTL): 1/3 pregnancies following BTL are ectopic. Increased risk if bipolar coagulation done
- Risk factors and associated Odds ratios are listed in Table 2-11

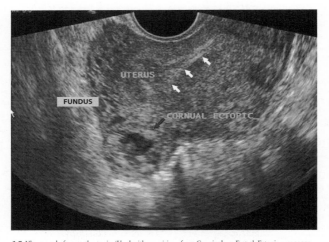

Figure 2-7 Ultrasound of cornual ectopic. (Used with permission from Cunningham F, et al. Ectopic pregnancy. In: Cunningham F, et al., eds. *Williams Obstetrics*, 23rd ed. New York, NY: McGraw-Hill; 2010.)

TABLE 2-11 RISK FACTORS FOR ECTOPIC PREGNANCY

Risk Factors for Ectopic Pregnancy	ODDS Ratio (95% CI)
Previous ectopic	12.5 (7.5, 20.9)
Previous tubal surgery	4.0 (2.6, 6.1)
Smoking >20 cigarettes per day	3.5 (1.4, 8.6)
Prior STI with confirmed PID and/or positive Chlamydia	3.4 (2.4, 5.0)
Three or more prior SABs	3.0 (1.3, 6.9)
Age ≥40 years	2.9 (1.4, 6.1)
Prior medical or surgical abortion	2.8 (1.1, 7.2)
Infertility over 1 year	2.6 (1.6, 4.2)
Lifelong sexual partners—more than 5	1.6 (1.2, 2.1)
Previous IUD use	1.3 (1.0, 1.8)

Location: See Figure 2-8 for sites and frequencies

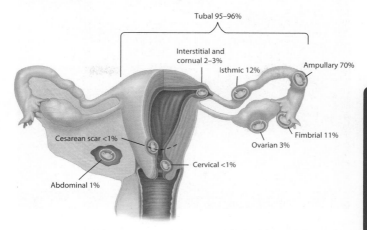

Figure 2-8 Sites and frequencies of ectopic pregnancies. (Used with permission from Hoffman BL, et al. Chapter 7. Ectopic pregnancy. In: Hoffman BL, et al., eds. *Williams Gynecology*, 2nd ed. New York, NY: McGraw-Hill; 2012.)

Diagnosis

- *Classic presentation:* Abdominal pain (97%), vaginal bleeding (79%), adnexal mass (study: approximately 14% of patients with classic presentation had ectopic)
- *Labs:* Quantitative β-hCG, CBC, Type and Screen (if Rh negative, give RhoGAM), complete metabolic panel (CMP) (need AST/ALT, creatinine if giving methotrexate)
- *β-hCG:* The **minimum rise for a potentially viable IUP is 53% per 2 days**. Intervention when β-hCG rises less than 66% over 2 days may result in interruption of a viable IUP. In 85% of viable IUPs, β-hCG rises by at least 66% every 48 hours during the first 40 days of pregnancy
- *Progesterone level:* Generally, progesterone of 20–25 ng/mL is highly predictive (95–100%) of a normal IUP; levels less than 5 ng/mL are nearly 100% predictive of an abnormal pregnancy. Most women with an ectopic have progesterone level between these concentrations at presentation, limiting the diagnostic usefulness of progesterone
- *Sonograms:* Traditionally, the discriminatory level of β-hCG (lowest level gestational sac should be visible) is noted to be about 6500 mIU/mL (7–8 weeks) for transabdominal sono; 1500–2000 mIU/mL (5–6 weeks) for transvaginal. More recent data suggests that although pregnancies may be detected at lower β-hCG thresholds, the discriminatory levels may be higher. See Table 2-12
  - *Intraperitoneal fluid on ultrasound:* Free peritoneal fluid suggests intra-abdominal bleeding (as little as 50 mL of fluid can be detected on transvaginal ultrasound in the cul-de-sac of Douglas). See Figure 2-9. Fluid in right-upper-quadrant (Morison's pouch) indicates significant hemorrhage (seen with about 400–700 mL hemoperitoneum)

TABLE 2-12 β-hCG DISCRIMINATORY LEVELS

	Discriminatory β-hCG (seen 99% of the time)
Gestational sac	3 510 mIU/mL
Yolk sac	17 716 mIU/mL
Fetal pole	47 685 mIU/mL

Used with permission from Connolly A, Ryan DH, Stuebe AM, et al. Reevaluation of discriminatory and threshold levels for serum β-hcG in early pregnancy. *Obstet Gynecol.* 2013;121:65–70.

Keys to Recognizing an IUP

- *"Double sac or double decidual sign"* (Figure 2-10). Two rings surround gestational sac (GS)—inner sac is decidua capsularis (DC); outer layer is the decidua parietalis (DP). Present at approximately 4.5 weeks. Not visible in all early pregnancies. Do NOT diagnose IUP with this finding

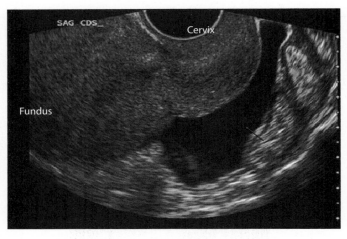

Figure 2-9 Fluid collection in cul-de-sac of Douglas, suggestive of ruptured ectopic. (Used with permission from Hoffman BL, et al. Chapter 7. Ectopic pregnancy. In: Hoffman BL, et al., eds. *Williams Gynecology*, 2nd ed. New York, NY: McGraw-Hill; 2012.)

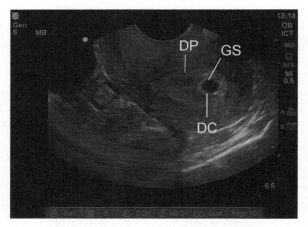

Figure 2-10 Early ultrasound—double decidual sign. The double decidual sign comprises two rings surrounding the gestational sac (GS): the decidua capsularis (DC) and the decidua parietalis (DP). (Used with permission from Fritz DA. Chapter 6. Emergency bedside ultrasound. In: Stone C, Humphries RL, eds. *Current Diagnosis & Treatment Emergency Medicine*. 7th ed. New York, NY: McGraw-Hill; 2011.)

- *Gestational sac*
  - Mean sac diameter (MSD) = (L + W + D)/3
  - Should see live pregnancy when MSD >18 mm
  - Should see yolk sac when MSD 8–10 mm
  - General rule: EGA in days = MSD + 30
- *IUP*
  - Well-defined gestational sac with a yolk sac, confirming IUP (Figure 2-11)
  - Fetal pole is first seen on transvaginal ultrasound about 6 weeks. When approximately 5 mm, fetal heart beat can be detected (9 mm transabdominal)
  - Average fetal heart rate is 110 bpm at 6 weeks; 170 bpm by 8 weeks; 160 at week 14. If less than 100, poorer prognosis

Ectopic Pregnancy Evaluation Algorithm:

- If patient presents with a positive pregnancy test and abdominal cramping and/or vaginal bleeding, an algorithm may be followed (Figure 2-12)

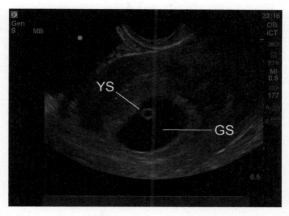

Figure 2-11 Gestational sac with yolk sac. (Used with permission from Fritz DA. Chapter 6. Emergency bedside ultrasound. In: Stone C, Humphries RL, eds. *Current Diagnosis & Treatment Emergency Medicine*. 7th ed. New York, NY: McGraw-Hill; 2011.)

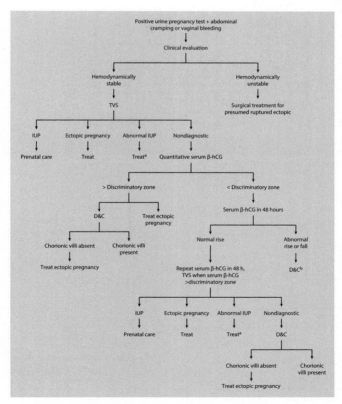

Figure 2-12 Ectopic pregnancy evaluation—algorithm. a (in superscript), expectant management, D&C, or medical management; b (in superscript), serial serum β-hCG levels may be appropriate if a normal uterine pregnancy or if completed abortion is suspected clinically. (Used with permission from Hoffman BL, et al. Chapter 7. Ectopic pregnancy. In: Hoffman BL, et al., eds. *Williams Gynecology*, 2nd ed. New York, NY: McGraw-Hill; 2012.)

Treatment of Ectopic Pregnancy

- *Expectant management:* Consider **only** for patients with low and declining β-hCG. Women must be carefully informed of risks and followed closely. Overall success for expectant management is approximately 57% with major risk for morbidity in those who fail
- Rates of tubal patency (62–90%) and recurrence of ectopic (8–15%) are similar after medical and surgical treatment

Medical Management

- *Methotrexate (MTX):* Folic acid antagonist, inhibits DNA synthesis and repair and cell replication. Stop all folinic acid supplements if administering MTX. OBTAIN CONSENT!
  - Dose: *Methotrexate: 50 mg/m² intramuscular for single-dose treatment*
  - Success rate varies with β-hCG level (Table 2-13)
  - Contraindications to MTX are listed in Table 2-14

TABLE 2-13 SUCCESS RATES OF METHOTREXATE BY β-hCG LEVEL

β-hCG	Success Rate (%)
<1000	98
1000–1999	93–94
2000–4999	92–96
5000–9999	85–87
10 000–14 999	82
≥15 000	68

Data from Lipscomb GH, Mccord, ML, Stovall, TG, et al. Predictors of success of methotrexate treatment in women with tubal ectopic pregnancies. *NEJM.* 1999, 341:1974–1978; Menon S, Colins J, Barnhart KT. Establishing a human chorionic gonadotropin cut off to guide methotrexate treatment of ectopic pregnancy: a systematic review. *Fertil Steril.* 2007;87:481–484.

TABLE 2-14 CONTRAINDICATIONS TO METHOTREXATE

	ACOG	ASRM
Absolute contraindications	• Breast feeding • Overt or lab evidence of immunodeficiency • Preexisting blood dyscrasias (bone marrow hypoplasia, leukopenia, thrombocytopenia, significant anemia) • Known sensitivity to MTX • Active pulmonary disease • Peptic ulcer disease • Hepatic, renal, hematologic dysfunction • Alcoholism, alcoholic liver disease, or other chronic liver disease	• Breast feeding • Evidence of immunodeficiency • Moderate-to-severe anemia, leukopenia, or thrombocytopenia • Sensitivity to MTX • Active pulmonary or peptic ulcer disease • Clinically important hepatic or renal dysfunction • IUP
Relative contraindications	• Ectopic mass over 3.5 cm • Embryonic cardiac motion	• Ectopic mass over 4 cm on transvaginal ultrasound • Embryonic cardiac activity detected by ultrasound • Patient declines blood transfusion • Patient unable to follow-up • High initial β-hCG (over 5000)
Choice of regimen based on β-hCG level	• Multidose regimen may be appropriate if presenting β-hCG value over 5000 mIU/mL or if interstitial ectopic	• Single-dose regimen better in patients with a low initial β-hCG

Data from ASRM: American Society for Reproductive Medicine

- **Protocols**: Three regimens are available (Table 2-15)
  - Single dose protocol (Table 2-16)
  - Multiple dose protocol (Table 2-17)
- Complete resolution of ectopic takes between 2 and 3 weeks but can take as long as 6–8 weeks when pretreatment β-hCG levels are in higher ranges
- When declining β-hCG levels again increase, diagnosis is *persistent ectopic pregnancy*
- Inform patient of MTX treatment effects and side effects (Table 2-18)

TABLE 2-15 PROTOCOLS FOR METHOTREXATE ADMINISTRATION

Single-dose	Two-dose	Multi-dose
• Success rate: about 88% • Most common • Higher rate of failure	• Designed to increase success without more visits than single dose • Not been directly compared with other regimens	• Success rate about 93% • About 50% will not require full 8-day regimen

TABLE 2-16 SINGLE DOSE METHOTREXATE PROTOCOL

Day #	Lab Evaluation	Intervention
Pretreatment	β-hCG, CBC with differential, LFTs, Cr, Type and Screen	Rule out spontaneous abortion RhoGAM if Rh negative
1	β-hCG	MTX 50 mg/m² IM
4	β-hCG	
7	β-hCG	MTX 50 mg/m² IM if β-hCG decreased less than 15% between days 4 and 7, or less than 25% between day 1 and 7

β-hCG every week until β-hCG is less than 5 mIU/mL.

TABLE 2-17 MULTIPLE DOSE METHOTREXATE PROTOCOL

Day #	Lab Evaluation	Intervention
Pretreatment	β-hCG, CBC with differential LFTs, Cr, Type and Screen	Rule out spontaneous abortion RhoGAM if Rh negative
1	β-hCG	MTX 1 mg/kg IM
2		Leucovorin 0.1 mg/kg IM
3	β-hCG	MTX 1 mg/kg IM (if less than 15% decline from day 1 to 3; if over 15%, stop treatment and start surveillance)
4		Leucovorin 0.1 mg/kg IM
5	β-hCG	MTX 1 mg/kg IM (if less than 15% decline from day 3 to 5; if over 15%, stop treatment and start surveillance)
6		Leucovorin 0.1 mg/kg IM
7	β-hCG	MTX 1 mg/kg IM (if less than 15% decline from day 5 to 7; if over 15%, stop treatment and start surveillance)
8		Leucovorin 0.1 mg/kg IM

β-hCG every week until β-hCG is less than 5 mIU/mL.
Screening labs should be repeated 1 week after last dose of MTX.

TABLE 2-18 METHOTREXATE TREATMENT AND SIDE EFFECTS

MTX Treatment Effects	MTX Drug Side Effects
Increase in abdominal girth	Gastric distress, N/V
Increase in β-hCG during initial therapy	Stomatitis
Vaginal bleeding or spotting	Dizziness
Abdominal pain—during days 3–7, usually resolves within 4–12 hours post-onset. If severe/persistent, evaluate. Surgery if rupture suspected	Severe neutropenia (rare) Reversible alopecia (rare) Pneumonitis (rare)

- *Other information for patient*
  - Advise women not to use alcohol or NSAIDs (due to GI side effects)
  - Patient should receive antiemetic prophylaxis (ondansetron (*Zofran*) or compazine for 3 days)
  - Avoid sun exposure to limit risk of MTX dermatitis
  - Avoid intercourse until β-hCG is undetectable
  - Avoid pelvic exams and ultrasound during surveillance of MTX therapy
  - Avoid gas-forming foods; they produce pain
  - Avoid another pregnancy until β-hCG is undetectable
- **Sonography** of patients treated with MTX is complicated because most patients show a worsening appearance, with increased hemorrhage around ectopic. There may be an initial **increase** in size of tubal mass after MTX and an adnexal mass may be visible up to 3 months after treatment. The increase in tubal size and vascularity, despite the decreased β-hCG, represents a healing process and should not cause concern unless patient is clinically unstable or has persistent symptoms

Surgical Management
- Salpingostomy
  - Controversial; inadequate data, but it is thought that subsequent IUP rate is higher after linear salpingostomy. Should be considered as the primary treatment option for tubal pregnancy in the presence of disease in the contralateral tube and desire for future fertility
  - Persistent trophoblastic tissue can remain. Obtain weekly β-hCGs until normal
- Salpingectomy
  - Performed when tubal pregnancy is ruptured to control hemorrhage, recurrent, tube is damaged, patient desires no further fertility

SPONTANEOUS ABORTIONS (SABs)

- Over 80% of SABs occur in the first 12 weeks
- Causes:
  - Chromosomes abnormal in 50–60% of first trimester SABs (monosomy X (45,X), trisomy, triploidy)
  - Structural: Uterine synechiae, septate and bicornuate uteri, leiomyomas
  - Maternal disease: Infection, thyroid disease, diabetes, PCOS, thrombophilia
- Types of Abortions (Table 2-19)

Treatment Options for missed or incomplete abortions
(often depends on patient preference)

- Expectant: 66–76% effective (may take more than 4 weeks)
- Surgical (D&C): 97% effective
- Medical: 66–99% effective

Medical management with Misoprostol (PGE1)
- Median success 80% or higher for missed abortion
- Median success 92% for incomplete abortion
- Dose: Table 2-20
- *Contraindications*
  - Allergy to misoprostol or other prostaglandin
  - Suspicion of ectopic or pelvic infection

TABLE 2-19 TYPES OF ABORTIONS

Type	Fetal Tissue	Bleeding	Cramping	Internal Os
Inevitable	−	+	+	Open
Incomplete	+	+	+	Open
Complete	+	+	+/−	Closed
Early pregnancy failure (missed)	−	+/−	−	Closed
Septic	+/−	+/−	+/−	Open/Closed
Threatened	−	+	+/−	Closed

TABLE 2-20 MISOPROSTOL DOSING

Incomplete Abortion	Missed Abortion
Misoprostol 600 µg orally once *OR* Misoprostol 400 µg sublingual once	Misoprostol 800 µg vaginally once *OR* Misoprostol 600 µg sublingual once (may repeat every 3 hours × 2 more doses)

GYNECOLOGY

- Symptoms of hemodynamic instability
- Greater than 12 weeks uterine size
- Hemoglobin less than 10.0 mg/dL or hematocrit less than 30.0% (relative contraindication)
- *Post-treatment*
- Provide prescriptions for pain (may need narcotic, motrin), **antiemetic**
- Highest success rates with extended follow-up (7–14 days) to allow full expulsion
- Evaluate in 2 days to 1–2 weeks. If not completed and patient is stable, may choose expectant management or repeat misoprostol dose
- Surgical intervention not recommended in less than 7 days after treatment unless medically necessary
- *Side Effects*: INFORM PATIENT OF THESE!
- Bleeding: May be fairly heavy initially (slightly heavier than typical menses for 3–4 days), then spotting. **Call if soaking 1–2 pads per hour for over 2 hours**
- Cramping: Usually starts within 30 minutes to first few hours
- Nausea/Vomiting/Fevers and Chills (call if fever persists beyond 24 hours)
- Diarrhea (especially with oral misoprostol). Resolves in 2–6 hours

MEDICAL/SURGICAL ABORTIONS

Elective Pregnancy Termination

- Nearly half of the pregnancies in the United States are unintended; 40% of these are ended by abortion
- 19% of all pregnancies end in abortion. One-third of women have had an abortion by age 45
- Does **not** increase infertility, future SAB risk, breast cancer
- When do women have abortions?

Less than 8 weeks	63.9%
9–13 weeks	27.5%
14–15 weeks	3.3%
16–17 weeks	1.9%
18–20 weeks	1.9%
21 or more weeks	1.4%

Safety
- Less than 0.3% of abortion patients have a complication requiring hospitalization
- Risk of complication increases with increasing gestational age

Evaluation, Counseling, and Follow-up
- Confirm IUP and dating (CRL or BPD). Obtain Rh status. ±STI screening
- **Fertility returns immediately!** May ovulate within 2 weeks: Provide contraception!
- Pregnancy symptoms resolve within 1 week; normal menses resume within 6 weeks
- Follow-up appointment in 2–4 weeks: To confirm resolution of pregnancy (very early gestations), assess for complications, follow up contraception
- Average time for β-hCG to become nondetectable after first trimester surgical abortion is 31–38 days

Surgical Abortions

- D&C versus Dilation and Evacuation (D&E) (Table 2-21)

TABLE 2-21 SURGICAL ABORTIONS

Dilation and Curettage	Dilation and Evacuation
Less than 14 weeks	Over 14 weeks
Local anesthetic (paracervical) or IV sedation	Local anesthetic (paracervical) or IV sedation
Manual dilation with Pratt (tapered) or Hagar (blunt) dilators Consider buccal or vaginal misoprostol for cervical preparation (eg, nulliparous)	Requires increased dilation pre-op using osmotic dilators (Laminaria and Dilapan) often placed the day before procedure, and/or misoprostol or mifepristone
Evacuation with electronic vacuum aspiration (EVA) suction or manual vacuum aspiration (MVA)	Requires experienced surgeon Safest under ultrasound guidance Usually requires forceps (eg, Bierers)
Examine products of conception for placental villi at <7 weeks and fetal parts >7 weeks to include calvarium	Examine products of conception for placental villi at <7 weeks and fetal parts >7 weeks to include calvarium

Paracervical Block
- Clean cervix with betadine
- Draw up 10–20 mL of 1% lidocaine or 0.25% bupivacaine
- 10 mL of 1% lidocaine = 100 mg; maximum dose 4.5 mg/kg or 20 mL for 50 kg patient
- Place small wheal (1 cc) at 12 o'clock of cervix for tenaculum, then the rest in divided doses at 4 and 8 o'clock at cervical–vaginal junction
- Remember to first aspirate as cervical branches of uterine arteries are at 3 and 9 o'clock
- Patient may experience tinnitus or metallic taste in the mouth

Complications of Surgical Abortion
- Perforation
  - **If** suspected, STOP, do not apply suction, ultrasound abdomen, observe. If hypotension, tachycardia, bleeding, drop in hemoglobin → laparoscopy versus laparotomy
- Hematometra
  - **If** suspected (intense pain with boggy, enlarged uterus immediately after procedure), aspirate uterine clot, administer methylergonovine (*Methergine*)
- Post-abortal Endometritis
  - 42% reduction if given antibiotics (EVEN IF NEGATIVE GC/CT TESTING)
  - **Doxycycline 100 mg (IV/orally) before and 200 mg orally once after procedure**
- Treatment
  - Cefotetan 2 g IV once + Doxycycline 100 mg IV/orally twice daily for 14 days *OR*
  - Ceftriaxone 250 mg IM once + Doxycycline 100 mg orally for 14 days
  - ± Flagyl 500 mg twice daily for 14 days

Medical Abortions

- Effective up to 63 days (9 weeks) gestation
- Evidence-based protocol different from FDA protocol
- More subjective pain and bleeding with medical than surgical procedure
- Requires reliable patient for follow-up. Risk of teratogenicity if pregnancy continued

- Risk of fatal sepsis (*Clostridium sordellii*) 0.6:100 000
- Mifepristone: Approved in the United States in 2000. An antiprogesterone—binds to progesterone receptor with greater affinity than progesterone
  - Necrotizes the decidua
  - Softens the cervix
  - Increases uterine contractility (24–36 hours after administration) and prostaglandin sensitivity
- *Contraindications:*
  - Ectopic pregnancy, chronic corticosteroid use, chronic adrenal failure, porphyria, allergy to mifepristone or misoprostol, anticoagulation therapy, clotting disorder, IUD in place.
  - Anemia (hemoglobin less than 10.0 mg/dL) is a relative contraindication

Medical Abortion Protocols (Table 2-22)

- Other medical abortion protocols exist using misoprostol alone or MTX and misoprostol, but are less effective
- *Failed Medical Abortion:* Any outcome that requires surgical intervention (incidence approximately 5%). Continued pregnancy (gestational cardiac activity on TV sono 2 weeks after start of therapy), incomplete abortion, retained products of conception (POC), and patient request are possible reasons for D&C
- Incomplete AB or retained POCs may be managed with repeat misoprostol

TABLE 2-22 MEDICAL ABORTION PROTOCOLS

Protocol 1 (FDA Approved)	Protocol 2 (Evidence-Based)
Day 1: Mifepristone 600 mg orally	Day 1: Mifepristone 200 mg orally
Day 3: Misoprostol 400 µg orally (in office)	24–72 hours later (earlier dosing may be as effective but with more side effects):
Office follow-up on day 10–15	**Misoprostol 800 µg vaginal or buccal (at home)**
	Office follow-up between days 4–14 (for sono or confirmation of completion)

CONTRACEPTION

Types

- Hormonal = combined estrogen/progestin, progestin only
- Nonhormonal = barrier methods, sterilization, copper IUD, timed intercourse

Efficacy (Table 2-23)

Eligibility Criteria

- For a Summary Chart of U.S. Medical Eligibility Criteria for Contraceptive Use (ie, contraindications and recommendations for use of contraceptives according to medical conditions) see the following Web site:
  - http://www.cdc.gov/reproductivehealth/UnintendedPregnancy/USMEC.htm
- **For U.S. Selected Practice Recommendations (ie, recommendations and guidelines for how to initiate contraception and how to deal with common issues with contraception management), see the following Web site:**
  - http://www.cdc.gov/mmwr/preview/mmwrhtml/rr6205a1.htm?s_cid=rr6205a1_w

Combined Estrogen and Progesterone Contraceptives

- *Mechanism:* Ovulation suppression (90–95% of time). Also thicken cervical mucus, blocking sperm penetration and entry into the upper reproductive tract. Thin, asynchronous endometrium inhibits implantation. Tubal motility slowed
- *Contraindications:* Table 2-24

TABLE 2-23 PERCENTAGE OF WOMEN EXPERIENCING AN UNINTENDED PREGNANCY DURING THE FIRST YEAR OF TYPICAL USE AND THE FIRST YEAR OF PERFECT USE OF CONTRACEPTION AND THE PERCENTAGE CONTINUING USE AT THE END OF THE FIRST YEAR—UNITED STATES

Method	% of Women Experiencing an Unintended Pregnancy within the First Year of Use		% of Women Continuing Use at 1 Year
	Typical Use	Perfect Use	
No method	85	85	
Spermicides	28	18	42
Fertility awareness-based methods	24		47
Standard Days method		5	
Two Day method		4	
Ovulation method		3	
Symptothermal method		0.4	
Withdrawal	22	4	46
Sponge			36
Parous women	24	20	
Nulliparous women	12	9	
Condom			
Female	21	5	41
Male	18	2	43
Diaphragm	12	6	57
Combined pill and progestin-only pill	9	0.3	67
Evra patch	9	0.3	67
NuvaRing	9	0.3	67
Depo-Provera	6	0.2	56
Intrauterine contraceptives			
ParaGard® (copper T)	0.8	0.6	78
Mirena® (LNG)	0.2	0.2	80
Implanon	0.05	0.05	84
Female sterilization	0.5	0.5	100
Male sterilization	0.15	0.10	

LNG-IUS = levonorgestrel intrauterine system.
Data from Hoffman BL, et al. Chapter 5. Implantation and Placental Development. In: Hoffman BL, et al., eds. *Williams Gynecology*, 2nd ed. New York, NY: McGraw-Hill; 2012; Trussell, 2011.

Oral Contraceptive Pills (OCPs)

• Majority contain less than 50 μg ethinyl estradiol (EE); progestin varies
• Traditional packs have 21 active combined pills, with or without 7 placebo pills
• Newer formulations have varying numbers of active pills and hormone-free pills
  • *Yaz* and *Minastrin-24* have 24 days hormonal pills; 4 days of placebo pills
  • *Lo Loestrin Fe* has 24 days 10 μg EE and norethindrone, 2 days of 10 μg EE, and 2 days of ferrous sulfate
  • *Natazia* has 26 days of active hormones (four phases of varying doses of estradiol valerate and dienogest) and 2 days of placebo pills
  • Extended cycles
    • *Seasonale*—84 consecutive hormonal pills followed by 7 placebos
    • *Seasonique*—(10 μg EE in "placebos"); 84 active pills, 7 placebos
  • Continuous: *Lybrel* (EE 20 μg; levonorgestrel 0.9 mg); no hormone-free pills
• Rapid return of fertility after discontinuing. Average delay in ovulation is 1–2 weeks

TABLE 2-24 CONTRAINDICATIONS TO COMBINED ESTROGEN/ PROGESTERONE

Breast cancer
  Current [4]
  Past and no evidence of disease for 5 years [3]
	Gallbladder disease, current or medically treated [3]

Cirrhosis, severe, decompensated [4]	Viral hepatitis, acute or flare [3,4]
Hepatocellular adenoma or hepatoma [4]	Bariatric surgery (malabsorptive) [3]

DVT/PE
  Acute [4]
  h/o DVT, higher risk for recurrence [4]
  h/o DVT, lower risk for recurrence [3]
	Peripartum cardiomyopathy
	  Less than 6 months [4]
	  Over 6 months [3]
	  Moderate or severely impaired cardiac function [4]

Major surgery with prolonged immobilization [4]	Thrombogenic mutations [4]

Diabetes with nephropathy/retinopathy/ neuropathy; other vascular disease; or diabetes of more than 20 years duration [3,4]	Smoking
	  Age ≥35, <15 cigarettes/day [3]
	  Age ≥35, ≥15 cigarettes/day [4]

Migraine Headaches
  With aura, any age [4]
  Without aura, ≥35 years of age [3, initiation; 4 continuation]
  Without aura <35 years [2, initiation; 3, continuation]
	Drugs
	  Ritonavir-boosted protease inhibitors [3]
	  Certain anticonvulsants [3]
	  (phenytoin, carbamazepine, barbiturates, primidone, topiramate, oxcarbazepine, lamotrigine)
	  Rifampicin or rifabutin [3]

Hypertension
  Adequately controlled [3]
  Systolic 140–159 or diastolic 90–99 [3]
  ≥160/≥100 or with vascular disease [4]
	SLE with positive (or unknown) anti-phospholipid antibodies [4]

Ischemic heart disease (current or history) [4]	Multiple risk factors for CVD [3,4]
Valvular heart disease, complicated [4]	History of stroke [4]
Solid organ transplant, complicated [4]	Ulcerative colitis/Crohn's disease [2,3]

Postpartum (non-breast feeding)
  Less than 21 days [4]
  21–42 days with other risk factor for DVT (eg, age ≥35, c-section, smoker, preeclampsia, thrombophilia) [3]
	Postpartum (breast feeding)
	  Less than 21 days [4]
	  21–30 days [3]
	  30–42 days and other risk factor for DVT [3]

KEY

[2]: Advantages generally outweigh theoretical or proven risks
[3]: Theoretical or proven risks usually outweigh the advantages
[4]: Unacceptable health risk (method not to be used)

Data from CDC's U.S. medical eligibility criteria for contraceptive use, 2010: Revised recommendations for the use of contraceptive methods during the postpartum period. *MMWR Morb Mortal Wkly Rep.* 2011;60:878.

- 2 OCP Formulations
  - **Monophasic:** All active pills contain same amount of hormones
    - Preferable if interested in controlling cycle lengths or timing (medical reasons personal preference)
    - *"Bicycling" or "tricycling":* Skip placebos for one or two packs; then take placebos, have withdrawal bleed after 6 weeks (end of second pack) or 9 weeks (end of third pack)
    - *"Continuous use":* Only take active pills; no withdrawal bleeding. May need to transition by bicycling/tricycling. Counsel about breakthrough bleeding and spotting
  - One approach to spotting: Stop active pills on first day of spotting (after taking pills for at least 21 days). Take no pill for 2 or 3 days. Then restart pills daily until the next spotting

day (again as long as pill has been taken for at least 21 days). The number of days with breakthrough bleeding will decrease over time

- Studies of extended cycles: No increased risk of endometrial hyperplasia
- **Multiphasic:** Active pills contain varying amounts of progestin and estrogen throughout cycle
- *To start*
  - **Quick Start:** Start pills on day provider sees patient if reasonably certain patient is not pregnant. Better for compliance, especially with teens. Provide 7-day backup. Preferred starting method
  - **Sunday Start:** Recommend 7 days backup method if Sunday is more than 5 days after first day of menses
  - **First day of next period:** No backup contraception needed
- *Side effects:* Important to counsel, many are transient and will improve after a couple of cycles
  - *Estrogen related*: Bloating, headache, nausea, mastalgia, leukorrhea, hypertension, melasma/telengectasia
  - *Progestin related*: Mood swings, mastalgia, depression, fatigue, decreased libido, weight gain
  - About 30% have breakthrough bleeding in first 3 months—don't change pills
- *Missed Pills*
  - *One pill:* Take missed pill ASAP. Resume schedule. Backup not needed
  - *Two or more pills*
    - Take most recent missed active pill (discard other missed pills); continue taking 1 pill daily
    - Use condoms or abstinence for 7 days
    - If missed in week 3, finish active pills in current pack and start new pack the next day. Skip current pack's inactive pills. If unable to start a new pack immediately, use condoms or abstinence until finished 7 consecutive days of hormonal pills from new pack
    - If missed pills in first week and had sex, use emergency contraception (EC). Resume taking pills in pack the next day after finishing EC
- Special considerations regarding which pill to prescribe
  - *Endometriosis:* Continuous use is most effective in reducing symptoms
  - *Functional ovarian cysts:* Higher dose monophasic pills may be slightly more effective. Extended/continuous use of pills may also be more effective
  - *Androgen excess states:* All helpful but pills with higher estrogen/progestin ratios are preferable
  - *Note:* OCPs containing the progestin drospirenone have been associated with possible excess risk of VTE compared to OCPs with levonorgestrel

Nuva Ring (releases 0.12 mg etonogestrel/0.015 mg ethinyl estradiol per day)
- Leave in for 3 weeks; then remove for 1 week
- Can use continuously (change every 3 or 4 weeks) or shorten withdrawal bleed (leave out for less than 1 week)
- If removed (or falls out) rinse with warm water, replace. **If removed, do not leave out for more than 3 hours**
- Can leave in during intercourse
- Vaginitis and leukorrhea are more common

Ortho Evra Patch (6 mg norelgestromin/0.75 mg ethinyl estradiol)
- Delivers 20 µg ethinyl estradiol and 150 µg of the progestin, norelgestromin (the active metabolite of norgestimate) daily
- Place on lower abdomen, buttocks, upper outer arm or upper torso (not breasts)
- Delivers about 60% more estrogen over 21 days than 35 µg EE pill and three times more than the ring
- Possible increased risk in VTE
  - *INFO ON LABEL: "You will be exposed to about 60% more estrogen if you use ORTHO EVRA than if you use a typical birth control pill containing 35 micrograms of estrogen"*
  - Counsel patient about this risk and document the discussion. Strongly advise not to use if patient smokes
- Less effective in women over 90 kg (198 lbs). Counsel overweight women about possible decreased efficacy
- To start
  - Place patch on first day of next period. If start any other day, use backup for 7 days
  - If switching from pills, can do so at anytime in cycle. Do not wait to complete pack

Progestin-Only Contraceptive Methods

Progestin-Only Pills ("Mini Pills")
- Taken daily with no hormone-free days
- Lower progestin doses than combined pills (approximately 75% less)

- Norethindrone (*Micronor, Nor-QD*): 0.35 mg norethindrone
- Good for women with contraindications to estrogen; breast feeding women
- Must take at same time each day (over 3-hour delay considered a "missed pill")
  If more than 3 hours late, use a backup method for 48 hours

Etonogestrel Subdermal Implants (Implanon/Nexplanon) (68 mg etonogestrel)
- *Insertion* (Figure 2-13)
- Single implant is 4 cm long, 2 mm in diameter (size of a match). Nexplanon is radiopaque
- Initially, progestin released at 60 µg/day decreasing to 25–30 µg/day by end of year 3
- *Mechanism:* Ovulation suppression, thickening of cervical mucus
- Placed under skin of upper arm; need to take training course to administer
- Irregular menses may persist throughout life of implant. 29–51% of women complain of irregular bleeding (may be frequent or prolonged; usually light and well tolerated). 11% remove because of unfavorable bleeding
- Quick return to fertility: 94% ovulate within 3–6 weeks of removal

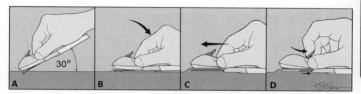

Figure 2-13 Nexplanon insertion. A sterile pen marks the insertion site, which is 8 to 10 cm proximal to the medial humeral condyle on the non-dominant upper arm. A second mark is placed 4 cm proximally along the arm's long axis in the sulcus between the triceps and biceps muscles. The implant is inserted just under the skin in order to avoid large blood vessels and nerves. The area is cleaned aseptically, and a 1-percent lidocaine anesthetic track is injected along the planned insertion path. **A.** The insertion device is grasped at its gripper bubbles found on either side, and the needle cap is removed outward. The device can be seen within the needle bore. The needle bevel then pierces the skin at a 30-degree angle. **B.** Once the complete bevel is subcutaneous, lower the applicator to a horizontal position. **C.** Importantly, the skin is tented upward by the needle as the needle is slowly advanced horizontally and subdermally. **D.** Once the needle is completely inserted, the lever on the top of the device is pulled backward toward the operator. This retracts the needle and thereby deposits the implant. The device is then lifted away from the skin. After placement, both patient and operator should palpate the 4-cm implant. (Used with permission from Cunningham F, et al. Contraception. In: Cunningham F, et al., eds. *Williams Obstetrics*, 24th ed. New York, NY: McGraw-Hill; 2013).

Depot Medroxyprogesterone Acetate (DMPA; Depo-Provera)
- Intramuscular dose 150 mg, subcutaneous dose 104 mg (*Depo-SubQ Provera 104*™). SubQ dose available in prefilled syringes; equivalent efficacy as conventional IM dose with 30% less progestin. Less painful; possible self-administration. Both given every 12 weeks
- Preferred start is during first 5 days of menses, but may start anytime in cycle if not pregnant but will need backup for 7 days
- Changing from Depo to other method: Start when convenient for patient. Ideally, near end of effectiveness of last injection. Don't wait until next menses to start OCPs

- Administer repeat doses anytime between 12 and 13 weeks (Can be given early when necessary)
  - The repeat *Depo-Provera* injection can be given up to 2 weeks late (15 weeks from the last injection) without requiring additional contraceptive protection
  - If patient presents more than 15 weeks from last injection
    - If pregnancy test is negative and patient has had unprotected sex in the last 5 days—advise that pregnancy test is not conclusive, but *Depo-Provera* (and other hormonal agents) will NOT affect fetus. If patient desires shot, administer and have her use backup for 7 days. Repeat pregnancy test in 2 weeks. Can also give EC
- Advantages of *Depo-Provera*
  - Amenorrhea: After 1 year, **50%**; after 5 years, 80% develop amenorrhea
  - May see improvement in endometriosis; decreased menstrual cramps
  - Reduces acute sickle cell crises by 70%
  - Excellent method for women on anticonvulsant drugs
- Disadvantages
  - May cause irregular menses during first several months
  - Possible increase in depression, anxiety, fatigue, mood changes (but can decrease). History of depression is not a contraindication
  - **Slow to return to baseline fertility**—average 10 months from last injection
  - Weight gain: Average of 5.4 lbs in first year and 16.5 lbs after 5 years
  - **Potential for decrease in Bone Mineral Density (BMD)** with prolonged use
    - *Depo-Provera* received a black box warning from FDA in 11/2004. ACOG and American Academy of Pediatrics **recommend no limit to use and no BMD testing.** Studies show lower BMD in Depo users than nonusers (loss of 0.5–3.5% at hip and spine after 1 year; 5.7–7.5% loss at 2 years; and 5.2–5.4% after 5 years). However, recovery of BMD occurs after stopping *Depo-Provera*
    - Explain warning to *Depo-Provera* users and discuss alternatives
    - Advise calcium supplementation: 1000 mg (> age 18) to 1300 mg (adolescents) daily
    - Encourage regular exercise and avoid smoking

Breastfeeding—Lactational Amenorrhea Method

- Effective only under specific conditions
  - Women breast-feeding exclusively (at least 90% of baby's nutrition)
  - Woman is amenorrheic
  - Infant less than 6 months old
- Probability that ovulation will precede the first menstrual period in a lactating woman is 33–45% during first 3 months; 64–71% from months 4 to 12; and 87% after 12 months

IUDs

Progestin IUD (Mirena®) (52 mg/unit levonorgestrel)
- See Figure 2-14 for insertion instructions
- Releases initially 20 μg/day levonorgestrel; progressively decreases to half that amount after 5 years
- Effective for up to 5 years
- Mechanism: Cervical mucus becomes thicker; changes in uterotubal fluid impair sperm migration; alteration of endometrium prevents implantation
- Menorrhagia improves (70–90% less blood loss; versus 50% with pills)
- Amenorrhea develops in approximately 20% of users by 1 year and 60% by 5 years
- Irregular bleeding (spotting) expected for approximately 3–6 months
- Expulsion rate: 3–6% if using for contraception; 9–14% if for menorrhagia
- **May be used by women with history of ectopic pregnancy**
- Return of fertility is immediate

Progestin IUD (Skyla®) (13.5 mg/unit levonorgestrel)
- Follow instructions as outlined for *Mirena®* insertion
- Releases initially 14 μg/day levonorgestrel; falls to 6 μg/day after 3 years
- Effective for up to 3 years
- Mechanism same as *Mirena®*
- Amenorrhea develops in approximately 6% of users by 1 year and 12% by 3 years
- Irregular bleeding (spotting) expected for approximately 3–6 months
- Expulsion rate: 3%
- *Skyla's®* insertion tube diameter is smaller (3.8 mm) compared to *Mirena's®* (4.4 mm)

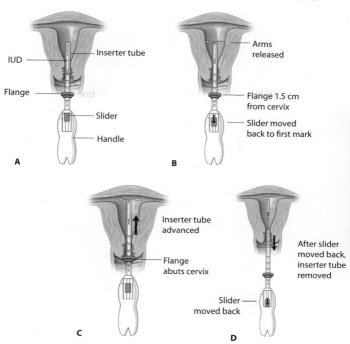

Figure 2-14 Mirena/Skyla® IUD insertion **A.** Gently sound uterus. Push slider forward as far as possible to load IUD into insertion tube. DO NOT move slider downward at first as this may release the strings prematurely. The IUD cannot be reloaded after the slider is moved below the mark. Set flange to depth measured by sound. After grasping cervix with tenaculum or ring forcep, apply gentle traction and gently insert IUD into uterus. **B.** Continue to hold slider in forward position and advance insertion tube until flange is 1.5-2 cm from external os. Hold inserter steady and pull slider back to first mark to release arms of the IUD. Wait 10 seconds to allow arms to completely deploy. **C.** Gently push inserter into uterus until flange touches cervix (IUD should be at fundus). **D.** While holding inserter firmly, release IUD by pulling slider down all the way. Threads release automatically. Continue to hold slider all the way down as inserter is removed. Cut threads to leave 3-4 cm visible. (Used with permission from Cunningham F, et al. Contraception. In: Cunningham F, et al., eds. *Williams Obstetrics*, 24th ed. New York, NY: McGraw-Hill; 2013).

Copper IUD (ParaGard®) (380 mm² exposed copper wire)
• See Figure 2-15 for insertion instructions
• Provides protection for 10 years according to label (actually 12 years)
• Mechanism: Works primarily as a spermicide
• Average monthly blood loss may increase and up to 15% have IUD removed for menorrhagia
• Can use as **emergency contraception** up to 5 days after sex—99% effective

Post-Pregnancy IUD Insertion
• Can be placed immediately after first or second trimester abortion (slight increased risk of expulsion after second trimester)
• *Immediate postpartum*
  • Preferably within 10 minutes of placenta expulsion but may be inserted up to 48 hours after vaginal delivery
  • May be placed at time of cesarean section
  • Higher expulsion rate: 7–20% at 6 months
  • Advise patients they may need to come back to have strings trimmed
• *Contraindications* (particular to postpartum insertion): Chorioamnionitis or endometritis, history of post-abortal or postpartum sepsis, hemorrhage (relative contraindication)

IUD Insertion Protocol—Selected Points
Counseling and Consent
• Risks: Pregnancy (1–8:1000 the first year), infection within the first 20 days after insertion (9.6:1000), uterine perforation (1:1000), and expulsion (3–10:100 higher if immediate postpartum)

1. Load ParaGard into insertion tube: Fold the horizontal arms against stem and push tips into inserter tube. Insert no further than necessary to insure retention

2. Introduce solid white rod into insertion tube from bottom until it touches the bottom of ParaGard

3. Adjust blue flange to the uterine depth (from sound)

4. Rotate insertion tube so horizontal arms and long axis of blue flange are in the same horizontal plane

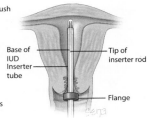

5. Insert through cervical canal until ParaGard almost touches fundus. The blue flange should almost be at the cervix (see figure)

6. To release arms: Hold solid white rod steady; withdraw insertion tube no more than 1 cm. Then, gently move insertion tube (not inserter rod) toward fundus, until slight resistance is felt. At no time during insertion is the inserter rod advanced forward

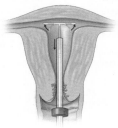
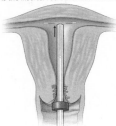

7. Hold the insertion tube steady; withdraw solid white rod

8. Slowly withdraw the insertion tube from cervical canal

9. Cut threads to leave 3–4 cm visible

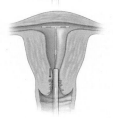

Figure 2-15 ParaGard® IUD insertion. (Used with permission from Cunningham F, et al. Contraception. In: Cunningham F, eds. *Williams Obstetrics*, 23rd ed. New York, NY: McGraw-Hill; 2010.)

IUD Insertion Protocol—Selected Points (*Continued*)

- *Absolute Contraindications*
  - Possible or confirmed pregnancy
  - Severe distortion of uterine cavity (eg, submucosal fibroid or anatomic abnormalities)
  - PID (acute diagnosis or within 3 months)
  - Postpartum and post-abortal infections (acute or within 3 months)
  - Current sexually transmitted infection
  - Untreated cervicitis or vaginitis
  - Active genital actinomycoses infection
  - Wilson's disease or copper allergy (for ParaGard®)
  - Allergy to levonorgestrel, acute liver disease or tumor, breast cancer (for Mirena/Skyla®)
- *Relative Contraindications*
  - Risk factors for STIs, including nonmonogamous relationship
  - History of previous IUD problem (perforation, expulsion, significant pain)
  - Abnormal uterine bleeding of unknown etiology (ie, need workup first)
  - Current anemia or history of menorrhagia-associated anemia (for ParaGard®)
  - History of progestin intolerance (Mirena®, Skyla®)
  - Patient would not accept possible amenorrhea (Mirena®, Skyla®)

Pre-Procedure Considerations

- Because a patient's greatest risk of developing PID is within the first 20 days of insertion, medical providers should take the following steps to minimize infection
  - Screen for GC/CT if
    - 25 years of age or less
    - 25 years of age with risk factors for acquiring STIs
    - Signs of cervicitis
  - For low-risk patients, GC/CT testing can be deferred or performed at time of insertion. Testing prior to insertion of an IUD is **not** required
  - For all women less than age 25 and any woman with a new sexual partner, regardless of age, an IUD may be inserted if she has had negative GC/CT within the past 3 months
- Treat symptomatic bacterial vaginosis (BV). The timing of IUD insertion, whether to insert an IUD during the same visit or at a later visit when cure is documented, is at the physician's discretion. No evidence-based recommendations in this clinical setting
- Routine prophylactic antibiotics do not reduce the occurrence of PID and are **not** indicated
- Assuming no contraindications exist, administer an oral NSAID, such as ibuprofen 600 mg or naproxen 500 mg, about 30–60 minutes prior to IUD insertion. Note, however, that studies have not proven this to be effective in reducing discomfort
- Consider administering misoprostol 400 μg vaginally 12–24 hours prior to insertion if history of previous difficult cervical dilation/IUD insertion (400 μg sublingually 1–3 hours prior to insertion is another option). Can also consider a paracervical block

Timing of Insertion/Pregnancy Testing

- Document a negative pregnancy test for all women of reproductive age
- The IUD can be inserted within 5 days of the start of menses, regardless of recent intercourse (lowest expulsion rates if placed at midcycle)
- The IUD can be inserted at anytime during the cycle if
  - She is consistently using a reliable contraceptive method, *OR*
  - She has been abstinent since her last menses
  - Otherwise, patient should refrain from unprotected intercourse and return in 2 weeks for a second negative pregnancy test prior to insertion

IUD Insertion

- Bimanual exam to determine size and position of uterus
- Cleanse cervix with antiseptic; administer paracervical block, if indicated
- Grasp lip of cervix with tenaculum (or ring forcep), apply gentle traction
- Sound uterus
- See Figures 2-14 and 2-15

FEMALE STERILIZATION

Bilateral Tubal Ligation

- Failure rates of various methods listed in Table 2-25

TABLE 2-25 FAILURE RATES OF BILATERAL TUBAL LIGATION METHODS

Method	% Pregnant in 10 Years
Postpartum partial salpingectomy (best performed within 8 hours post-delivery)	0.75
Silastic bands (Falope rings)	1.77
Interval partial salpingectomy	2.0
Unipolar cautery	0.37
Bipolar cautery	2.48
Hulka clip (spring clip)	3.65
Filshie clip	0.9–1.2

Used with permission from Peterson HB, Xia Z, Hughes JM, et al. the risk of pregnancy after tubal sterilization: Findings from the U.S. collaborative Review of Sterilization. *Am J Obstet Gynecol.* 1996;174:1161–1170.

Falope Rings
• Apply at least 3 cm from uterotubal junction

Filshie Clips
• Apply to isthmic portion; 1–2 cm from cornua

Bipolar Cautery
• At least three separate coagulations performed, destroying more than 3 cm isthmus, more than 2.5 cm from cornu. If closer, increased ectopic rate

Pomeroy
• Fallopian tube identified along its full length to fimbriae. An avascular, mid-isthmic portion is grasped with a Babcock clamp. As loop of the tube is pulled up, the knuckle is doubly ligated with 2-0 plain catgut (or chromic). Dome of knuckle is then excised.
• Severed ends retract and months later are widely separated (Figure 2-16)

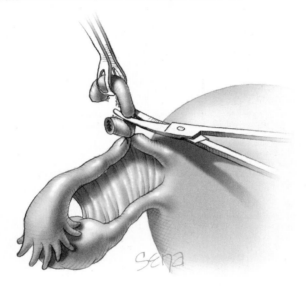

Figure 2-16 Pomeroy method of tubal ligation. (Used with permission from Cunningham F, et al. Sterilization. In: Cunningham F, et al., eds. *Williams Obstetrics*, 23rd ed. New York, NY: McGraw-Hill; 2010.)

Parkland
• Identify tube. An avascular, mid-isthmic portion is grasped with a Babcock clamp. The mesosalpinx is perforated with a small hemostat or cautery and tube is separated from the adjacent mesosalpinx for about 2.5 cm.
• The freed tube is then ligated at both ends with 2-0 absorbable sutures (plain catgut or chromic), and the intervening segment is excised (Figure 2-17)

Irving
• Similar to Parkland, except the ties on the proximal tubal segment are left long. A 1-cm incision is made into the uterine serosa on the posterior uterine wall. Using a hemostat, a 1–2 cm tunnel is made in the myometrium parallel to the serosa. The free ends from the proximal tie are threaded onto a curved needle and driven deep into the myometrial tunnel, exiting onto the uterine serosa. Needle is removed and sutures are pulled—pulling the tubal stump into the tunnel. Sutures are tied outside serosa.
• Tunnel opening is closed using 2-0 absorbable suture (Figure 2-18)

Essure
• Irreversible. Can be performed hysteroscopically in the operating room or in office (less than 1 hour) (Figure 2-19)
• Hysteroscopically, a 4-cm nickel titanium stainless steel coiled spring is released into the tubal ostia; tubal blockage by encouraging local tissue growth and scarring
• 94% will have successful bilateral placement of inserts at first attempt (should discuss back up plan for what will be done if cannot place both inserts at time of hysteroscopy)
• Takes 3 months to occlude tubes. HSG must be done after 3 months to confirm tubal occlusion. Alternate contraception should be used until confirmation.
• At 3 months, 3.5% of patients have patent tubes. When repeat HSG is done at 6 months, all are occluded
• Failure rate: 0.1% at 5 years

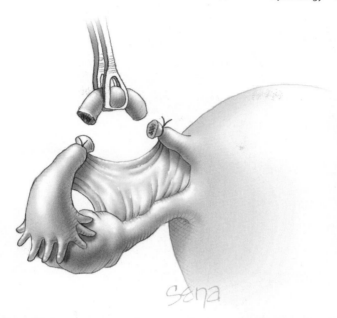

Figure 2-17 Parkland method of tubal ligation. (Used with permission from Cunningham F, et al. Sterilization. In: Cunningham F, et al., eds. *Williams Obstetrics*, 23rd ed. New York, NY: McGraw-Hill; 2010.)

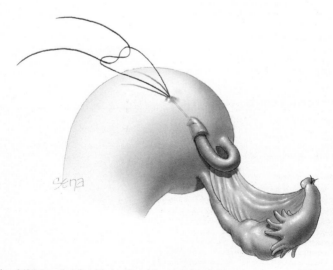

Figure 2-18 Irving method of tubal ligation. (Used with permission from Hoffman BL, et al. Chapter 41. Surgeries for benign gynecologic conditions. In: Hoffman BL, et al., eds. *Williams Gynecology*, 2nd ed. New York, NY: McGraw-Hill; 2012.)

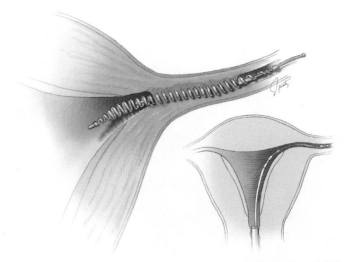

Figure 2-19 Essure. (Used with permission from Hoffman BL, et al. Chapter 42. Minimally invasive surgery. In: Hoffman BL, et al., eds. *Williams Gynecology*, 2nd ed. New York, NY: McGraw-Hill; 2012.)

Regret After Tubal Ligation

- 20% of women 30 years of age or younger at time of BTL and 6% of those over 30 years of age express regret
- Regret after postpartum BTL is greater than after interval BTL
- 1% of BTL patients seriously pursue re-anastomosis. "Success" rates for reversal vary from 70% to 80% (clips and rings easiest to reverse—less tubal damage)
- *Young age* most important factor in regret

Risk of Ectopic Pregnancy

- If a BTL patient gets pregnant, she has a higher risk of that pregnancy being ectopic. Still, the majority of pregnancies are intrauterine
- **Ectopic rate = 7.3/1000** (one-third of pregnancies are ectopic)

EMERGENCY CONTRACEPTION (EC)

Types of EC

Copper IUD (ParaGard®)

- Appropriate in women who meet standard criteria for IUD. Most effective if inserted within 5 days after unprotected intercourse

Oral Formulations:

Progestin only regimen

- **Plan B:** Two tabs containing 0.75 mg levonorgestrel
- **Plan B One-Step:** One tab containing 1.5 mg levonorgestrel
- **Next Choice:** Two tabs containing 0.75 mg levonorgestrel
- **Next Choice One Dose:** One tab containing 1.5 mg levonorgestrel
- **Progestin-only EC pills** can be provided over the counter for ages 17 and older
- Progestin-only pills more effective than combined pills with less side effects
  - WHO Study: 1.1% of 967 women using *Plan B* for EC became pregnant
  - Combined contraceptive pills have a 2–3% failure rate
- Two ways to take *Plan B/Next Choice*
  - **Take two pills (1.5 mg levonorgestrel) ASAP—(failure rate 1.5%)**
    Is now recommended; likely better compliance
  - Take first pill, then take second pill 12 hours later (failure rate 1.8%)

Selective progesterone receptor modulator
- *Ella* one tab (30 mg ulipristal acetate)
- More effective than progestin-only pills, especially if 72–120 hours after unprotected intercourse or if overweight. Requires a prescription; may not be as available in pharmacies

Combined estrogen-progestin regimen (Yuzpe method)
- Many approved regimens containing at least 100 μg EE and 0.5 mg levonorgestrel, taken as two doses 12 hours apart (see http://ec.princeton.edu)
- Mechanism: Prevent pregnancy (delays ovulation); does not disrupt an implanted pregnancy
- Take ideally within 72 hours but may be taken for up to *120 hours* after unprotected sex

Information about EC pills
- Up to 98% of patients will menstruate by 21 days after the treatment
- Pregnancy test if no period in 3 weeks
- Patient should restart their regular birth control pills immediately
- Consider providing patient a prescription for ECs PRIOR to need for them

SEXUALLY TRANSMITTED INFECTIONS (STIs): CDC GUIDELINES

Pelvic Inflammatory Disease (PID)

Pathogens
- *Neisseria gonorrhoeae* (GC) and *Chlamydia trachomatis* (CT)
- Bacteria that compromise vaginal environment: anaerobes, *Gardnerella vaginalis, Haemophilus influenzae,* enteric gram-negative rods, and *Streptococcus agalactiae,* enteric organisms
- Less common: Cytomegalovirus (CMV), *Mycoplasma hominis, Ureaplasma urealyticum,* and *M. genitalium*

Diagnosis
- Obtain *Nucleic Acid Amplification Tests (NAAT)* for GC/CT; screen for HIV
- Consider imaging to evaluate for tubo-ovarian abscess (TOA)

Minimum criteria for PID diagnosis	Specific criteria for PID diagnosis
· Uterine tenderness *OR* · Adnexal tenderness *OR* · Cervical motion tenderness	· Endometrial biopsy showing endometritis
	· TV sono or MRI—thickened, fluid-filled tubes with or without free pelvic fluid or tubo-ovarian complex
	· Laparoscopic abnormalities consistent with PID

- Additional Supporting Criteria for Diagnosis
  - Oral temperature >101°F (>38.3°C);
  - Cervical/Vaginal muco-purulent discharge
  - Presence of WBCs on wet prep
  - Elevated erythrocyte sedimentation rate (ESR)
  - Elevated C-reactive protein
  - Lab documentation of cervical infection with GC/CT

Criteria for Hospitalization
- Surgical emergencies can't be excluded (ie, appendicitis)
- Patient is pregnant
- Does not respond clinically to oral therapy
- Unable to follow/tolerate out-patient regimen
- Severe illness, nausea/vomiting, fever
- TOA
- **No available data suggest adolescents benefit from hospitalization for treatment of PID**

Treatment

All regimens must be effective against GC/CT, because negative screening does not preclude infection

Parenteral Treatment

Parenteral Regimen A
Cefotetan 2 g IV every 12 hours OR
Cefoxitin 2 g IV every 6 hours
  PLUS
Doxycycline 100 mg orally or IV every 12 hours

Note: Because of pain with infusion, doxycycline should be administered orally when possible, even when patient is hospitalized. Oral and IV provide similar bioavailability

Parenteral Regimen B
Clindamycin 900 mg IV every 8 hours
  PLUS
Gentamicin loading dose IV or IM (2 mg/kg) with maintenance dose (1.5 mg/kg) every 8 hours. May use single daily dosing (3–5 mg/kg)

Alternative Parenteral Regimens
Ampicillin/Sulbactam (Unasyn) 3 g IV every 6 hours
  PLUS
Doxycycline 100 mg oral or IV every 12 hours

- **One study supports azithromycin 500 mg IV for 1–2 doses, then 250 mg orally for 5–6 days alone or combined with 12 days of metronidazole**
- Although most trials have used parenteral therapy for at least 48 hours after substantial clinical improvement, this is arbitrary. Clinical experience should guide decisions regarding transition to oral medications, which usually can be within 24–48 hours of improvement. If TOA, then at least 24 hours of inpatient observation is recommended
- Continue treatment with doxycycline (100 mg orally twice daily) to complete 14 days. If TOA, add clindamycin or metronidazole for effective anaerobic coverage

Oral Treatment
- Consider unless patient meets criteria for IV antibiotics as above
- If no response to oral regimen within 72 hours, reevaluate, confirm diagnosis and admit for IV antibiotics

Recommended Oral Regimen
Ceftriaxone 250 mg IM single dose
  PLUS
Doxycycline 100 mg orally twice daily for 14 days
  WITH or WITHOUT
Metronidazole 500 mg orally twice daily for 14 days
  OR
Cefoxitin 2 g IM in a single dose and **Probenecid** 1 g orally administered concurrently in a single dose
  PLUS
Doxycycline 100 mg orally twice daily for 14 days
  WITH or WITHOUT
Metronidazole 500 mg orally twice daily for 14 days
  OR
Other parenteral third-generation **cephalosporin** (eg, **ceftizoxime, cefotaxime**)
  PLUS
Doxycycline 100 mg orally twice daily for 14 days
  WITH or WITHOUT
Metronidazole 500 mg orally twice daily for 14 days

Alternative Oral Regimens
- Amoxicillin/clavulanate (Augmentin) + doxycycline (GI symptoms might limit compliance)
- Azithromycin ± ceftriaxone
- CDC no longer recommends fluoroquinolones to treat gonorrhea associated conditions (resistance)
  - If parenteral cephalosporin therapy is not feasible, and if community prevalence and individual risk of GC is low, may consider either
  - **Levofloxacin** 500 mg orally once daily for 14 days OR
  - **Ofloxacin** 400 mg orally twice daily for 14 days
      WITH OR WITHOUT
      Metronidazole 500 mg orally twice daily for 14 days
- If NAAT positive for GC, parenteral cephalosporin is recommended. If culture is positive, base therapy on susceptibility results

Follow-up
- Symptoms and objective findings should improve within 3 days of treatment
- Failure to improve should prompt additional diagnostic testing, adjustment of antibiotics, and may require surgical intervention, especially if TOA
- Repeat testing for GC and CT 3–6 months after treatment if documented infection with these pathogens
- Sex partners
  - Treat all partners who had sexual contact with the patient within 60 days prior to the onset of symptoms
  - If patient's last intercourse was more than 60 days before diagnosis, the most recent sex partner should be treated
  - Treat with regimens effective against both GC and CT, regardless of etiology of PID
- Abstain from intercourse until treatment is completed and symptoms are gone

Special Considerations
- Pregnancy: Pregnant women with suspected PID should be hospitalized and treated with parenteral antibiotics
- HIV: Increased incidence of TOA
- IUD: Risk of PID with IUD usually confined to the first 3 weeks after insertion. No evidence suggests IUD should be removed if acute PID. Close clinical follow-up is mandatory

Chlamydial Infections
- Most frequently reported infectious disease in the United States

Diagnosis
- NAAT are preferred tests (higher sensitivity)
- Can be diagnosed by testing urine or swabs from endocervix or vagina
- Liquid-based cytology (paps) may also be sent for NAAT, but are less sensitive

Treatment
Recommended Regimens (either)
    Azithromycin 1 g orally in a single dose
    Doxycycline 100 mg orally twice daily for 7 days

Alternative Regimens (any of the following)
    Erythromycin base 500 mg orally four times daily for 7 days
    Erythromycin ethylsuccinate 800 mg orally four times daily for 7 days
    Ofloxacin 300 mg orally twice daily for 7 days
    Levofloxacin 500 mg orally once daily for 7 days
- Use Azithromycin if there is any question of compliance
- Erythromycin is less efficacious and has more frequent GI side effects
- Ofloxacin and Levofloxacin are as efficacious as Doxycycline, but more expensive

Follow-up
- Patients treated should abstain from sexual intercourse for 7 days after single-dose therapy or until completion of a 7-day regimen and until all sex partners are treated
- Except in pregnant women, test-of-cure is not recommended after treatment unless compliance is in question or reinfection is suspected
- Non-culture tests conducted at less than 3 weeks after treatment could yield false-positive results because of continued excretion of dead organisms
- Repeat testing 3 months after treatment is advised because of high rate of reinfection
- Sex partners: Treat all partners who had sexual contact with the patient within 60 days prior to the onset of symptoms OR the most recent sex partner if last intercourse more than 60 days prior

Special Considerations
- **Pregnancy**
  - Preferably use Azithromycin; Doxycycline, Ofloxacin, Levofloxacin are contraindicated
  - Repeat testing (preferably by NAAT) 3 weeks after completion of therapy
  - Women under age 25 and those at increased risk should also be retested in the third trimester
  - Women diagnosed in the first trimester should receive a test of cure AND be retested in 3 months
  - Erythromycin esolate contraindicated due to neonatal hepatotoxicity

Recommended Regimens in Pregnancy (either)
   Azithromycin 1 g orally for 1 dose
   Amoxicillin 500 mg orally three times daily for 7 days

Alternative Regimens (any of the following)
   Erythromycin base 500 mg orally four times daily for 7 days
   Erythromycin base 250 mg orally four times daily for 14 day
   Erythromycin ethylsuccinate 800 mg orally four times daily for 7 days
   Erythromycin ethylsuccinate 400 mg orally four times daily for 14 days

Gonococcal Infections

Diagnosis
• NAAT are preferred tests (higher sensitivity)
• Can be diagnosed by testing urine or swabs from endocervix or vagina

Treatment (Uncomplicated Infections of Cervix, Urethra, and Rectum)
• Patients with GC are often coinfected with CT. Routine dual therapy without testing for CT can be cost-effective. Because most GC in the United States are susceptible to doxycycline and azithromycin, routine co-treatment might also hinder the development of antimicrobial-resistant GC

Recommended Regimens (either)
   Ceftriaxone 250 mg IM single dose
   Cefixime 400 mg* orally for 1 dose
      OR

Single-dose injectable cephalosporin (any of the following)
   Ceftizoxime 500 mg IM
   Cefoxitin 2 g IM + Probenecid 1 g orally
   Cefotaxime 500 mg IM
      PLUS
   Azithromycin 1 g orally for 1 dose
      OR
   Doxycycline 100 mg orally twice daily for 7 days

   *Cefixime does not provide as high nor as sustained a bactericidal level as ceftriaxone (cures 97.5% of uncomplicated GC infections versus 99.2%). Advantage of cefixime is oral route

Alternative Regimens (any of the following)
   Spectinomycin* 2 g IM for 1 dose
   Cefpodoxime 400 mg orally or **Cefuroxime** 1 g orally may be effective
   Azithromycin** 2 g orally for 1 dose

   *Not currently available in the United States
   **Restrict use to limited circumstances due to concerns for development of resistance

Note: *In April 2007, due to increase in fluoroquinolone-resistant gonorrhea, CDC no longer recommends fluoroquinolones—only if susceptibility is documented by culture*

Follow-up
• Patients should abstain from intercourse until treatment is completed and symptoms resolve
• Patients treated for uncomplicated GC do not need a test of cure
• Patients with persistent symptoms should be evaluated by culture (with antibiotic susceptibility)
• Repeat testing for all patients at 3 months after treatment is advised
• Sex partners: Treat all partners who had sexual contact with the patient within 60 days prior to the onset of symptoms OR the most recent sex partner if last intercourse more than 60 days prior

Special Considerations
• *Pregnancy:* Preferably treat with a cephalosporin. Patients who cannot tolerate a cephalosporin should be given azithromycin 2 g. Co-treat for presumed CT with azithromycin or amoxicillin
• Children weighing 45 kg or less: Treat with Ceftriaxone 125 mg IM for 1 dose

Genital Herpes Simplex Virus (HSV)

- Chronic condition; typical painful vesicular lesions or ulcerations are often absent making clinical diagnosis nonsensitive and nonspecific
- Most cases of recurrent genital HSV are caused by HSV-2, but HSV-1 is increasing
- Recurrence and shedding are less frequent in HSV-1 infections

Diagnosis

- **Virologic Tests**
  - **Cell culture:** Low sensitivity, about 25% false negative rate. Sensitivity of culture declines as lesions heal, usually within a few days of onset
  - **PCR:** More sensitive, increasing availability. Preferred for detection of HSV in CSF
  - Cytologic detection of cellular changes of HSV is insensitive and nonspecific, both in genital lesions (Tzanck prep) and cervical Paps, and should not be relied on for diagnosis
- **Type-specific Serologic Tests**
  - **HSV IgG I and II:** Antibodies to HSV develop during first few weeks following infection and persist indefinitely. IgM testing is not useful
  - Serologic screening for HSV-1 and HSV-2 is not indicated in the general population
  - May be helpful with recurrent symptoms and negative cultures, clinical diagnosis of genital herpes without lab confirmation, or partner with genital herpes
  - Consider screening in women presenting for STI evaluation (especially if multiple partners), or HIV-infected
  - Almost all HSV-2 infections are sexually acquired; therefore, type-specific HSV-2 antibodies imply anogenital infection. HSV-1 antibody is more difficult to interpret
  - Persons with HSV-2 positive screening should be counseled on possible asymptomatic viral shedding and offered suppressive therapy

Treatment

- Used for symptomatic relief; will not eradicate the virus completely

First Clinical Episode of Genital Herpes

- Typically more severe, prolonged, and can cause neurologic sequelae. All primary outbreaks should be treated with antiviral therapy

Recommended Regimens (any of the following)

    Acyclovir 400 mg orally three times daily for 7–10 days
    Acyclovir 200 mg orally five times daily for 7–10 days
    Famciclovir 250 mg orally three times daily for 7–10 days
    Valacyclovir 1 g orally twice daily for 7–10 days

    Note: Treatment may be extended if healing is incomplete after 10 days of therapy

Recurrent Genital Herpes

- Can treat each recurrence or prescribe daily suppression to reduce frequency of outbreaks
- Suppression can reduce frequency of outbreaks by 70–80% and can decrease length of recurrences
- Episodic therapy should be started within 1 day of lesions onset or during prodrome

Recommended Regimens—Suppression (any of the following)

    Acyclovir 400 mg orally twice daily
    Famciclovir 250 mg orally twice daily
    Valacyclovir 500 mg orally once daily
    Valacyclovir 1 g orally once daily

- Famciclovir is less effective for suppression
- Valacyclovir 500 mg once daily has been shown to decrease HSV-2 transmission in heterosexual, discordant partners

Recommended Regimens—Episodic Treatment (any of the following)

    Acyclovir 400 mg orally three times daily for 5 days
    Acyclovir 800 mg orally twice daily for 5 days
    Acyclovir 800 mg orally three times daily for 2 days
    Famciclovir 125 mg orally twice daily for 5 days
    Famciclovir 1000 mg orally twice daily for 1 day

Famciclovir 500 mg orally once, then 250 mg twice daily for 2 days
Valacyclovir 500 mg orally twice daily for 3 days
Valacyclovir 1 g orally once daily for 5 days

Follow-up
- Inform patients that sexual HSV transmission can occur at anytime; use of male latex condoms and suppressive therapy may decrease rates of transmission
- Asymptomatic viral shedding is more frequent in genital HSV-2 infection than genital HSV-1 infection and is most frequent in the first 12 months of acquiring HSV-2
- Provide a prescription for suppressive or episodic therapy

Special Considerations
- Pregnancy
  - Primary and recurrent outbreaks are treated the same as nonpregnant population
  - Safety of systemic Acyclovir, Valacyclovir, and Famciclovir in pregnancy not established
  - Acyclovir and Valacyclovir more commonly used
  - Suppression with Acyclovir 400 mg orally three times daily or Valacyclovir 500 mg orally twice daily is recommended for women with a history of genital HSV from 36 weeks gestation until delivery (earlier if preterm labor)
  - No data support the use of antiviral therapy among HSV seropositive women without a history of genital HSV
  - Risk of transmission to neonate is high (30–50%) if genital HSV is acquired near delivery and low (less than 1%) if history of recurrent HSV at term or acquired genital HSV during first half of pregnancy
  - At time of labor, women should be asked about any prodromal symptoms and carefully examined for lesions. If any symptoms/lesions are present, cesarean is recommended
  - See OB section for further detail
- HIV
  - Episodes may be more prolonged and severe; lesions may be more atypical
  - Symptoms may worsen following initiation of antiretroviral therapy
  - Suppression is still effective at decreasing symptoms, but the extent of its effect on viral shedding in HIV positive patients is unknown

Chancroid
- Sporadic outbreaks; painful genital ulcer with tender lymphadenopathy
- Caused by *H. ducreyi*

Diagnosis
- Definitive Diagnosis: Identification of *H. ducreyi* on special culture media, not widely available and sensitivity when used is <80%
- Probable Diagnosis: If all of the following are present
  - One or more painful genital ulcers
  - Negative serologic test for >7 days after onset of ulcers
  - No evidence of *Treponema pallidum* infection by dark field exam of ulcer exudate
  - Presentation, appearance of ulcers, and lymphadenopathy typical for chancroid
  - Ulcer exudate tests negative for HSV

Treatment
Recommended Regimens (any of the following)
  Azithromycin 1 g orally in a single dose
  Ceftriaxone 250 mg IM once
  Ciprofloxacin 500 mg orally twice daily for 3 days
  Erythromycin base 500 mg orally three times daily for 7 days

Follow-up
- Symptoms should improve within 3 days of treatment initiation and physical signs should improve by 7 days
- Fluctuant lymphadenopathy may require incision and drainage
- Test for HIV at time of diagnosis and again with syphilis testing 3 months later
- Sex partners: Treat all partners who had sexual contact with the patient within 10 days prior to the start of the patient's symptoms

Special Considerations
- Pregnancy: Avoid ciprofloxacin; no adverse outcomes related to pregnancy reported
- HIV: More likely to have treatment failure; limit use of azithromycin or ceftriaxone if compliance with follow-up is in question

Syphilis

- Clinical findings depend on stage of disease
  - Primary: Chancre
  - Secondary: Rash, mucocutaneous lesions, lymphadenopathy
  - Tertiary: Cardiac, gummatous lesions
  - Neurosyphilis: Neurologic/ophthalmic involvement at any stage
  - Latent: No symptoms, serologic diagnosis only
- Caused by *T. pallidum*

Diagnosis

- Definitive Diagnosis: Identification of *T. pallidum* in lesion exudate or tissue by dark-field exam, direct fluorescent antibody test, or PCR. Majority not readily available
- Presumptive Diagnosis: Two positive serologic tests
  - **Non-treponemal tests** (detect markers of cellular damage caused by disease): VDRL, RPR; used for screening but limited by high false-positive rate
  - **Treponemal tests** (detect antibodies that are a direct result of infection):
    - FTA-ABS, TP-PA
    - Enzyme immunoassay (EIA)/Chemiluminescence immunoassay (CIA) tests. Automated initial screening test (eg, syphilis trep test (STT)). Should be confirmed with either the VDRL or RPR tests
- Test Interpretation (examples)
  - STT+, RPR+, FTA-ABS−: False-positive result
  - STT+, RPR−, FTA-ABS+: Previously treated; contact health department
- Evaluation of CSF only indicated if neurologic signs are present or treatment failure for primary/secondary syphilis is documented

Treatment Overview

- Parenteral Penicillin G is used for all stages
- Potential reaction: **Jarisch–Herxheimer reaction** (a response to release of endotoxins after destruction of spirochetes; fever, myalgias, headache, etc occurring typically within 24 hours of administration). Usually occurs with early syphilis. Can use antipyretics for symptoms, but no prevention method known

Primary and Secondary Syphilis
Recommended Regimen for Adults
    Benzathine penicillin G 2.4 million units IM in a single dose

Follow-up

- Repeat clinical evaluation and serologic testing at 6 and 12 months following treatment
- Follow-up serologic testing should involve the same test and same lab if possible
- Test all patients for HIV at the time of diagnosis
- Titers of non-treponemal tests are used to determine reinfection or treatment failure; treponemal test titers do not correlate with disease activity. Evidence of reinfection/treatment failure include
  - Clinical signs/symptoms of disease that recur or persist despite treatment
  - Four fold increase in non-treponemal test titer compared with baseline or maximum titer (ie, 1:4 to 1:16; or 1:8 to 1:32)
- In the event of reinfection/treatment failure
  - Retest for HIV
  - Perform CSF analysis
  - If no evidence of neurosyphilis: Benzathine penicillin G 2.4 million units IM for 3 weeks
- If at 6–12 month evaluation, titers do not rise, but fail to decline, consider repeat testing for HIV, CSF evaluation, and continue close follow-up. Re-treat if compliance is in question
- Sex partners
  - Primary: Treat all partners within 3 months + duration of symptoms
  - Secondary: Treat all partners within 6 months + duration of symptoms
  - Early latent: Treat all partners within 12 months + duration of symptoms
  - Unknown latent: If high titer (over 1:32), assume early and treat as above
  - Late latent: Long-term partners should have frequent clinical/serologic testing

Latent Syphilis

- Defined as "early latent" if seropositive and at least one of the following:
  - Seroconversion or greater than or equal to fourfold increase in serum titer within 1 year
  - Definite symptoms of primary or secondary syphilis
  - Sex partner with primary, secondary, or early latent syphilis
  - Only possible exposure for conversion was within the past year

- Otherwise, defined as "late latent" or "unknown duration"
- Examine all for signs of disease

Recommended Regimens for Adults
  Early Latent Syphilis
    Benzathine penicillin G 2.4 million units IM in a single dose
  Late Latent Syphilis or Latent Syphilis of Unknown Duration
    Benzathine penicillin G 2.4 million units IM weekly for 3 weeks

Follow-up
- Repeat serologic testing at 6, 12, and 24 months
- Test all patients for HIV at the time of diagnosis
- Indications for CSF testing
  - Neurologic disease or evidence of tertiary syphilis
  - Developing signs or symptoms of syphilis
  - Greater than or equal to fourfold increase in titer
  - Initial titer of 1:32 or higher that fails to decline by fourfold or more within 1–2 years of treatment

Tertiary Syphilis and Neurosyphilis
- Care should be coordinated with Infectious Disease specialist
- See CDC guidelines for further detail on treatment and follow-up recommendations

Special Considerations
- **Penicillin Allergy:** Limited data; the following regimens may be used in nonpregnant patients

Alternative Regimens for Nonpregnant Adults (either)
  Doxycycline 100 mg orally twice daily for 28 days
  Tetracycline 500 mg four times daily for 28 days
    If compliance is in question, desensitize and then treat with PCN as above
- Pregnancy
  - Screening recommended for all women in first trimester with repeat screening at 28–32 weeks and delivery in areas of higher prevalence and high-risk populations
  - Women who test positive should be considered to have active disease and be treated unless prior treatment and appropriate decline in titers has been documented
  - All pregnant women diagnosed with syphilis need treatment with PCN; if allergic, must be desensitized. **Alternatives are unacceptable**
  - PCN is effective for preventing maternal transmission to fetus and treating fetal infection
  - Women treated during late second and third trimesters are at risk for preterm labor/fetal distress if treatment causes the Jarish–Herxheimer reaction—resembles sepsis

Genital Warts
- Majority caused by HPV 6 and 11
- Typically asymptomatic pedunculated, flat or papular, non-erythematous skin growths occurring near the vaginal introitus, but may occur in the vagina, on the cervix, etc. May also have some associated pain/pruritis

Diagnosis
- Primarily based on clinical findings
- Biopsy is indicated in cases of treatment failure, uncertain diagnosis, atypical appearance, or immunocompromised status

Treatment
- For patient symptoms or cosmetic purposes; untreated warts may resolve on their own
- Treatment can result in resolution of warts, but may not eradicate HPV entirely
- Several treatment options exist; selection will depend on the number/size/location of warts, cost of treatment, side effects of treatment, patient preference, and provider experience
- See Table 2-26 for treatment options
- Patient-applied options should only be selected if the patient can identify and reach all warts and are felt to be reliable to comply with the treatment regimen; it may be helpful for primary applications to be performed under supervision of a provider in the office

Follow-up
- Counseling
  - Genital warts are very common and can be spread by vaginal, oral, or anal intercourse
  - Genital warts are NOT associated with future development of cervical cancer
  - The diagnosis of HPV is NOT indicative of sexual infidelity

- HPV does not affect future fertility and is not a risk factor for preterm birth
- Genital warts can recur after treatment of any kind
- Sex partners: Male condom use may decrease transmission but is not fully protective

TABLE 2-26 TREATMENT OPTIONS FOR GENITAL WARTS

Medication/Therapy	Mechanism/Dosage/Advantages	Disadvantages
Patient-Applied Medications		
Podofilox 0.5% solution or gel	Anti-mitotic; Apply twice daily for 3 days, no medications for 4 days; repeat cycle up to three times Max 0.5 mL/day Inexpensive	Limited to wart area of 10 × 10 cm Mild–moderate pain or irritation after treatment
Imiquimod 5% cream	Immune-enhancer Apply at bedtime 3 days per week for up to 16 weeks. Wash area with soap and water 6–10 hours after application	Local irritation/induration/ulceration may be common Can weaken condoms/diaphragms Hypopigmentation may result
Sinecatechins 15% ointment	Green-tea extract with active catechins Apply 0.5 cm ointment three times daily to each wart for up to 16 weeks Do not wash off and avoid sexual contact while ointment is on	Can cause pain/erythema/vesicular rash/ulceration Can weaken condoms/diaphragms NOT for immune-compromised patients, patients with clinical genital HSV
Provider-Administered Therapy		
Liquid nitrogen or cryoprobe cryotherapy	Induces thermal cellular destruction Consider topical or injected local anesthetic if area is large	Requires provider training Post-treatment pain, possible blistering/necrosis
Podophyllin resin 10–25% in a compound tincture of benzoin	Cytotoxic agent; allow to air-dry after applying to each wart. Apply once per week up to 6 weeks. Consider bordering area with petroleum jelly to prevent local skin irritation. Wash off 1–4 hours after application	Systemic absorption can cause multisystem failure and rarely death. Limit to wart area of <10 × 10 cm and use <0.5 mL; do not use on open lesions
Trichloroacetic acid (TCA) or bichloroacetic acid (BCA) 80–90%	Destroys cellular proteins; allow to air-dry after applying to each wart. Apply once per week up to 6 weeks. Consider bordering area with petroleum jelly to prevent local skin irritation. White coating will develop after application	Pain with application; can be neutralized with soap or sodium bicarbonate
Surgical removal	Removal or ablation after local anesthesia by excision, curettage, or electrosurgery. CO_2 laser reserved for extensive or resistant warts—procedure performed in OR	Requires provider training May cause scarring

Special Considerations
- Pregnancy
  - Warts may increase and become more friable
  - Treatment options include cryotherapy, TCA/BCA, or surgical excision. Excision is normally reserved until postpartum unless necessary
  - Rare cases of respiratory papillomatosis in infants may occur, but the mode of transmission is unclear and cesarean may not be protective and should not be recommended due to warts alone
  - Cesarean only recommended if warts occlude vaginal introitus or bleeding from warts is of concern

- HIV: Immunocompromised patients have increased risk of squamous cell carcinoma. Biopsy any suspicious lesions prior to treatment
- Cervical Warts: Biopsy to exclude HSIL. Further management by a specialist
- Vaginal Warts: Can use cryotherapy with liquid nitrogen or TCA/BCA
- Anal Warts: Can use cryotherapy with liquid nitrogen or TCA/BCA or surgical excision
- Intra-anal Warts: Management by a specialist

HIV

- Acute retroviral syndrome: Often occurs before antibody testing is positive; can include fever, rash, malaise, and lymphadenopathy. Occurs in 50–80% infected patients
- If untreated, time from initial infection to AIDS can vary from months to years, median 11 years
- All persons who present for STI screening should be screened for HIV; notification of testing and option to decline ("opt-out") should be verbally communicated

Diagnosis

- Screening: HIV-1 and HIV-2 antibody serologic tests [enzyme immunoassay (EIA) or rapid test]. Positive screening results should be confirmed with follow-up testing
- Confirmatory tests: Additional antibody testing (Western Blot, indirect immunofluorescence assay), or virologic test (HIV-1 RNA assay)
- HIV antibody detected in 95% of patients within 3 months of infection
- HIV-1 RNA assay can detect infection in persons with negative antibody screening

Treatment

- Patients should be followed and managed by providers up-to-date and skilled in care of HIV-infected individuals
- The mainstay of treatment is close follow-up and antiretroviral therapy
- Counseling/support regarding medical, psychological, and reproductive implications is integral to care
- Some forms of antiretroviral therapy may interact with various types of contraception; medical eligibility criteria for contraceptive use is available on both WHO and CDC Web sites

HIV Follow-up

- Additional testing for all newly diagnosed female patients
  - Physical and gynecologic exam
  - Screen for GC, CT, and trichomonas, and perform Pap
  - CBC, CMP, lipid panel, Hepatitis C, Toxoplasma Antibody, Hepatitis A and B, Syphilis
  - HIV viral load, CD4 count, HIV genotypic resistance testing
  - PPD, urinalysis, chest x-ray
  - Consider serologic testing for HSV-2 if status unknown
- Vaccinate for Hepatitis A and Hepatitis B if indicated
- Partners (sex partners and persons sharing injection devices)
  - Notification is essential and confidential; can be accomplished via direct communication by the patient (with or without a health care provider present) OR by provider referral in which case trained health department personnel communicate with partners and the confidentiality/identity of the patient is protected
  - All partners should be tested for infection and counseled
  - Post-exposure prophylaxis can be offered to partners exposed within preceding 72 hours

Special Considerations

- Pregnancy
  - All pregnant women should be tested upon presentation for prenatal care and consider again in the third trimester; counseling with the option to opt out must be provided
  - See Section 1 on Obstetrics for further detail on managing HIV during pregnancy

Hepatitis C (HCV)

- Most common chronic blood-borne infection in the United States
- Transmission more common via injection drug use/needle-sharing, rarely sexually transmitted
- Clinical presentation is asymptomatic to mild illness with signs of active liver disease appearing more commonly in the setting of chronic infection

Diagnosis

- Screening: Anti-HCV serology (detects antibodies to Hepatitis C)
  - On average, anti-HCV will be positive approximately 8–9 weeks from exposure
- Confirmatory testing: HCV RNA serology (ie, RT-PCR)
  - Can generally be detected within 1–3 weeks following exposure
  - Liver function tests should also be performed; elevated ALT is evidence of chronic liver disease

Treatment

- Pegylated interferon and Ribavirin are standard therapy for chronic HCV
- Care should be provided by specialists in the field of HCV
- Outcomes are improved in the setting of early diagnosis and treatment

Follow-up
- Counseling should be provided regarding avoidance of alcohol and other hepatotoxic drugs/substances
- Vaccinations for Hepatitis A and Hepatitis B should be considered
- Chronic HCV
  - Will develop in 70–80% of HCV-infected individuals
  - 60–70% of patients with chronic HCV will develop active liver disease
  - Long-term risks include cirrhosis and hepatocellular carcinoma
- Prevention and Partners
  - No vaccination or post-exposure prophylaxis is available
  - Spread of infection from a long-term heterosexual partner is rare, but sexual spread may be more common among individuals with multiple partners or HIV

Special Considerations
- Pregnancy
  - Perinatal transmission rate approximately 6%, mainly occurring during/near the time of delivery; increased risk with higher HCV viral loads and in patients co-infected with HIV
  - No obstetrical intervention has been shown to decrease this risk
  - Infants born to HCV-positive mothers should be tested
  - Breast feeding is safe and should only be avoided in the case of cracked or bleeding nipples
- HIV
  - Sexual transmission is more common
  - All HIV-infected individuals should be screened for Hepatitis C
  - 25% of HIV-infected patients also have HCV
- Additional Risk Factors for HCV
  - Blood transfusion or solid organ transplant before July 1992
  - Persons with signs or symptoms of liver disease
  - Patients on long-term dialysis
  - Recipients of clotting factor concentrates made before 1987

Hepatitis B (HBV)

- Infection may be limited or chronic; time from exposure to onset of symptoms is approximately 6 weeks to 6 months
- 50% patients with newly acquired HBV are symptomatic
- 1% patients with HBV may suffer from acute liver failure and death
- Transmission by blood/bodily fluids; sexual transmission accounts for most cases in the United States

Diagnosis (Table 2-27)
- Requires serologic testing; screen by testing for Hepatitis B surface antigen (HbsAg)
- If HbsAg +, test: Total anti-HBc and IgM anti-HBc

TABLE 2-27 HEPATITIS B LAB TEST INTERPRETATION

Interpretation	HbsAg	Total Anti-HBc	IgM Anti-HBc	Anti-HBs
Never infected	−	−	−	−
Early acute infection; transient (up to 18 days) after vaccination	+	−	−	−
Acute infection	+	+	+	−
Acute resolving infection	−	+	+	−
Immune due to natural infection	−	+	−	+
Chronic infection	+	+	−	−
False (+) (ie, susceptible); previous infection; low-level chronic infection; passive transfer to infant born to HBsAg (+) mother	−	+	−	−
Immune if concentration is ≥10 mIU/mL; passive transfer after HBIG administration	−	−	−	+

- Note that both patients with acute and chronic HBV will test positive for HbsAg; if IgM antibody to Hepatitis B core Ag (IgM anti-HBc) is present, infection is acute
- Antibody to HbsAg (anti-HBs) is a marker of immunity or past infection

Treatment

- Supportive therapy and close follow-up only; no specific treatment options to date
- Due to risks from chronic disease, patients with chronic HBV should be followed by a specialist

Follow-up

- Counseling should be provided regarding avoidance of alcohol and other hepatotoxic drugs/ substances
- Chronic HBV
  - Increased risk with younger age of exposure (ie, 90% of infants, 2–6% of adults)
  - Long-term risks include cirrhosis and hepatocellular carcinoma
- Partners/contacts: All unvaccinated partners or household members should be vaccinated. Non-immune sex partners should be instructed on latex condom use until immunity can be confirmed

Special Considerations

- Pregnancy
  - Test all pregnant women for HbsAg
  - Vaccinate all HbsAg negative patients who have not previously been vaccinated
- Prevention: Hepatitis B vaccination and/or Hepatitis B immune globulin (HBIG)
  - Vaccination given to adults generally in three doses over 0–6 months, but several schedules are available; missed doses should be given ASAP
  - HBIG will provide temporary protection (approximately 3–6 months)
  - Pre-exposure vaccination should be provided to the following groups:
    - All infants
    - Children under 18 who have not been vaccinated
    - Adults who have not been vaccinated and are at high risk of infection or seek vaccination
  - Pre-vaccination testing with anti-HBc should be considered in high-risk adult groups
  - Post-vaccination testing with anti-HBs should be performed in HIV positive, immunocompromised patients, sex/needle-sharing partners of HbsAg+ individuals
  - Post-exposure prophylaxis: Vaccination alone or in combination with HBIG
    - Unvaccinated patient exposed to bodily fluids from HbsAg+ individual: Vaccine + HBIG ASAP
    - Unvaccinated patient exposed to bodily fluids from patient with unknown HbsAg status: Vaccine only ASAP (eg., sexual assault victims)
  - Vaccine + HBIG are also recommended for all infants born to mothers who are HbsAg positive or unknown status
  - HBIG may also be used in patients who have not responded to vaccination

Hepatitis A (HAV)

- Limited disease; does NOT result in chronic liver disease
- Incubation period approximately 15–50 days
- Symptoms consistent with acute viral hepatitis (fatigue, N/V, abdominal pain, etc) and occur more frequently in adults than children. Symptoms may relapse within 6 months following initial illness
- Transmission primarily fecal-oral through contaminated food/water or person-person

Diagnosis

- Requires serologic testing; IgM antibody to HAV indicates acute infection

Treatment

- Supportive therapy and close follow-up only

Special Considerations

- Prevention: Hepatitis A vaccination and/or Hepatitis A immune globulin (IG)
  - Vaccination given to adults in two doses over 0–(6–12) months and should be offered to
    - Substance abusers (IV and non-IV)
    - Patients with chronic liver disease
    - Men sexually active with other men (MSM) and their partners
  - Pre-vaccination testing may be considered in high-prevalence populations
  - Post-vaccination testing is not necessary
  - Post-exposure prophylaxis

- Exposed unvaccinated patients should be vaccinated ASAP
- Hepatitis A IG should be given instead to the following exposed/nonimmune patients
  - Over 40 years of age if exposed (risk for more severe symptoms)
  - Children under 12 months of age
  - Immunocompromised patients
- Exposed unvaccinated patients who are substance abusers, chronic liver disease, or MSM should receive both vaccine and IG concurrently
- Patients with HIV or chronic liver disease may not respond as well to vaccination

Bacterial Vaginosis (BV)

- Most common cause of vaginal discharge with odor, though patients may also be asymptomatic
- More prevalent in women who douche, have multiple sexual partners or a new partner, and those who do not use condoms
- Not clear that BV results from sexual activity as women who have never been sexually active may be affected
- Caused by anaerobic bacteria that replace *Lactobacillus* (ie, *G. vaginalis, Mycoplasma, Ureaplasma, Prevotella, Mobiluncus*)

Diagnosis
- Gram stain (gold standard) OR Amsel's Diagnostic Criteria (three out of four of the following):
  - pH vaginal fluid over 4.5
  - Whiff test: Fishy odor of discharge before or after addition of 10% KOH
  - Clue cells on saline wet prep
  - Thin, white, homogeneous discharge coating vagina
- Should not be diagnosed from a cervical Pap test; low sensitivity

Treatment
- Recommended for symptomatic relief in nonpregnant women

Recommended Regimens (any of the following)
    Metronidazole 500 mg orally twice daily for 7 days
    Metronidazole gel 0.75%, one full applicator (5 g) intravaginally, once daily for 5 days
    Clindamycin cream 2%, one full applicator (5 g) intravaginally at bedtime for 7 days

Alternative Regimens (any of the following)
    Tinidazole 2 g orally once daily for 2 days
    Tinidazole 1 g orally once daily for 5 days
    Clindamycin 300 mg orally twice daily for 7 days
    Clindamycin ovules 100 g intravaginally nightly for 3 days

Follow-up
- BV increases risk of other STIs; consider screening
- Women should avoid intercourse or use condoms 100% of the time during treatment
- Counsel patients on avoiding alcohol during treatment with Metronidazole and 24 hours following completion; if Clindamycin is used, counsel on potential weakening of condoms/diaphragms
- Recurrence is common; can consider Metronidazole gel two times per week for 4–6 months after multiple recurrences
- Sex partners: Treatment of male sex partners does not decrease risk of recurrence

Special Considerations
- Pregnancy
  - Treat all symptomatic women. Oral therapy is preferred (any of the following)
    - Metronidazole 500 mg orally twice daily for 7 days
    - Metronidazole 250 mg orally three times daily for 7 days
    - Clindamycin 300 mg orally twice daily for 7 days
  - BV can be associated with PPROM, PTL, chorioamnionitis, endometritis, but the only certain benefit of treatment is to decrease symptoms
  - Asymptomatic women: Data insufficient for clear recommendations; may be beneficial to treat women at high risk for preterm delivery
  - Avoid vaginal clindamycin cream due to reported adverse outcomes later in pregnancy
- Gynecologic Surgery: BV can increase risk of post-op infection (ie, cuff cellulitis). Consider treatment preoperatively or upon diagnosis

Trichomoniasis

- Symptomatic infection may result in foul-smelling vaginal discharge with yellow or green discoloration and vaginal discomfort, although may be asymptomatic
- Caused by protozoan *T. vaginalis*

Diagnosis

- Wet mount of vaginal discharge and microscopy: Most commonly used, sensitivity 60–70%
- Culture may be useful if disease is suspected but not confirmed on microscopy
- OSOM Trichomonas Rapid Test (immunochromatographic technology) and Affirm VP III (nucleic acid test); both yield more rapid results, over 80% sensitive, over 90% specific, but may yield false positives
- PCR testing: Available for urinary, vaginal, and endocervical samples, highly sensitive and specific
- NAAT: APTIMA testing can use same swab to test for Trichomoniasis, Chlamydia, and Gonorrhea concurrently; sensitivity 74–98%, specificity 87–98%

Treatment
Recommended Regimens (either)
   Metronidazole 2 g orally once
   Tinidazole 2 g orally once
Alternative Regimen
   Metronidazole 500 mg orally twice daily for 7 days
- Metronidazole gel is not recommended as it is much less efficacious than oral preparations
- *Avoid alcohol for 24 hours after metronidazole and 72 hours after tinidazole*

Follow-up

- May consider re-screening in 3 months due to high risk of reinfection
- Patients should avoid intercourse until treatment is completed and symptoms have resolved
- Sex partners: All sex partners should be treated
- Treatment failure: Low levels of metronidazole resistance have been reported; if treatment fails (NOT reinfection) consider Metronidazole 500 mg orally twice daily for 7 days, and if no response, Metronidazole or Tinidazole 2 g orally daily for 5 days

Special Considerations

- Pregnancy: Vaginal trichomoniasis associated with preterm delivery, PROM, low birth weight, but treatment has not been shown to reduce morbidity. In addition some studies have shown worse outcomes following treatment during pregnancy, but data have not been strong enough to draw definitive conclusions. Recommendations are as follows:
  - Symptomatic: Counsel and consider treatment with Metronidazole 2 g orally once. Safety of Tinidazole in pregnancy has not been established
  - Asymptomatic: Counsel on risks/benefits and consider delaying treatment until over 37 weeks gestation
- Breast-feeding: Will need to pump and dispose of breast milk for 12–24 hours after treatment with Metronidazole, 3 days after treatment with Tinidazole
- Allergy to Metronidazole/Tinidazole: Refer to a specialist for possible desensitization

Vulvovaginal Candidiasis (VVC)

- Symptoms may include vaginal discharge with pruritis, dysuria, dyspareunia, vulvar/vaginal burning, or discomfort
- Clinical signs: Redness/swelling/pain of vulva, thick curd-like vaginal discharge
- Commonly caused by *Candida albicans* but may be caused by other *Candida* spp. or yeasts
- Classified as Uncomplicated VVC versus Complicated VVC

Uncomplicated VVC

- Includes the following cases:
  - Sporadic/Infrequent *OR*
  - Mild–moderate *OR*
  - Occurring in nonimmunocompromised patient *OR*
  - Likely caused by *C. albicans*

Diagnosis

- Can be made in a patient with the above signs/symptoms and wet prep or Gram stain of the discharge that demonstrates yeast or culture/additional test positive for yeast
- Associated with a normal vaginal pH (<4.5)

- 10% KOH wet mount of discharge and microscopy: Disrupts cellular material making yeast buds/pseudohyphae easier to visualize
- Consider culture in patients who have symptoms with a negative wet mount. Consider a trial of treatment despite negative wet mount in patients with other clinical signs if culture is unavailable
- 10–20% of women will routinely have yeast vaginally; asymptomatic patients do not need treatment

Treatment

Recommended Regimens

OTC-Intravaginal Agents	Prescription-Intravaginal Agents
Butoconazole 2% cream 5 g for 3 days	**Butoconazole** 2% cream 5 g once (sustained release)
Clotrimazole 1% cream 5 g for 7–14 days	**Nystatin** 100 000-unit tab for 14 days
Clotrimazole 2% cream 5 g for 3 days	**Terconazole** 0.4% cream 5 g for 7 days
Miconazole 2% cream 5 g for 7 days	**Terconazole** 0.8% cream 5 g for 3 days
Miconazole 4% cream 5 g for 3 days	**Terconazole** 80 mg suppository for 3 days
Miconazole 100 mg vaginal supp for 7 days	
Miconazole 200 mg vaginal supp for 3 days	**Oral Agent**
Miconazole 1200 mg vaginal supp for 1 day	**Fluconazole** 150 mg orally once
Tioconazole 6.5% ointment 5 g once	

Note: Inform patients that creams and suppositories may weaken condoms and diaphragms.
OTC: over-the-counter

- For patients with external symptoms, especially those opting for treatment with an oral agent, consider concurrent prescription of an antifungal/steroid topical agent (ie, Mycolog II)

Follow-up

- Reexamine if symptoms persist or recur within 2 months
- Sex partners: Do not need to be treated. VVC is not acquired through intercourse. Rarely male partners may have erythema/pruritis/irritation of the glans of the penis (Balanitis) which may be treated with topical antifungals

Special Considerations

- Treatment with oral azoles may cause liver function test abnormalities and can interact with other medications (ie, warfarin, oral hypoglycemic agents, Ca^{++} channel blockers, etc)
- *Note:* Pregnancy and HIV fall under Complicated VVC; see below

Complicated VVC

- Includes the following cases:
  - Recurrent
  - Severe
  - Occurring in immunosuppressed, pregnant, debilitated, or uncontrolled diabetic patient
  - Caused by non-*C. albicans*

Recurrent VVC

- Four or more episodes of symptomatic VVC in a year
- Diagnosis: Obtain vaginal cultures to confirm diagnosis and identify non-*C. albicans* yeasts
- Non-*C. albicans* yeasts may not respond as well to routine treatment and may not produce clear pseudohyphae, etc on microscopy (ie, *C. glabrata*)
- Treatment: Consider longer duration of therapy
  - Topical therapy for 7–14 days OR
  - Fluconazole 100 mg or 150 mg or 200 mg every 3 days for 3 doses
- Follow-up: Maintenance therapy with Fluconazole 100 mg or 150 mg or 200 mg every week for 6 months is preferred. Alternatives include intermittent topical treatments
- 30–50% of patients will have recurrence after maintenance has ended

Severe VVC

- Characterized by severe signs: Vulvar edema, excoriations, fissures, extensive erythema
- Treatment: Topical azole for 7–14 days or Fluconazole 150 mg orally every 3 days for 2 doses

Non-albicans VVC

- More difficult to treat; avoid use of Fluconazole, treat 7–14 days with an alternative oral or topical azole
- Recurrent episodes: Treat with Boric acid (in a gelatin capsule) 600 mg per vagina daily for 2 weeks

Patients Requiring Special Consideration
- Pregnancy: Use only topical azole regimens for 7 days
- HIV: Treatment should not differ
- Other debilitated/compromised patients (uncontrolled diabetics, chronic steroid users) require more prolonged treatment courses (7–14 days) and modification of conditions if possible

Differential Diagnosis of Vaginal Discharge (Table 2-28)

TABLE 2-28 DIFFERENTIAL DIAGNOSIS OF VAGINAL DISCHARGE

Characteristic	Normal	Bacterial Vaginosis	Trichomoniasis	Candidiasis
Discharge color	White to slate gray	Dirty gray	Dirty gray to green	White
Consistency	Homogeneous liquid to pasty	Liquid	Liquid	Pasty
Odor	None	Fishlike	Foul	None
pH	3.8–4.2	≥5	≥5	<4.5
Whiff test	Negative	Positive	±	Negative
Clue cells	Absent	Positive	±	Negative

WELL WOMAN CARE GUIDELINES

Guidelines: See Table 2-29 for guidelines by age group

IMMUNIZATIONS

Human Papillomavirus (HPV)
- Males and females ideally at ages 11–12; otherwise, recommended for females and males ages 13–26
  - Gardasil (quadrivalent 6, 11, 16, 18)—three doses given at 0, 2, 6 months OR
  - Cervarix (bivalent 16, 18)—three doses given at 0, 1, 6 months
- If doses are missed or the schedule is interrupted, can resume without restarting the series
- *Contraindications:* Severe allergic reaction to prior dose or component

Tetanus Diphtheria Pertussis (Tdap)
- Should be given once to persons over 11 years of age who have not received it previously
  - Td booster every 10 years to follow
- Should be given to pregnant women in every pregnancy between 27 and 36 weeks regardless of time since last Tdap/Td
- *Contraindications:* Severe allergic reaction to prior dose or component

Influenza
- Annual vaccine for all over 6 months of age
- *Contraindications:*
  - Inactivated: Severe allergic reaction to prior dose or component, egg protein allergy
  - Recombinant: Severe allergic reaction to prior dose or component
  - Live attenuated: Severe allergic reaction to prior dose or component, egg protein allergy, immunosuppression, asthma, diabetes, heart disease, kidney disease, pregnancy

Hepatitis B (HBV)
- Three doses (0, 1, 6 months) at any age if not received as a child; adults at risk
  - More than one sex partner, MSM, people who inject drugs, infected sex partner
  - Chronic kidney or liver disease, less than 60 years old with diabetes mellitus, HIV-infected
  - Health care workers, household contacts of people with HBV, travel to endemic area
- Can give during pregnancy
- *Contraindications:* Severe allergic reaction to prior dose or component

Meningococcal Vaccine
- Routinely given to adolescents first at 11–12 years of age, second (booster) at age 16
- Two doses at least 2 months apart for individuals with functional asplenia, complement deficiencies, or who are microbiologists, international travel to endemic areas, military recruits, etc
- *Contraindications:* Severe allergic reaction to prior dose or component

TABLE 2-29 WELL WOMAN CARE GUIDELINES BY AGE GROUP

	13–18 Years Old	19–39 Years Old	40–64 Years Old	65+ Years Old
History	Chief complaint Past medical and surgical history, medications, allergies, social history, family history, nutrition, physical activity Use of complementary/alternative medicine Tobacco/alcohol/drug use Violence/depression screening Sexual practices	As outlined for 13- to 18-year-old group *Plus* Urinary and fecal incontinence	As outlined for 13- to 18-year-old group *Plus* Urinary and fecal incontinence	As outlined for 13- to 18-year-old group *Plus* Urinary and fecal incontinence
Physical exam	Vital signs, height, weight, BMI Tanner staging Pelvic exam when indicated Skin	Vital signs, height, weight, BMI Neck: Lymph nodes, thyroid Breasts (age 22+), axillae, abdomen Pelvic exam Skin	Vital signs, height, weight, BMI Neck: Lymph nodes, thyroid Oral cavity Breasts, axillae Abdomen, pelvic exam, skin	Vital signs, height, weight, BMI Neck: Lymph nodes, thyroid Oral cavity Breasts, axillae Abdomen Pelvic exam, skin
Labs/Imaging	STI testing if sexually active High-risk groups: CBC Urine culture STI/HIV/HCV testing Genetic testing/counseling Rubella titer assessment	Cervical cancer screening (see separate section) STI testing High-risk groups: CBC Urine culture Mammography Fasting glucose Genetic testing/counseling Rubella titer assessment	Cervical cancer screening (see separate section) Mammography Lipid profile assessment (every 5 years starting age 45) Colorectal cancer screening (age 50) Thyroid stimulating hormone test (every 5 years starting age 50) HIV testing Fasting glucose (every 3 years starting age 45)	Cervical cancer screening (see separate section) Urinalysis Mammography Lipid profile assessment (every 5 years) Colorectal cancer screening Thyroid stimulating hormone test (every 5 years) Fasting glucose (every 3 years) DEXA

(Continued)

TABLE 2-29 WELL WOMAN CARE GUIDELINES BY AGE GROUP (*Continued*)

	13–18 Years Old	19–39 Years Old	40–64 Years Old	65+ Years Old
	TB skin testing	TB skin testing	High-risk groups:	High-risk groups:
	Lipid profile assessment	Lipid profile assessment	CBC	CBC
	Fasting glucose testing	Fasting glucose testing	Urine culture	STI/HIV/HCV testing
	Colorectal cancer screening	Colorectal cancer screening	STI/HCV testing	TB skin testing
	(if Familial Adenomatous Polyposis (FAP))	Thyroid stimulating hormone test	TB skin testing	
		DEXA	DEXA	
Counseling	Contraception	As outlined for 13- to 18-year-old group	As outlined for 13- to 18-year-old group	As outlined for 13- to 18-year-old group
	STI prevention	*Plus*	*Plus*	*Plus*
	Date-rape prevention	Preconception/genetic counseling	Preconception/genetic counseling as	Sexual function
	Exercise and diet	Breast self-awareness	needed	Breast self-awareness
	Bone health		Menopause	
	Seatbelts, firearms		Sexual function	
	School/Occupational hazards		Breast self-awareness	
	Exercise/Sports involvement			
	UV protection			
	Tobacco/Drug cessation			

Hepatitis A Vaccine (HAV)

- Two doses (0, 6 months) at any age if not received as a child; adults at risk
  - Travel to endemic areas (ideal to give more than 1 month in advance)
  - MSM, people who inject drugs
  - Chronic liver disease, patients treated with clotting factor concentrates
  - Individuals who work with HAV, exposed to HAV, or who desire protection
- *Contraindications:* Severe allergic reaction to prior dose or component

Pneumovax

- One dose for all adults 65 years of age or older or younger adults who are at risk for invasive pneumococcal disease
- *Contraindications:* Severe allergic reaction to prior dose or component

Measles Mumps Rubella (MMR)

- Most people will have received two doses of MMR as a child
- Adults who should receive MMR
  - Eighteen years of age or older born after 1956 should receive at least one dose of MMR unless previously vaccinated or have had all three diseases
  - Health care workers, students entering college, and international travelers should have received two doses of MMR
  - Women of reproductive age should be screened for immunity to rubella and if not immune should receive MMR or a Rubella vaccine
- *Contraindications:* Severe allergic reaction to prior dose or component, severe immunodeficiency, pregnancy

Varicella

- Two doses of varicella vaccine (at least 28 days apart) should be given to any adult WITHOUT evidence of immunity
- All pregnant women should be screened for immunity and vaccinated immediately in the postpartum period, if needed
- Evidence of immunity
  - Health care provider documentation of disease or vaccination
  - U.S. birth before 1980 EXCEPT in pregnant or immune-compromised patients or health care workers
  - Lab evidence of immunity or active disease
- *Contraindications:* Severe allergic reaction to prior dose or component, severe immunodeficiency, pregnancy

Zoster

- One dose for all adults 60 years of age or older, regardless of prior disease
- *Contraindications:* Severe allergic reaction to prior dose or component pregnancy, severe immunodeficiency

CERVICAL CANCER SCREENING

Background

- Infection with HPV is necessary to develop squamous cervical neoplasia
  - HPV types 16 and 18 cause 70% of cervical cancer
- Lifetime risk of HPV is approximately 80%
- Prevalence of HPV higher in younger women who are also more likely to clear the infection; women less than 21 years old clear HPV in 8–24 months
- Infections in older women likely reflect persistent infections
- MUST use an FDA-approved HPV test to use HPV results to stratify follow-up
- Consider uploading "*papapp.org*" as a shortcut on your smartphone. Excellent resource

Timing of Screening (Table 2-30)

Who May Require More Frequent Paps?

- HIV-infected: CDC recommends paps every 6 months in first year of diagnosis, then annually
- Previously treated for CIN 2,3 or cancer: Continue age-based screening for 20 years
- Immunocompromised (transplant patients, chronic steroid users)
- Women exposed to DES (diethylstilbestrol) in utero

When to Stop Screening?

- Over 65 years of age if three consecutive negative cytology or two consecutive negative co-test results in prior 10 years
- Continue screening in women over age 65 treated for CIN2+ in the last 20 years or with any condition as outlined above

TABLE 2-30 SCREENING METHODS FOR CERVICAL CANCER

Population	Recommended Screening Method	Comment
Women younger than 21 years	No screening	
Women aged 21–29 years	Cytology alone every 3 years	
Women aged 30–65 years	HPV and cytology co-testing (preferred) every 5 years	Screening by HPV testing alone is not recommended
Women older than 65 years	No screening is necessary after adequate negative prior screening result	Women with a history of CIN 2, CIN 3, or adenocarcinoma in situ should continue routine age-based screening for at least 20 years
Women who underwent total hysterectomy	No screening is necessary	Applies to women without a cervix and without a history of CIN 2, CIN 3, adenocarcinoma in situ, or cancer in the past 20 years
Women vaccinated against HPV	Follow age-specific recommendations (same as unvaccinated women)	

CIN, cervical intraepithelial neoplasia; HPV, human papillomavirus.
Used with permission from Salslow D, Solomon D, Lawson HW, et al. American Cancer Society, American Society for colposcopy and cervical Pathology, and American Society for clinical Pathology screening guidelines for the prevention and early detection of cervical cancer. *CA Cancer J Clin.* 2012;62:147–172.

When to Stop Screening Post-hysterectomy?
- Stop if total hysterectomy for benign indications (confirm pathology) and no prior high-grade CIN
- If total hysterectomy and history of CIN 2,3, screen with cytology alone every 3 years for 20 years after initial post-treatment surveillance period (utility of HPV not clear in this setting)
- Women with history of cervical cancer post total hysterectomy need screening indefinitely

HPV Testing

- To stratify risk to women 21 or older with ASCUS and postmenopausal women with LSIL
- As an adjunct to cytology for primary screening if over 30 years old
- As co-testing in women following colposcopy for abnormal paps

Management of Abnormal Paps

- Cervical cancer screening may be reported as abnormal for a variety of reasons including insufficient sampling, HPV positivity, or the presence of squamous or glandular cytologic atypia
- New data suggest risk of cancer is far less for women under age 25; consequently less invasive management is now recommended for women ages 21–24
- Adolescents (less than 21 years of age) should NOT be screened, but if they are, guidelines should be followed for the 21–24 age group
- If colposcopy is indicated, endocervical sampling (ECC) is acceptable in all cases except pregnancy; ECC should be performed if no lesions are seen or colposcopy is inadequate
  - ECC can be performed by endocervical brush or curette; use of the curette followed by brush may yield improved sampling
- The sensitivity of colposcopy for CIN2+ is low; perform multiple biopsies to improve detection if multiple or large lesions are present

Unsatisfactory Cytology
- Causes: Obscuring blood, inflammation, etc; try to modify conditions prior to repeat
- *Recommendations*
  - HPV negative ($\geq$30 years) or HPV unknown (any age)
    - Repeat cytology in 2–4 months
      - If negative, return to routine screening
      - If unsatisfactory again, refer to colposcopy
  - HPV positive ($\geq$30 years)
    - Perform colposcopy *OR*
    - Repeat cytology in 2–4 months
      - If negative, repeat cytology and HPV testing in 1 year
      - If unsatisfactory again, refer to colposcopy

Normal Cytology with Insufficient or Absent Transformation Zone (TZ)
- Prior recommendations were to repeat cytology in 6–12 months; however
  - Women with an absent TZ on cytology DO NOT appear to have a higher risk of CIN3+
  - HPV testing can be interpreted independent of TZ sampling
  - In women with history of CIN2+, absent TZ is NOT associated with increased incidence of cervical dysplasia
- *Recommendations*
  - **21–29 years old**: Routine screening
  - **≥30 years old**
    - HPV negative: Routine screening
    - HPV unknown: Perform HPV testing if possible *OR* repeat cytology in 3 years
    - HPV positive
      - Repeat cytology and HPV testing in 1 year *OR*
      - Perform genotyping for HPV 16 and 18 and manage accordingly (see below)

Normal Cytology with Positive HPV Testing
- These recommendations apply to women ≥30 years of age as HPV should not be used for screening purposes in younger women
- In women with HPV persistent at 1 year, approximately 21% will go on to develop CIN2+ by 30 months
- *Recommendations*
  - Option #1: Repeat cytology and HPV testing in 1 year
    - If cytology negative and HPV negative, repeat cytology and HPV in 3 years
    - If cytology is negative and HPV is positive, perform colposcopy
    - If cytology is abnormal regardless of HPV status, perform colposcopy (this means if the repeat is ASCUS, negative HPV, colposcopy is still recommended)
  - Option #2: Perform genotyping for HPV 16 and 18
    - If HPV 16 or 18 is positive, perform colposcopy
    - If HPV 16 and 18 are negative, repeat cytology and HPV in 1 year

Atypical Squamous Cells of Undetermined Significance (ASCUS)
- Most common abnormal cytology, lowest risk of CIN3+
- *Recommendations* (differ based on age, pregnancy status)
  - **21–24 years of age**
    - HPV negative: Repeat cytology in 3 years
    - HPV unknown or positive: Repeat cytology in 1 year (colposcopy NOT recommended)
      - If repeat is cytology negative, ASCUS or LSIL, repeat cytology again in 1 year
      - If 1- and 2-year cytologies are normal, return to routine screening
      - If 1-year cytology was abnormal and 2-year is normal, repeat cytology in 1 year. Need two consecutive normal results to return to routine screening
      - If 2-year cytology is abnormal, perform colposcopy
      - If repeat cytology is ASC-H, AGC, or HSIL+, perform colposcopy
  - **25–64 years of age**
    - HPV negative: Repeat cytology and HPV in 3 years
    - HPV unknown: Perform HPV testing if possible *OR* repeat cytology in 1 year
      - If repeat cytology is negative, repeat cytology in 3 years
      - If repeat cytology is abnormal, perform colposcopy (see below)
    - HPV positive: Perform colposcopy
  - **≥65 years of age**
    - Manage the same as 25- to 64-year-old age group
    - ASCUS, negative HPV is not an acceptable pap result to end screening. Repeat cytology and HPV if possible in 1 year. If both are negative, may stop screening
  - **Pregnant**
    - Manage as per age-related guidelines
    - If colposcopy is indicated by guidelines, it is OK to defer until 6 weeks postpartum

Low-Grade Squamous Intraepithelial Lesion (LSIL)
- LSIL incidence of disease similar to that of ASCUS, +HPV
- Reflex HPV is not indicated with LSIL due to high incidence of HPV with this cytologic result, but HPV performed as co-testing in women 30 years of age and older is useful for triage
- *Recommendations*
  - **21–24 years of age**
    - HPV status should be unknown; reflex testing is not acceptable
    - Repeat cytology in 1 year (colposcopy NOT recommended)
      - If repeat cytology is negative, ASCUS or LSIL, repeat cytology in 1 year
      - If 1- and 2-year cytologies are normal, return to routine screening
      - If 1-year cytology was abnormal and 2-year is normal, repeat cytology in 1 year. Need two consecutive normal results to return to routine screening

• If 2-year cytology is abnormal, perform colposcopy
• If repeat cytology is ASC-H, AGC, or HSIL, perform colposcopy
- **25 years of age to menopause**
  - HPV negative: Repeat cytology and HPV in 1 year *OR* perform colposcopy
    - If repeat cytology and HPV both are negative, repeat both in 3 years
    - If repeat cytology or HPV are abnormal/positive, perform colposcopy
  - HPV unknown or positive: Perform colposcopy
- **Postmenopausal**
  - HPV negative: Repeat cytology in 1 year
  - HPV unknown
    - Perform HPV testing and manage accordingly *OR*
    - Repeat cytology at 6 and 12 months *OR*
    - Perform colposcopy
  - HPV positive: Perform colposcopy
- **Pregnant**
  - Manage per age-related guidelines. If colposcopy is indicated by guidelines, it is preferable to perform during pregnancy, but OK to defer until 6 weeks postpartum

Atypical Squamous Cells, Cannot Exclude High-Grade Lesion (ASC-H)

• Incidence of disease higher than LSIL/ASCUS but lower than HSIL
• HPV reflex not useful in management; even ASC-H, HPV *negative* carries a 2% 5-year cancer risk
• Colposcopy is recommended for all women and follow-up is identical to women with HSIL

High-Grade Squamous Intraepithelial Lesion (HSIL)

• Incidence of CIN2+ is approximately 60%. Immediate colposcopy is recommended
• HPV should not be used to delay management, but if performed can help in decision making for colposcopy versus immediate Loop Electrosurgical Excision Procedure (LEEP) for women over 24 years of age
• HPV positive HSIL carries higher incidence of CIN3+ and higher 5-year cancer risk
• *Recommendations*
  - **21–24 years of age**
    - Perform colposcopy with ECC; immediate LEEP is not acceptable
  - **≥25 years of age**
    - Option #1: Immediate LEEP
    - Option #2: Perform colposcopy with ECC
      - Inadequate colposcopy: Perform LEEP
  - **Pregnant**
    - Perform colposcopy; ECC and immediate LEEP are unacceptable

Atypical Glandular Cells (AGC) on Cytology

• AGC associated with broad range of diagnoses: Polyps, adenocarcinomas of the cervix, uterus, fallopian tubes, ovaries, etc, but most commonly with CIN
• Reported as *AGC-NOS* (not otherwise specified) or *AGC-favor neoplasia*, atypical endometrial cells, or cytologic *Adenocarcinoma In Situ (AIS)*
• Workup of atypical endometrial cells alone differs (see below)
• Cancer risk higher in women over 35 years of age
• HPV testing does not alter management
• *Recommendations (AGC-NOS, AGC-favor neoplasia, AIS)*
  - <35 years of age: Colposcopy and ECC (consider endometrial sampling if risk factors for endometrial cancer)
  - ≥35 years of age: Colposcopy, ECC, and endometrial sampling
  - Pregnant: Perform colposcopy; cannot perform ECC or endometrial sampling
• *Follow up for all ages*
  - Initial cytology AGC-NOS
    - No CIN 2+, AIS or cancer: Repeat cytology and HPV testing at 1 and 2 years
      - If all repeat testing is negative, repeat cytology and HPV in 3 years
      - If any repeat test is positive, perform colposcopy
    - CIN 2+ but no AIS or cancer: Follow age-related guidelines for CIN2/3
  - Initial cytology AGC-favor neoplasia or AIS
    - If no invasive disease is identified, perform excisional procedure (preferably cold-knife conization (CKC) to permit interpretation of margins)

Atypical Endometrial Cells on Cytology

• Perform ECC and endometrial sampling; can delay colposcopy and only perform if no endocervical/endometrial abnormalities are detected

Benign Endometrial Cells on Cytology
- Considered normal in asymptomatic premenopausal women
- Perform endometrial sampling in postmenopausal women due to association with endometrial cancer *OR* premenopausal women with abnormal uterine bleeding
- Benign glandular cells are occasionally reported in women post-hysterectomy and do not require further workup

Management of Histologic/Colposcopic Findings Following Abnormal Screening Tests

- Follow-up may vary based on age, the preceding abnormal pap, and dysplasia identified (ie, CIN 1 versus CIN 2/3)

No Lesion Detected OR CIN 1
- **21–24 years of age**
  - Initial pap ASCUS or LSIL
    - Repeat cytology at 1 year
      - If cytology is normal/ASCUS/LSIL, repeat cytology again in 1 year
      - If 2-year cytology is normal, return to routine screening
      - If 2-year cytology is abnormal, perform colposcopy
      - If cytology is ASC-H or HSIL, perform colposcopy
  - Initial pap ASC-H or HSIL
    - Repeat colposcopy and cytology every 6 months (up to 2 years)
      - If cytology is negative twice and no high-grade changes on colposcopy, return to routine screening
      - If HSIL persists for 2 years with no CIN 2/3 identified, perform LEEP
      - Manage all other abnormal cytology results per guidelines (see above)
      - If colposcopy is inadequate perform LEEP
  - Treatment of persistent CIN 1 in this age group is NOT recommended
- **≥25 years of age**
  - Initial pap normal cytology/persistent +HPV, +HPV 16/18, ASCUS, or LSIL
    - No Lesion or CIN 1 identified
      - Repeat cytology and HPV testing at 1 year
        If both cytology and HPV are negative, repeat age appropriate screening in 3 years; if negative, return to routine screening
        Note: Two consecutive normal results are needed to return to routine screening
        If cytology or HPV are positive, repeat colposcopy
        If CIN 1 persists for 2 or more years, can opt to continue follow-up or treat with an ablative or excisional procedure
        　　Excision is recommended in this case if colposcopy is inadequate or the patient has been previously treated
  - Initial pap ASC-H or HSIL
    - Perform LEEP *OR*
    - Re-review specimens and colposcopic findings with pathology to ensure correct initial diagnosis *OR*
    - Repeat cytology and HPV testing at 1 and 2 years
      - If cytology and HPV negative twice, repeat age appropriate testing in 3 years
      - If HPV positive or cytology positive (<HSIL), perform colposcopy
      - If cytology +HSIL at either 1- or 2-year mark, perform LEEP
      - If colposcopy is inadequate, perform LEEP
- CIN 1 on an ECC does not require immediate excision and may be followed as above with the addition of a repeat ECC at 1 year

CIN 2, CIN 3, CIN 2/3
- Management does not vary based on the preceding abnormal pap, but may vary based on age
- CIN 2 and 3 may be difficult to distinguish and may therefore be referred to as CIN 2/3
- Treatment is generally recommended for most women
  - Excision (LEEP, CKC): Recommended if colposcopy is inadequate, dysplasia is recurrent, or ECC+ or CIN2+
  - Alternative treatment: Ablation
  - Follow-up after treatment
    - Ablation, specimen margins < CIN2, ECC is < CIN2
      - Repeat cytology and HPV testing at 1 and 2 years
        If both cytology and HPV remain negative at 2 years, repeat cytology and HPV in 3 years
        　　If both cytology and HPV are negative, return to routine screening for a total of 20 years following treatment
      - If any cytology or HPV test is abnormal during follow-up, perform colposcopy and ECC

- Specimen margins positive CIN2+ or ECC is CIN2+ (performed at the time of excision)
  - Repeat cytology and ECC in 4–6 months (preferred) OR
  - Repeat excisional procedure OR
  - Offer hysterectomy if repeat excisional procedure is not possible
- EXCEPTION #1: "Young Women"
  - Can consider observation with colposcopy and cytology every 6 months as an alternative to treatment in cases of CIN 2 or CIN 2/3
  - If colposcopy is inadequate or CIN 3 is specified, treatment is recommended
  - Follow-up
    - If colposcopy and cytology are negative twice, repeat cytology and HPV in 1 year
      - If both cytology and HPV are negative, repeat cytology and HPV in 3 years
      - If any test is abnormal, perform colposcopy
    - If colposcopic findings worsen or persist at 1 year or HSIL persists at 1 year, repeat colposcopy and biopsy
    - If CIN2 or CIN 2/3 persists at 2 years or CIN 3 is identified at anytime during follow-up, treatment is recommended
    - Follow-up after treatment is the same for the general and "younger" populations
- EXCEPTION #2: Pregnant Women
  - If CIN2+ is identified during pregnancy, follow with colposcopy and cytology every 3 months during pregnancy with repeat biopsy only if the lesion worsens or cytology suggests an invasive cancer
    - Alternative: Defer follow-up until 6 or more weeks postpartum
    - Excisional procedures should only be considered if invasion is suspected

Adenocarcinoma In Situ (AIS)

- Hysterectomy is recommended for all women who have completed childbearing
- Conservative management with excision and observation is an option, understanding that the disease is often multifocal with skip lesions such that negative margins may not indicate absence of further disease
  - Excision with CKC and concurrent ECC is preferred
    - If margins or ECC are positive for any dysplasia, re-excision is recommended
    - Colposcopy + cytology and HPV testing at 6 months is an acceptable alternative; HPV negativity following treatment indicates a lower risk for persistent/recurrent disease

VULVAR DERMATOSES

- May be asymptomatic, but commonly present with vulvar pruritis; differential diagnosis
  - *Acute*: Fungal infection, trichomoniasis, molluscum contagiosum, scabies, allergic dermatitis
  - *Chronic*: Contact/atopic dermatitis, atrophy, lichen sclerosus, lichen planus, lichen simplex chronicus, psoriasis, VIN, vulvar cancer, Paget's disease, Crohn's disease, Behçet's disease

Diagnosis

- History
  - Length of presence of symptoms, possible associated medical co-morbidities
  - Vulvar irritants: Dyes, antiseptics, wipes, semen, saliva, detergents, pads, topical medications, vasoline
- Exam: Look for lesions, surrounding skin change, associated discharge
- Low threshold for biopsy! (punch, shave, or snip)

Vulvar care

- Avoid tight-fitting clothing, scented lotions/detergents/soaps, douching, chronic pad wearing;
- Wear cotton underwear or no underwear; pat vulva dry after bathing

Common Dermatoses

Vulvovaginal Atrophy

- Presentation: Skin is pale, thin, and dry; may be friable, generally minimal discharge, but severe atrophy may result in purulent discharge, skin fissures, etc
- Management
  - Topical estrogen: *Estring, Vagifem, Premarin*
  - Vaginal moisturizers: *Replens, Gyne-moistrin, Moist again, K-Y, Luvena*
  - Vaginal lubrication (with intercourse): Water-based (*K-Y, Astroglide*), silicone-based (*Millennium*, etc)

Lichen Sclerosus

- Presentation: White plaques/patches, may coalesce; obliteration of anatomy, labial fusion, fissures; failure to treat may result in disease progression; malignancy (squamous cell carcinoma) develops in approximately 4%
- Management: Clobetasol 0.05% ointment (cream may be irritating) nightly for 6–12 weeks; follow-up exam, then maintenance two times per week; should be examined yearly at a minimum

Lichen Planus

- Presentation: Chronic discharge, intense pruritis, bright, erythematous papules, possible white striae; possible erosions, labial agglutination

- Management: High-potency topical corticosteroids (Clobetasol, hydrocortisone suppository, etc) for initial approximately 12-week period followed by maintenance dosing; disease progression can otherwise result in adhesions with progression to vaginal obliteration; less clear association with malignancy

Vulvar Intraepithelial Neoplasia (VIN)

- Presentation: Pruritis, ulceration, warty growth, white patch, skin thickening (varies); perform vulvar colposcopy (soak gauze with 3% acetic acid, apply to area for approximately 5 minutes), biopsy acetowhite areas/those with increased vascularity, etc; caused by HPV
- Management options
  - Wide local excision/vulvectomy
  - Laser ablation
  - Topical medicine (imiquimod—*Aldara*)

VULVAR CYSTS/ABSCESSES

Bartholin's Gland Cyst/Abscess

- Location: Drain at 4 and 8 o'clock within vaginal orifice
- Cysts generally benign; may regress spontaneously; treat if symptomatic or if persistent in women 40 years of age or older (small risk of adenocarcinoma)
- *Management*
  - Incision and Drainage (I&D) (biopsy base if over 40 years of age)
  - I&D/possible biopsy/Word catheter (Figure 2-20)
    - Fill catheter balloon with approximately 3 cc saline and leave in place 2–4 weeks to promote epithelialization of tract
  - Marsupialization
  - Excision (definitive); risks extensive blood loss
  - Consider culture and oral antibiotics if infected (clindamycin or trimethoprim/sulfamethoxazole (*Bactrim*), etc)
  - Consider sitz baths for vulvar care

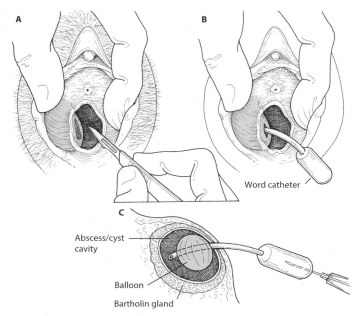

Figure 2-20 Bartholin's abscess—insertion of the Word catheter. **A.** Make a 0.5-cm-long stab incision on the mucosal surface of the labia minora. **B.** The cavity has been evacuated and the Word catheter inserted. **C.** The balloon is inflated with saline. (Used with permission from Kelly EW, Magilner D. Chapter 147. Soft tissue infections. In: Tintinalli JE, et al., eds. *Tintinalli's Emergency Medicine: A Comprehensive Study Guide.* 7th ed. New York, NY: McGraw-Hill; 2011.)

Gartner's Duct Cyst

- Location: Remnants of mesonephric ducts; found most commonly within lateral vaginal wall; may also present as predominantly anterior or posterior vaginal cysts
- May communicate with a ureterocele; consider MRI with contrast for characterization prior to excision of vaginal cyst

Skene Gland Cyst/Abscess

- Location: Inferior/para-urethral ductal drainage; cysts typically more anterior in location; located at distal urethra; often distort meatus
- Differential diagnosis: Urethral diverticulum

Hidradenitis Suppurativa

- Chronic, papular abscesses forming proximal to aprocine glands; managed with antibiotics, topical care, or surgical excision

Epidermal Inclusion Cyst

- Benign, well-circumscribed, superficial masses of labia/mons

Vulvar Abscess

- Risk factors: Obesity, shaving, diabetes/immunocompromised states, poor hygiene
- Diagnosis: Painful vulvar mass; examine to determine extent of involvement/stability of patient; consider imaging with CT scan with and without contrast, especially if diabetic or immunocompromised—increased risk of necrotizing fasciitis
- *Management*
  - Conservative follow-up/oral antibiotics (trimethoprim/sulfamethoxazole, cefazolin, clindamycin): Abscess less than 2 cm, unable to drain (no fluctuant area), stable; warm compresses, sitz baths
  - I&D: For abscesses over 2 cm, superficial fluctuance, immunocompromised; consider admission, IV antibiotics, drainage in OR, packing for larger abscesses, unstable patients

Gynecologic Oncology

PERIOPERATIVE CONSIDERATIONS AND COMPLICATIONS

Bowel Obstruction

Small Bowel Obstructions (SBO)

- Workup may include imaging (abdominal x-ray, CT scan), CBC, CMP, lactate level
- Trial of conservative (nonsurgical) management appropriate if no evidence of perforation, ischemia, or strangulation
  - Bowel rest and **decompression with nasogastric (NG) tube** are appropriate first steps
  - Start GI prophylaxis with Ranitidine (*Zantac*) 50 mg IV every 8 hours or proton pump inhibitor [eg, pantoprazole (*Protonix*)]
  - Replace NG tube output [1 cc NS (or LR) per cc NG tube output every 4 hours] and replete electrolyte losses

Note: *If obstruction occurs acutely within 1 week of surgery, high likelihood of requiring surgical intervention*

- If conservative management fails
  - Consider risks/benefits of surgical intervention: Consent for exploratory laparotomy, possible bowel resection, possible bypass, possible ostomy
  - Consider preoperative Gastrografin enema to rule out concurrent large bowel obstruction (LBO)
  - Surgery not appropriate in patients with poor prognostic criteria (ie, diffuse intra-abdominal carcinomatosis, multifocal obstruction, poor performance status, or massive ascites)

Note: *For women with ovarian cancer and bowel obstruction, data show 90% relieved with surgery, but major morbidity (fistulas and anastomotic leaks) occurred in 32% and perioperative death in 15%. Re-obstruction rate of 10–50%*

- If the patient is not a surgical candidate, consider percutaneous endoscopic gastrostomy (PEG) tube
  - Octreotide (100-300 µg subcutaneously 2-3 times daily) can decrease gastric secretions and slow intestinal mobility → decreases nausea/vomiting associated with SBO
  - Obstruction at cancer diagnosis and mucin histology are associated with recurrent obstructions

Large Bowel Obstruction (LBO)

- Rare in ovarian cancer patients
- In general, considered a surgical emergency
- Surgical management generally involves creation of an ostomy
- Endoscopic management with rectal stent is possible in select patients (stable, no peritoneal signs, partially obstructed, poor surgical candidate)

Closed Loop Obstruction

- In general, considered a surgical emergency
- Commonly due to adhesions. Occurs when two points along the small bowel are obstructed at the same junction, causing necrosis and edema of the internal segment
- May look like a gasless abdomen on plain films. CT usually diagnostic and may show ground glass haziness in mid-abdomen, displacement of adjacent bowel, dilated clumps of edematous bowel, or classic U or C signs (pathognomonic)

Constipation

First-Line Medications

- Bisacodyl (*Dulcolax*) 10 mg orally daily or 10 mg per rectum daily
- Docusate sodium (*Colace*) 100 mg orally twice daily
- Mineral oil 15–45 mL/day
- Cascara 325 mg orally nightly

Second-Line/More Aggressive Medications

- Polyethylene glycol (*MiraLax*) 240–720 mL/day
- Lactulose 15–30 mL twice daily
- Sorbitol 120 mL of 25% solution daily
- Glycerin 3 g per rectum daily or 5–15 mL enemas

Remember: *All patients on around-the-clock opiates should be on a bowel regimen*

Antimotility Agents

- Consider in patients with high-output ileostomies or short bowel syndrome in order to avoid dehydration and other electrolyte abnormalities, including hypocalcemia, hypomagnesemia, or hypokalemia
- Be mindful of stoma outputs greater than 1000 cc/day
- Loperamide (*Imodium*) 2 mg orally three times daily
- Diphenoxylate/atropine (*Lomotil*)—requires narcotic prescription—2.5 mg orally three times daily
- Tincture of opium 6 mg orally four times daily—sometimes in drop form (2 drops three times daily may be sufficient)—requires narcotic prescription

Note: Patient education on self-management is crucial

Electrolyte Abnormalities

Potassium

Hypokalemia (serum potassium <3.5 mEq/L)

Causes

- **Transcellular shift:** Metabolic alkalosis, insulin, β agonists
- **Extrarenal:** Decreased K intake, GI losses including vomiting and diarrhea
- **Renal:** Diuresis, hyperaldosterone (primary, secondary), increased glucocorticoids (Cushing's syndrome), renal tubule disease (renal tubular acidosis)

Signs and Symptoms

- Diffuse muscle weakness; change in mental status
- ECG changes: Earliest change is flattened T waves, followed by inversion, U waves may be visible, ST-segment depression, arrhythmias
- Check magnesium as *hypo*magnesemia can cause refractory hypokalemia. Magnesium level must be corrected for potassium repletion to be effective

Treatment

- *<3 mEq/L:* 40 mEq KCl IV minibag over 4 hours (administer twice)
- *3.0–3.5 mEq/L:* 40 mEq KCl IV minibag over 4 hours once, or 40 mEq potassium chloride (*KDur*) orally every 4 hours
- *<2.5 mEq/L:* Obtain ECG and replace as above
- Do not replace faster than 10 mEq/h.
- Serum K rises approximately 0.1 for every 10 mEq given

Hyperkalemia

Causes

- **Transcellular shift:** Metabolic acidosis, insulin deficiency, β blockers, tissue damage
- **Extrarenal:** Excessive potassium intake
- **Renal:** Hypoaldosteronism, acute or chronic renal failure
- **Other:** Decreased volume, K-sparing diuretics
- Pseudo-hyperkalemia may be caused by blood draw secondary to hemolysis

Signs and Symptoms

- ECG changes: Increased T wave amplitude, prolonged PR interval, increased QRS duration, loss of P waves, sine wave pattern, ventricular fibrillation, asystole (Figure 3-1)

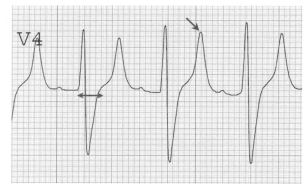

Figure 3-1 EKG in hyperkalemia. (Used with permission from Ritchie JV, Juliano ML, Thurman R. Chapter 23. ECG Abnormalities. In: Knoop KJ, Stack LB, Storrow AB, Thurman R., eds. *The Atlas of Emergency Medicine*. 3rd ed. New York, NY: McGraw-Hill; 2010.)

Treatment

- Calcium gluconate 1 g over 2-3 minutes (decreases membrane excitability)
- Insulin/Glucose (shifts into cells)
  - Ex: Insulin 10 units followed by 1 amp D50, then D5-NS at 50 cc/h for 6 hours
  - *OR* 4 units insulin after 1 L bolus D5
- Kayexalate (binds potassium)
- Dialysis

Calcium

Hypocalcemia

- Ca <8.4 mg/dL. Calcium gluconate 1 gram over 2 hours, or CaCO$_3$ 650 mg orally three times daily
- Need to correct Ca for serum albumin: for every 1.0 decrease in albumin less than 4.0, add 0.8 to Ca to replace for corrected calcium <8.4 mg/dL

Hypercalcemia

Differential Diagnosis

- Primary hyperparathyroidism, malignancy, thyrotoxicosis, chronic kidney disease, milk alkali syndrome, hypervitaminosis D, sarcoidosis, lithium, thiazide diuretics, pheochromocytoma, adrenal insufficiency, rhabdomyolysis/acute renal failure, theophylline toxicity, familial hypocalciuric hypercalcemia, metaphyseal chondrodysplasia, congenital lactase deficiency
- In cancer, hypercalcemia is often associated with advanced disease and poor outcomes
- Labs
  - Serum parathyroid hormone (PTH) (if elevated, primary hyperparathyroidism is diagnosis). There is an increased frequency of primary hyperparathyroidism in the oncology population, so this is reasonable to evaluate
  - If serum PTH is low/normal, send PTH-related protein and vitamin D metabolites (calcidiol and calcitriol) to evaluate for hypercalcemia of malignancy and vitamin D intoxication.
  - Consider bone scan if you suspect malignancy
  - Additional labs that may be useful if picture still unclear: Serum and urinary protein electrophoresis (for possible multiple myeloma), TSH, vitamin A, serum phosphate, urinary 24 hour calcium

Treatment

- Patients who are symptomatic, have an acute rise, or who have a calcium concentration over 14 mg/dL (3.5 mmol/L) require treatment
  - Isotonic saline at 200–300 cc/h (corrects hypovolemia and urinary salt wasting), tapered down to urine output of 100–150 mL/h. Monitor carefully especially in patients with edema/heart/kidney problems. If edema develops, stop IV fluids and consider loop diuretic
  - Calcitonin 5 IU/kg IM every 12 hours, but can increase to 6–8 IU/kg every 6 hours. Tachyphylaxis develops in 48 hours. Nasal calcitonin is not efficacious
  - Bisphosphonates (maximal effect occurs in 2–4 days)

Magnesium

- *Replacement* (keep Mg above 1.7 mEq/L)
  - *<1 mEq/L:* MgSO$_4$ 6 g IV minibag over 6 hours
  - *1.1–1.3 mEq/L:* MgSO$_4$ 4 g IV minibag over 4 hours
  - *1.4–1.6 mEq/L:* MgSO$_4$ 2 g IV minibag over 2 hours
  - Oral: Magnesium oxide 400 mg orally three times daily

Phosphorus

- *Replacement*
  - Phos <2.7 mg/dL: K-phos or Na-phos 15–20 mmol IV minibag over 6 hours. If taking orally, Neutra-Phos 250 mg orally three times daily
- Neutra-Phos contains approximately 8 mmol Phos/250 mg and 7 mEq K/250 mg
- Hyperphosphatemia may be seen in patients with chronic kidney disease. These patients should typically be on calcium acetate (*PhosLo*)

Sodium

Hyponatremia (Figure 3-2)

- Calculate serum osmolality: $2 \times Na + glucose/18 + BUN/2.8$
  - Osm >295 (Hypertonic): Hyperglycemia or mannitol treatment
  - Osm 280–295 (Normal): Increased lipids
  - Osm <280 (Hypotonic): Evaluate volume status, check urine Na
- Prevent central pontine myelinolysis—don't correct too quickly
- **Syndrome of Inappropriate Antidiuretic Hormone Secretion (SIADH):** A condition when excess ADH is excreted, typically resulting in decreased urine output, hyponatremia
  - Treatment: Find the underlying cause that can be due to CNS disturbances of malignancy (especially lung). Treat the underlying cause and correct the sodium slowly with normal saline

Quick Reference Materials

- IV fluid formulations and electrolyte content (Table 3-1)
- Quick Management Guide (Table 3-2)

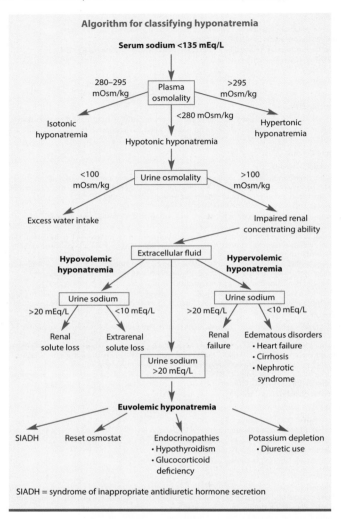

Figure 3-2 Hyponatremia. (Reprinted with permission from Douglas I. Hyponatremia: why it matters, how it presents, how we can manage it. *Cleve Clin J Med* 2006; 73(suppl 3):S4-S12. Copyright © 2006 Cleveland Clinic Foundation. All rights reserved.)

TABLE 3-1 IV FLUID FORMULATIONS

Solution	pH	Na⁺ (mEq/L)	Cl⁻ (mEq/L)	K⁺ (mEq/L)	Ca⁺² (mg/dL)	Lactate (mEq/L)	Glucose (g/L)	Osm (mOsm/L)
0.9% NS	5.0	154	154	0	0	0	0	308
LR	6.5	130	109	4	3	28	0	275
D₅W	4.0	0	0	0	0	0	50	252
D₅ ½ NS (0.45% NS)	4.5	77	77	0	0	0	50	406

TABLE 3-2 ELECTROLYTE ABNORMALITIES:
QUICK MANAGEMENT GUIDE

Cause	EKG Changes	Management
Hypokalemia (<3.5 mEq/L)		
Transcellular shift Diuretics Renal loss NG tube Magnesium depletion Diarrhea Insulin	T wave inversion/ flattening U waves ST depression	Replete Mg and K
Hyperkalemia (>5.5 mEq/L)		

Transcellular shift
Acidosis
Beta blockers
Digoxin
NSAIDs
Heparin
ACE inhibitors
Succinylcholine
Transfusion
Renal insufficiency
Adrenal insufficiency
Potassium-sparing diuretics
	Peaked T waves
	Flattened P waves
	
	More severe
	  Prolonged PR
	  Prolonged QRS
	  Asystole
		Membrane antagonism
		  Calcium gluconate (if unstable)
		  Calcium chloride (if severe)
		
		Transcellular shift
		  Insulin/glucose (if stable)
		  Beta 2 adrenergic antagonist
		  NaHCO₃
		
		Enhanced clearance
		  Dialysis
		  Lasix
		  Kayexalate

Hypocalcemia (< 8.4 mg/dL)		
Magnesium depletion Sepsis Alkalosis Blood transfusion Aminoglycosides Heparin Renal failure Pancreatitis Hypoparathyroidism Tumor lysis syndrome	Prolonged QT Ventricular tachycardia	Replete calcium
Hypercalcemia (>12 mg/dL)		
Hyperparathyroidism Malignancy	Shortened QT interval	Administer NS Lasix Hydrocortisone Bisphosphonate Calcitonin Mithramycin (Plicamycin) Dialysis DO NOT GIVE D5W

(Continued)

TABLE 3-2 ELECTROLYTE ABNORMALITIES:
QUICK MANAGEMENT GUIDE (*Continued*)

Cause	EKG Changes	Management
Hyponatremia (<135 mEq/L)		

Hypovolemic
  Extrarenal loss (*Urine Na < 10*)
  Vomiting, diarrhea
  Renal loss (*Urine Na >20*)
  Renal tubular acidosis
  Diuretics, adrenal insufficiency
 	
Normovolemic
  Water intoxication (*Urine Na < 10*);
  SIADH (*Urine Na >20, Urine Osm >100*)
  Steroid deficiency, stress, sepsis
 	
Hypervolemic
  Heart, liver (*Urine Na < 20*), kidney failure (*Urine Na >20*)
		Hypovolemic
		  NS or hypertonic saline if symptomatic
		Normovolemic
		  Fluid restriction, demeclocycline
		Hypervolemic
		  Fluid restriction or IV fluids ± Lasix
		  Rapid correction: Demyelination

Hypernatremia (>145 mEq/L)		

Hypovolemic
  Loss of hypotonic fluid
 	
Normovolemic: (ADH defect)
  Diabetes insipidus, head injury, nephrogenic
Hypervolemic: Salt, NaHCO$_3$ infusion
		Hypovolemic: Slow fluids with NS/albumin, then free water
		Normovolemic: Free water
		Hypervolemic: Lasix versus observation
		Rapid correction → cerebral edema

Hypomagnesemia		
Lasix Aminoglycosides Cisplatin Alcohol Diabetes Acute myocardial infarction Diarrhea	Torsades de pointes Prolonged QT	Magnesium repletion
Hypermagnesemia		
Renal insufficiency Hemolysis Diabetic ketoacidosis Adrenal insufficiency Hyperparathyroidism Lithium intoxication		Dialysis Calcium gluconate NS/Lasix
Hypophosphatemia		
Glucose loading Sepsis Respiratory alkalosis Diabetic ketoacidosis Beta receptor agonists		Phosphate repletion (Na-Phos or K-Phos) *Very important in liver resection*
Hyperphosphatemia		
Associated with hypocalcemia		

Imaging for Oncology Patients

- CT Scan: Sensitive to tumors approximately 1–2 cm
- PET Scan: Sensitive to approximately 8 mm
- Contrast Dye Allergy
  - Pre-treat with Prednisone 40 mg orally 24 hours before scan, 12 hours before, and immediately before scan
- Elevated Creatinine: Be particularly careful in patients with glomerular filtration rate (GFR) < 60mL/min or creatinine 1.5 or above (especially if diabetic). If there are no contraindications to volume expansion, pre-treat with IV isotonic bicarbonate (6 mL/kg) 1 hour prior to the procedure and 1 mL/kg/h for 6–12 hours following the procedure (longer for patients with severe renal impairment). If isotonic saline (1 mL/kg/h) is used, this can also be administered 6 hours prior to and 6 hours after the procedure

Pulmonary Embolism (PE)

- Clinical suspicion: Dyspnea, tachycardia, hypoxia, sense of impending doom
- *Workup*
  - Arterial Blood Gas (ABG)—look for A-a gradient *[A-a grad = 148 − 1.2 (Pa_{CO_2}) − Pa_{O_2}]*
    - Equation presumes patient is breathing room air at sea level ($F_{IO_2} = 0.21$)
    - A-a gradient is influenced by age and inspired oxygen. A normal gradient rises with age. Can be as high as 25–35 mm Hg for patients over age 40
    - *For patients on supplemental O_2, the normal A-a gradient increases 5–7 mm Hg for every 10% increase in F_{IO_2}*
  - ECG if tachycardic
  - Chest x-ray to look for another cause of desaturation
  - Spiral CT of chest
- Lower extremity Dopplers to evaluate for DVT
  - **Wells Criteria:** Determine likelihood of PE (>4 points—very likely)

• Clinical signs/symptoms of DVT	3 points
• Other causes of desaturation unlikely	3 points
• Heart rate over 100 bpm	1.5 points
• Immobilization >3 days *OR* surgery in past 4 weeks	1.5 points
• Previous DVT/PE	1.5 points
• Hemoptysis	1 point
• Malignancy	1 point

- *Treatment*
  - LMWH or UFH drip are equivalent treatment; then transition to warfarin (*Coumadin*) if appropriate (start 5 mg orally daily for 2 days, then adjust according to INR)
  - *LMWH:* Enoxaparin (*Lovenox*) 1 mg/kg SQ every 12 hours
    - LMWH doesn't require monitoring or dose adjustment but has longer half-life (which makes it more difficult to have lines placed, epidurals pulled, etc)
  - *UFH*
    - BE CAREFUL BEFORE STARTING HEPARIN BOLUS ON POST-OP PATIENT DUE TO BLEEDING RISK!! CONSIDER STARTING MAINTENANCE DOSE ONLY
    - *To Start UFH Treatment*
      - Baseline labs: aPTT/PT/INR, CBC, basic metabolic panel
      - Monitor CBC daily until UFH is discontinued
      - If CBC is normal for 7 consecutive days, can decrease frequency of obtaining lab to not less than every 3 days up to day 14. If stable at that point, can obtain weekly
      - See Table 3-3 for UFH Nomogram

TABLE 3-3 UFH NOMOGRAM

Heparin Nomograms	aPTT Goal
Standard: Atrial fibrillation, VTE, arterial thromboembolism, mechanical valve, obstetric VTE prophylaxis, peripheral vascular disease	50–80 seconds
Low: Age over 70, pulmonary hypertension, ischemic stroke in patient with atrial fibrillation, patient with acute coronary syndrome (including those on GP IIB/IIIA inhibitors or fibrinolytics)	50–65 seconds
High: Vascular surgery patients	65–80 seconds
Postsurgical: Ventricular assist device patients, organ transplant patients (main difference between this nomogram and low goal is the lack of bolus)	50–65 seconds

- Anti-Xa UFH activity
  - Measures anticoagulant activity of UFH directed against factor Xa
  - Not affected by lupus anticoagulant, factor VIII or XII activity, warfarin levels
  - No lot-to-lot variations
  - Studies have shown that patients monitored with Anti-Xa UFH activity can achieve therapeutic levels more quickly and require fewer monitoring tests compared to patients monitored with aPTT
  - Therapeutic range remains constant (0.3–0.7 IU/mL)
  - Drawn every 6 hours after initiation of therapy (or dose change) until two therapeutic levels are obtained, then daily
  - CAREFUL: There are Anti-Xa LMWH tests (for monitoring LMWH) and Anti-Xa UFH tests (for monitoring UFH)
- **Transitioning**
  - *Transition from UFH to LMWH*
    - Discontinue UFH concurrently with first dose of LMWH
  - *UFH or LMWH to Warfarin Transition*
    - During treatment of acute thrombosis, UFH (or LMWH) is continued for at least 5 days and the INR needs to be in goal range for at least 24 hours before UFH (or LMWH) is discontinued
      - *Remember: Warfarin dose is not reflected in INR for 2–3 days post dose change; daily increases in dose are not recommended*
- **Choice of long-term anticoagulant**
  - Warfarin relies on a steady intake of vitamin K, and cancer patients have wide fluctuations in their dietary habits for a variety of reasons (chemotherapy, bowel obstructions, etc). Some data suggest that cancer patients have improved outcomes with LMWH compared to warfarin. However, LMWH is very expensive
  - See Table 3-4 for trials on anticoagulation

TABLE 3-4 ANTICOAGULATION TRIALS

Trials	Conclusions
CLOT trial	RCT—dalteparin associated with half the risk of recurrent VTE in cancer patients compared to warfarin
CANTHANOX trial	RCT—warfarin associated with a statistically significant increased risk of bleeding and twice the risk of recurrent VTE (but this was not statistically significant) when compared with Lovenox.
Cochrane review	LMWH compared to vitamin K antagonists (ie, warfarin)—LMWH associated with less recurrent VTE, but no change in overall survival or bleeding

RCT, randomized controlled trial.

Blood Transfusions

Blood Products
- **Packed Red Blood Cells (PRBCs):** Most plasma has been removed; total volume of 1 unit of PRBCs is about 250–300 cc; hematocrit should increase by 3% or hemoglobin by 1 g/dL
- **Platelets:** 1 "pack" (6 units) should raise the count by 5000–8000.
- When to transfuse platelets
  - Part of resuscitation with PRBCs
  - Platelets less than 10 000 (to prevent spontaneous hemorrhage)
  - Platelets less than 50 000 if about to undergo procedure, are actively bleeding, or have a qualitative platelet disorder
  - Platelets less than 100 000 (in patients with CNS injury, multisystem trauma, undergoing neurosurgery, or who require an intrathecal catheter)
  - Normal platelet count but ongoing bleeding and a reason for platelet dysfunction (congenital disorder, chronic aspirin therapy, uremia)
- **Cryoprecipitate:** Contains Factor VIII, Factor XIII, von Willebrand's Factor, and fibrinogen. One unit is about 10 cc
- **Fresh Frozen Plasma (FFP):** Contains clotting factors. FFP must be thawed in a 37 degree C waterbath. This usually takes about 30 minutes. FFP has only a 24-hour shelf life; therefore, it is best ordered the same day it will be used. One unit is about 150–250 cc

Transfusion
- When transfusing PRBCs
  - **Premedicate with (prior to each unit)**
    - Tylenol 650 mg orally/rectally once
    - Diphenhydramine (*Benadryl*) 25 mg orally/IV once
  - Each unit should be run in over 3–4 hours

- Premedication does not necessarily decrease febrile non-hemolytic transfusion reactions
- Patients with cardiac risk factors may need furosemide (*Lasix*) (10–20 mg) in between units to prevent volume overload (avoid *Lasix* in the sulfa-allergic patients)
- When replacing large volumes of PRBCs, replace platelets and FFP accordingly
- For acute blood loss anemia, contemporary protocols suggest a 1:1 or 1:2 replacement of PRBCs: FFP
- In an emergency, anyone can receive type O PRBCs (preferably O negative), and type AB individuals can receive PRBCs of any ABO type. People with type O blood are "universal donors," and those with type AB blood are "universal recipients." In addition, AB plasma donors can give to all blood types

Risks of Transmission (Table 3-5)

TABLE 3-5 RISKS OF TRANSMISSION

Hepatitis C virus	1:1.6 million
Hepatitis B virus	1:180 000
Human immunodeficiency virus	1:1.9 million
Fatal red cell hemolytic reaction	1:250 000-1.1 million
Delayed red cell hemolysis	1:1 000–1 500
Transfusion-related acute lung injury (TRALI)	1:5 000
Febrile red cell nonhemolytic reaction	1:100
Allergic (urticarial reaction)	1:100
Anaphylactic reaction	1:150 000

Used with permission from Jones HW, Rock JA. control of pelvic hemorrhage. in Rock JA, Jones HW (eds.) *Te Linde's Operative Gynecology*. 9th ed. Philadelphia, PA: Lippicott Williams and Wilkins, 2003.

CRITICAL CARE

Mechanical Ventilation—The Basics

Conventional Mechanical Ventilation
- Improves gas exchange and decreases the work of breathing
- Classified by manner in which inspiration is terminated. Most common are
  - Volume—cycled
  - Pressure—cycled
  - Flow—cycled
  - Time—cycled
- Majority of postsurgical patients will be on volume-cycled ventilation with pressure support

Volume-Cycled Ventilation
- Inspiratory phase terminated after delivery of a preset tidal volume
- Physician sets inspiratory flow, tidal volume, and respiratory rate
- Airway pressure and inspiratory time are patient related
- Three common modes of volume-cycled ventilation
  - **CMV: *Controlled Mechanical Ventilation***
    The minute ventilation is completely a function of the preset respiratory rate and tidal volume. Patient's efforts do not contribute to ventilation. Suitable for a patient making no respiratory effort
  - *A/C: Assist-Control*
    The ventilator responds to patient's inspiratory effort by supplying a preset tidal volume. A control mode backup ensures against hypoventilation
  - *IMV: Intermittent Mandatory Ventilation*
    A preset tidal volume and respiratory rate triggers automatically at timed intervals. Most of these mechanical breaths are synchronized with an inspiratory effort by the patient [synchronized intermittent mandatory ventilation (SIMV)]

Flow-Cycled Ventilation
- Triggered by patient's inspiration; tidal volume and respiratory rate are **not** set
- Inspiration is terminated when a set flow rate is reached
- Pressure support [eg, positive end expiratory pressure (PEEP)] is a flow-cycled ventilation
- Preset pressure is sustained until the patient's inspiratory flow tapers to a set percentage of its maximum value
- Pressure support decreases the work of breathing; requires the patient to initiate their own breath
- Useful in combination with SIMV when weaning a patient

Settings
- Tidal volume: Approximately 8 mL/kg ideal body weight. Inversely proportional to $Paco_2$. This does not apply to patients on an acute respiratory distress syndrome (ARDS) protocol. $Paco_2$ is affected by minute ventilation and tidal volume
- Respiratory Rate: Product of respiratory rate and tidal volume is minute ventilation. Usually between 12 and 16 per minute
- Trigger mode: Ventilator senses negative airway pressure and responds with a "triggered" breath. Usual sensitivity is –1 to –3 cm H_2O
- PEEP: Improves V/Q matching and therefore gas exchange
- Fio_2: Always attempt to minimize while maintaining SaO_2
- Flow rate: Adjusted to provide appropriate I/E ratio, typically 1:3

ARDS Criteria
- Hypoxemic respiratory failure
- Chest x-ray typically reveals bilateral alveolar infiltrates
- Often accompanied with acute respiratory alkalosis and high A-a gradient
- Pulmonary Capillary Wedge Pressure (PCWP) less than 18 is classic; however, not on updated criteria
- Pao_2/Fio_2 less than 300
- Attempt to keep plateau pressures less than 30 cm H_2O
  - Keep tidal volumes low
  - Increase PEEP before Fio_2
- Refer to ARDSnet.org for protocol

Weaning Parameters
- Certain goals must be met prior to weaning patients off the ventilator
- First and foremost, a patient's level of alertness should be assessed prior to extubation—a patient should be alert enough to handle their own secretions and be able to mentate
- Assessing how a patient will do on minimal ventilator settings for a period of time prior to extubation is important—Minimal ventilator settings at our institution are pressure support 5, PEEP 5, Fio_2 40%
- Assessing a patient's volume status prior to extubation is equally important. Patients who have required liters of fluid for resuscitation may benefit from *Lasix* to diurese some of this fluid (and hence increase lung compliance) prior to extubation
- Tobin/RSBI
  - RSBI: Rapid Shallow Breathing Index (ratio of respiratory frequency/tidal volume) of less than 105 breaths/L/min has been associated with weaning success. Patients breathing in large tidal volumes and not hyperventilating will likely have lower RSBIs and an increased chance of weaning off sedation
  - Ideally their respiratory rate is under 25 breaths/min
- NIF: Negative Inspiratory Force more negative than −20 mm Hg is ideal. The NIF measures the strength of respiratory muscles. Tested by asking patients to suck up air through the ET tube
- A positive cuff leak (air moving through the trachea when the cuff is deflated) indicates that laryngeal edema is most likely NOT present; thus, the airway will not be compromised if extubated
- Vital Capacity: For weaning this should be 10–15 mL/kg of ideal body weight, tidal volume 2–3 mL/kg of ideal body weight

Acid–Base Issues

Acid–Base Pearls
- Sepsis: Anion gap metabolic acidosis
- Renal Tubular Acidosis: Non-anion gap metabolic acidosis
- Urinary diversion: Non-anion gap metabolic acidosis
- Vomiting is least likely to produce acidosis
- Prolonged NG tube use can lead to persistent metabolic alkalosis
- Normal values
  - pH: 7.35–7.45
  - HCO_3: 22–26
  - $Paco_2$: 38–42
- Patient Evaluation
  - Acidemic or Alkalemic?
    - Check pH: <7.38 is acidemic; >7.42 is alkalemic
  - Overriding problem respiratory or metabolic?
    - Check $Paco_2$, HCO_3 (Table 3-6)
- If metabolic acidosis present, is there an anion gap? (Check albumin)
  - Anion Gap = Na − (HCO_3 + Cl)
  - Gap: >12; non-gap: <12
  - See Table 3-7

TABLE 3-6 METABOLIC PARAMETERS

HCO₃	PaCO₂	PaCO₂	HCO₃
<24	>40	<40	>24
Metabolic Acidosis	Respiratory Acidosis	Respiratory Alkalosis	Metabolic Alkalosis

TABLE 3-7 METABOLIC ACIDOSIS: ANION GAP VERSUS NON-GAP

Anion Gap (accumulation of organic acid, H+)	Non-anion Gap (loss of HCO₃)
(MUDPILES)	**(HEART CCU)**
Methanol/Metformin	**H**ypoaldosterone/Addison's Disease
Uremia/**Renal failure**	**E**xpansion with IV fluids
Diabetic ketoacidosis	**A**cid ingestion
Paraldehyde	**Renal tubular acidosis**
Iron, isoniazid, inhalants, isopropyl alcohol	**T**urds (diarrhea)
Lactic acidosis, **sepsis**	**C**hronic pyelonephritis
Ethylene glycol	**C**arbonic anhydrase inhibitors (acetazolamide)
Salicylates, aspirin, solvents	**U**rinary diversions, GI losses
Treatment	
Treat underlying cause	Give HCO₃ (if PaCO₂ is less than 20)

- In metabolic disturbances, is the respiratory system compensating?
  - In metabolic acidosis
    - **Check expected Paco₂:** $[1.5 \times HCO_3] + 8 \pm 2$
    - If Paco₂ < predicted, there is a coexisting respiratory alkalosis
    - If Paco₂ > predicted, there is a coexisting respiratory acidosis
  - In metabolic alkalosis
    - If Paco₂ < 40, there is a coexisting primary respiratory alkalosis
    - If Paco₂ > 50, there is a coexisting primary respiratory acidosis
  - If a gap metabolic acidosis, are there other metabolic disturbances present?
    - Check corrected HCO₃: Measure HCO₃ + (anion gap−12)
      - If >24 there is a coexisting primary metabolic alkalosis
      - If <24 there is a coexisting non-gap metabolic acidosis

Acute Renal Failure

- Calculate Fractional Excretion of Sodium (FENa)
- Determines if renal failure is due to prerenal, postrenal, or intrinsic renal pathology (Table 3-8)
- FENa (%) = $[(Urine\ Na \times Plasma\ Cr/Plasma\ Na \times Urine\ Cr) \times 100]$
  - Prerenal: FENa <1%: low volume, pump failure
  - Postrenal: Obstruction (cervical cancer, ureteral injury, etc)
  - Intrinsic: Tubular (granular casts, Urine Na >40, BUN/Cr <15; from ischemia, drugs, rhabdomyolysis); interstitial (white blood cells, eosinophils; from drugs, pyelonephritis); glomerular (RBCs, RBC casts, proteinuria; from post-strep, connective tissue diseases); vascular (vasculitis, DIC, malignant hypertension)

Remember: *Renally dose Vancomycin. Obtain Vancomycin levels after the third dose and 1 hour prior to the fourth dose*

TABLE 3-8 CAUSES OF RENAL FAILURE

	Prerenal	Postrenal	Intrinsic Renal
FENa	<1%		>2–3%
Bun: Creatinine	>20:1	10–20:1	<10:1

Hemodynamics

• Hemodynamic parameters (Table 3-9)
• Types of shock (Table 3-10).

TABLE 3-9 HEMODYNAMIC PARAMETERS

Parameter	Normal Value
Systemic Vascular Resistance (SVR)	800–1200 dynes/s/cm^5
Cardiac Output (CO)	4–8 L/min
Mean Arterial Pressure (MAP)	70–105 mm Hg
Central Venous Pressure (CVP) or Right Atrial Pressure	2–8 mm Hg
Pulmonary Capillary Wedge Pressure (PCWP)	5–12 mm Hg
Pulmonary Artery Pressure (PAP)	15–30 mm Hg

TABLE 3-10 TYPES OF SHOCK

	Mechanism	Measurements	Management	Miscellaneous
Septic shock	Vascular tone is lost in arteries and veins (increased vascular capacitance)	Low PCWP High CO Low SVR Low CVP Low PCWP	Antibiotics Volume Dopamine or norepinephrine *No dobutamine*	TNF-alpha Initiator = IL2
Hemorrhagic shock	Decreased volume, decreased ventricular filling	Low CO High SVR Low CVP	VOLUME! NaHCO$_3$ if acidotic *Avoid pressors*	
Cardiogenic shock	Decreased cardiac function (decreased CO) leads to venous congestion	High PCWP Low CO High SVR High CVP	Dobutamine	ECHO can help differentiate

CERVICAL CANCER

General

• Most common gynecologic malignancy in the world
• Second most frequently diagnosed cancer worldwide after breast cancer
• Third most common gynecologic malignancy in the United States and third most common cause of gynecologic cancer death
• 0.68% lifetime risk of cervical cancer (1 in 147 women) in the United States
• Half of women diagnosed are 35 to 55 years old
• Mean age at diagnosis is 48 years; bimodal distribution with peaks at 35–39 and 60–64 years
• Overall 5-year survival rate (SEER data 1999–2006): 70.2%. If localized, 91%
• Incidence by Race: Hispanic > Black > White > American Indian > Asian/Pacific Islander

Etiology

• Infection: HPV 16, 18, 31, 33, 45, 51–53; HSV, chlamydia likely cofactors
  • HPV 16 accounts for 40–70% of invasive cervical cancers
  • HPV 18 is less prevalent but may be associated with cervical cancers that rapidly progress

Risk Factors

- First intercourse less than age 16 (first intercourse over age 20 reduces risk)
- Multiple partners
- Increased parity
- Cigarette smoking
- Immunosuppression (HIV, Fanconi anemia, chronic steroids, transplant)
- Low socioeconomic status

Types

- *Squamous cell carcinoma:* Keratinizing, nonkeratinizing, verrucous, condylomatous, papillary, lymphoepithelioma-like
- *Adenocarcinoma:* Mucinous (endocervical/intestinal/signet ring type), endometrioid (endometrioid AC with squamous metaplasia), clear cell, serous, minimal deviation (endocervical/ endometrioid type), mesonephric, well-differentiated villoglandular
- *Other epithelial:* Adenosquamous, glassy cell, mucoepidermoid, adenoid cystic, adenoid basal, carcinoid-like tumor, small cell, undifferentiated

Signs/Symptoms

- Early: Asymptomatic
- Late: Constitutional (anorexia, weight loss, weakness); vaginal bleeding (irregular, postcoital) serosanguineous or yellow discharge; pain (abdominopelvic, low back, dyspareunia); urinary frequency; lower extremity edema; hydronephrosis/acute renal failure; hemoptysis
- Laboratory findings: Anemia, thrombocytosis, elevated creatinine

Diagnosis

- Screening: Pap and HPV testing [see current American Society for Colposcopy and Cervical Pathology (ASCCP) guidelines]
- Diagnosis: Colposcopy with biopsy, endocervical curettage (ECC), excisional procedures (cold knife cone (CKC), loop electrosurgical excision procedure (LEEP))
- Assessing disease status: Ultrasound, abdomen/pelvis CT, MRI, PET/CT

Malignant Spread

- Cervical cancer spreads via
  - Direct invasion into cervical stroma, corpus, vagina, and parametrium
  - Lymphatic spread into cardinal ligament (causing ureteral obstruction), parametrial lymph vessels, lymph nodes of obturator, external iliac, and hypogastric vessels; parametrial, inferior gluteal, and presacral nodes; common iliac, para-aortic, inguinal, supraclavicular nodes (usually left)
  - Hematogenous
  - Intraperitoneal

Staging—CLINICAL (not surgical)

- FIGO standards
  - Permitted: Inspection, palpation, colposcopy, ECC, biopsies of cervix including conization, bladder, rectum, hysteroscopy, cystoscopy, proctoscopy, intravenous urography, and radiographic examination of the chest and skeleton
  - NOT included: Lymphangiograms, arteriograms, CT, MRI, PET, laparoscopy, laparotomy. (But, these may help plan treatment)
- *REVISED FIGO STAGING (2010)* (Table 3-11)
  - Remains a clinically staged disease
  - Use of diagnostic imaging techniques to assess size of primary tumor is encouraged but is not mandatory. Imaging studies improve assessment/treatment of disease, but >80% of cervical cancer occurs where PET/CT/MRI are not readily available
  - Examination under anesthesia, cystoscopy, sigmoidoscopy, and IV pyelography is optional and no longer mandatory
  - Diagnostic excision technique recommended is CKC not LEEP

TABLE 3-11 FIGO STAGING—CERVICAL CANCER

FIGO Staging—Cervical Cancer	
Stage I	**Cancer confined to the cervix**
IA	Invasive cancer which can be diagnosed only by microscopy, with maximum depth ≤5 mm and horizontal spread ≤7mm
IA1	Measured stromal invasion of ≤3 mm in depth and horizontal spread ≤7 mm
IA2	Measured stromal invasion of >3 mm but not >5 mm with horizontal spread ≤7 mm
IB*	Clinically visible lesions limited to cervix or preclinical cancers greater than stage IA2
IB1	Clinically visible lesion ≤4 cm in greatest dimension
IB2	Clinically visible lesion >4 cm in greatest dimension
Stage II	**Cancer invades beyond uterus, but not to pelvic wall or lower third of vagina**
IIA	Without parametrial invasion
IIA1	Clinically visible lesion, extends to the upper third of the vagina, ≤4 cm in greatest dimension
IIA2	Clinically visible lesion, extends to the upper third of the vagina, >4 cm in greatest dimension
IIB	With obvious parametrial invasion
Stage III†	**Cancer extends to pelvic wall and/or involves lower third of vagina and/or causes hydronephrosis or nonfunctioning kidney**
IIIA	Tumor involves the lower third of vagina, with no extension to pelvic wall
IIIB	Extension to pelvic wall and/or hydronephrosis or nonfunctioning kidney
Stage IV	**Cancer extends beyond the true pelvis or involves (biopsy-proven) the mucosa of bladder or rectum (bullous edema does not permit allotment to Stage IV)**
IVA	Spread or growth to adjacent organs (including bladder or rectum)
IVB	Spread to distant organs (liver, lung, distant lymph nodes)

*All macroscopically visible lesions—even with superficial invasion—are allotted to stage IB.
†On rectal examination, there is no cancer-free space between tumor and pelvic wall. All cases with hydronephrosis or nonfunctioning kidney are included, unless known to be due to another cause.
Reproduced, with permission granted by FIGO, from FIGO Committee on Gynecologic Oncology. Revised FIGO staging for carcinoma of the vulva, cervix, and endometrium. *Int J Gynecol Obstet* 2009;105(2):103–4.

Survival Statistics by Stage (Table 3-12)

TABLE 3-12 CERVICAL CANCER SURVIVAL BY STAGE

Stage	Five-Year Survival	Stage	Five-Year Survival
O	92.8%	IIIA	35.4%
IA	93.2%	IIIB	32.4%
IB	80.3%	IVA	16.1%
IIA	63.2%	IVB	14.5%
IIB	58.0%		

Used with permission from Edge S, Byrd DR, Compton, CC, et al. *AJCC Cancer Staging Manual*, 7th ed. Springer, 2010. National Cancer Database.

Surgical Management

• Primary surgical management is limited to stages I–IIA (Table 3-13)
• Advantages to surgical treatment, particularly for younger women: Allows for thorough pelvic/abdominal exploration, individualized therapy plan, and ovarian conservation with transposition out of radiation field

- Ovarian function conserved in fewer than 50% of patients with radiation
- Fertility sparing techniques (Table 3-14)
- Types of hysterectomies (Table 3-15) and differences among the types (Table 3-16) are shown in the tables

TABLE 3-13 SURGICAL MANAGEMENT OF CERVICAL CANCER

	Lymph Node (LN) and Recurrence Risk	Treatment	Miscellaneous
Microinvasive Disease (IA1)	0.5–1.2% LN Mets Recurrence: 1%	Simple Hyst (type I), CKC, or simple trachelectomy. Oophorectomy optional	
Adenocarcinoma	1.5% LN Mets Recurrence: 2.5%		
Stage IA2	5–7% LN Mets Recurrence: 3–5%	Can consider radical trachelectomy with lymphadenectomy and cerclage if fertility preservation is the goal	
Stage IB1	13–15% LN Mets 5 year survival: 90%		In IB–IIA tumors, surgery and radiation are equivalent in terms of survival
Stage IB2	24–44% LN Mets 5 year survival: 70–73%		
Stages IB–IIA			

TABLE 3-14 FERTILITY SPARING TECHNIQUES

Stage	Fertility Sparing Technique
IA1 with Lympho Vascular Space Involvement and IA2	• CKC biopsy with negative margins (preferably not fragmented) with 3 mm negative margins plus pelvic lymphadenectomy and para-aortic lymph node sampling (consider sentinel lymph node mapping) • If margins positive: Repeat CKC or trachelectomy • Radical trachelectomy plus pelvic lymphadenectomy and para-aortic lymph node sampling (consider sentinel lymph node mapping)
IB1	• Radical trachelectomy plus pelvic lymphadenectomy and para-aortic lymph node sampling (consider sentinel lymph node mapping)

TABLE 3-15 TYPES OF HYSTERECTOMIES

Class I	Extrafascial hysterectomy with pubocervical ligament excision	CIN, Stage IA1, IB
Class II	Wertheim's or modified radical with removal of medial half of cardinal and uterosacral ligaments and upper 1–2 cm of vagina, and pelvic lymphadenectomy	Stages IA2 to IB1
Class III	Meigs' or radical with removal of entire cardinal and uterosacral ligaments and upper one-third of vagina, and pelvic lymphadenectomy	Stages IB2 to IIA
Class IV	Extended radical with removal of all periureteral tissue, superior vesical artery, and three-fourth of vagina, and lymphadenectomy	Stages IB (bulky) to IIIB
Class V	Partial exenteration with removal of portions of distal ureter and bladder	Central recurrent cancer involving distal ureter or bladder

TABLE 3-16　DIFFERENCES AMONG HYSTERECTOMIES

	Simple Hysterectomy (Class I)	Modified Radical Hysterectomy (Class II)	Radical Hysterectomy (Class III)
Indications	Microinvasion up to Stage IA1	Stages IA1–IB1	Stage IB1-selected Stage IIA
Uterine artery		Ligated at the level of the ureter	Ligated at the origin
Ureters		Tunneled through the broad ligament	Tunneled through the broad ligament
Cardinal ligaments	Uterine/Cervical border	Divided where the ureter transits the broad ligament	Pelvic sidewall
Uterosacral ligaments	Cervical border	Partially divided	Sacral origin
Vagina	None	1-2 cm margins	Upper one-fourth to one-third
Rectum	None	Below cervix	Below middle vagina
Approach	Laparotomy, Laparoscopy, Robotic-Assisted Laparoscopy		

Pelvic Exenteration (Table 3-17)

• Potential contraindications: Triad of symptoms—unilateral leg swelling, hydronephrosis, sciatic pain (evidence of pelvic side wall involvement)

TABLE 3-17　PELVIC EXENTERATION

Type	Surgery	5-Year Survival Rate
Anterior exenteration	Radical cystectomy, hysterectomy, and vaginectomy	33–60%
Posterior exenteration	Abdominal perineal resection of rectum, radical hysterectomy, and vaginectomy	
Total exenteration	En bloc excision of the bladder, ureter, rectum, and vagina	20–40%

Radiotherapy

• Can be used for the majority of disease stages and for most patients, regardless of age, body habitus, or coexistent medical conditions (Table 3-18)
• Used concurrently with *Cisplatin (40 mg/m²)* as a radiosensitizer. Results in improved disease-free progression and survival compared to radiation alone

TABLE 3-18　RADIOTHERAPY FOR CERVICAL CANCER

External beam radiation therapy (EBRT)	Microscopic: 4500 cGy (180–200 cGy daily) Unresected adenopathy: Can use doses up to 1000–1500 cGy for grossly unresected adenopathy Clinically obvious tumors >6000 cGy	For most patients, concurrent chemotherapy with cisplatin or cisplatin plus 5-Fluorouracil is administered during EBRT
Brachytherapy	Intracavitary approach (intrauterine tandem) and vaginal colpostats (ovoid, ring, or cylinder) (Figure 3-3)	Critical for patients who are not surgical candidates Can be used without EBRT in early disease (stage ≤ IA2). With positive or close margins post-hysterectomy may be useful to use with EBRT as an adjunct

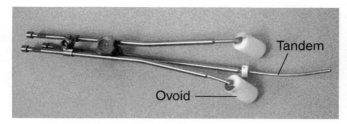

Figure 3-3 Reference points for radiotherapy. (Used with permission from Hoffman BL, et al. Chapter 28. Breech Delivery. In: Hoffman BL, et al., eds. *Williams Gynecology*, 2nd ed. New York, NY: McGraw-Hill; 2012.)

External Beam Radiation Therapy (EBRT)
- Should cover the gross disease (if present) and margins up to at least 3 cm, including presacral nodes and other nodes involved and/or at risk

Brachytherapy
- **Low-dose rate (LDR)** as inpatient over 3–4 days = 40–100 cGy/h. LDR procedures require insertion under anesthesia and hospitalization for radiation safety and patient immobilization. Uses ^{192}Ir or ^{137}Cs
- High-dose rate (HDR) as outpatient over three to five visits = 100 cGy/min. These HDR treatments may be completed under conscious sedation or less with cooperative patients with favorable vaginal anatomy. Uses Tandem and Ring. Uses ^{192}Ir or Cobalt
  - *Advantages*: Decreased treatment time and can be done as an outpatient; disadvantages include need for sedation
- HDR and LDR are equally effective to control tumor and are equivalent in terms of complications

Adjuvant radiation after radical hysterectomy
- High-risk early-stage disease (GOG 109)
  - Positive parametrium
  - Positive lymph nodes
  - Positive margins
- Intermediate-risk early-stage disease (GOG 92)
  - Radical hysterectomy and lymphadenectomy plus adjuvant radiation reduces the number of recurrences in stage IB disease at the cost of increased grade three and four adverse events
  - Lymphovascular Space Involvement (LVSI)
  - Deep stromal invasion (middle or deep third or >1/3 stromal invasion)
  - Tumor >4 cm

Complications of Radiation
- Skin erythema, desquamation, pigment changes, fibrosis, thinning, gland loss, necroses
- Vaginal discharge, shortening, bleeding, dyspareunia
- Radiation cystitis, colovesical, vesicovaginal fistulas
- Radiation enteritis
- Ovarian failure
- Insufficiency fractures, avascular necrosis of the femoral head

Chemotherapy

- Used to treat women with distant metastases, recurrent tumor, or those who have been previously treated with surgery or radiation and are not candidates for exenteration procedures
- Best candidates for chemotherapy are those with an excellent performance status and disease that is both outside of the field of radiation and not amenable to surgical resection
- Cisplatin/paclitaxel (*Taxol*)-current standard of care for recurrent, previously radiated cervical cancer in women who are not exenteration candidates based on GOG 204
- Recent data from GOG 240 shows an overall survival benefit and improved response rates with the addition of Bevacizumab (*Avastin*) to Cisplatin/Taxol in advanced/recurrent disease

Prognostic Factors

Prognosis is worse with:
- older age
- African-American race
- low socioeconomic status
- HIV or other immunocompromised status
- squamous cell histologic subtype
- poorly differentiated histologic grade
- higher FIGO stage
- greater number of positive lymph nodes
- bulky tumor volume
- greater depth of invasion
- LVSI
- pretreatment hemoglobin <12 g/dL

Recurrence (Table 3-19)

- If recurrence occurs, 50% occur within 1 year; 80% within 2 years after initial treatment.
- Recurrence tends to occur most often at the vaginal apex (22–56%), sidewall (28–37%), as opposed to distant metastasis (15–61%)
- Disease within 6 months after therapy = *persistent cancer*
- After 6 months = *recurrence*
- Symptoms: Pain, leg swelling, anorexia, vaginal bleeding, cachexia, psychiatric problems
- If recurs after initial surgical treatment, radiation is usually indicated
- If radiotherapy was the initial treatment, surgery may be indicated
- Distant metastases → palliative chemotherapy, radiation, or both
- Biopsy positive lymph nodes (fine needle aspiration with CT guidance) prior to treatment
- For small, centrally recurrent cervical cancer → pelvic exenteration

TABLE 3-19 RECURRENCE RATES—CERVICAL CANCER

Stage	Pelvic Recurrence Rates after Radiotherapy Alone
1B	10%
2A	17%
2B	23%
3	42%
4A	74%

Used with permission from Perez CA, Grigsby PW, Camel HM, et al. Irradiation alone or combined with surgery in stage IB, IIA, and IIB carcinoma of the uterine cervix: Update of a nonrandomized comparison. *Int J Radiat Oncol Biol Phys.* 1995;31:703–716.

Surveillance—National Comprehensive Cancer Network (NCCN) Guidelines
- Interval H&P every 3–6 months (2 years), 6–12 months (3–5 years), annually (>5 years)
- Annual paps
- Cervical/vaginal cytology annually for lower genital tract dysplasia
- Imaging as indicated by symptoms or examination
- Lab assessment as indicated by symptoms or examination
- Vaginal dilator after radiation therapy
- Patient education regarding recurrence
- Always encourage smoking cessation

Survival
- Stage Distribution and 5-Year Relative Survival by Stage at Diagnosis (Table 3-20)
- Survival Rates in women undergoing irradiation alone or irradiation combined with surgery in stages IB, IIA, and IIB cervical cancers (Table 3-21).

TABLE 3-20 STAGE DISTRIBUTION AND 5-YEAR RELATIVE SURVIVAL BY STAGE AT DIAGNOSIS: CERVIX UTERI CANCER

Stage at Diagnosis	Stage Distribution (%)	Five-Year Relative Survival (%)
Localized	47	91.5
Regional (spread to regional lymph nodes)	36	57.4
Distant (metastasized)	12	16.5
Unknown (unstaged)	4	53.2

Data from SEER 18 2005-2011. http://seer.cancer.gov/statfacts/html/cervix.html. Accessed May 4, 2015.

TABLE 3-21 RADIATION ALONE OR COMBINED WITH SURGERY AGE

Stage	Five-Year Survival Rate with Radiation	Five-Year Survival Rate with Surgery and Radiation	Ten-Year Survival Rate
IB (non-bulky)	90%	85%	84% with either modality
IB (bulky)	61%	66%	61% and 63% with RT versus RT and surgery, respectively
IIA (non-bulky)	75%	83%	66% and 71% with RT versus RT and surgery, respectively

Used with permission from Perez CA, Grigsby PW, Camel HM, et al. Irradiation alone or combined with surgery in stage IB, IIA, and IIB carcinoma of the uterine cervix: Update of a nonrandomized comparison. *Int J Radiat Oncol Biol Phys.* 1995;31:703–716.

OVARIAN CANCER

- Ranks fifth in cancer deaths among women, accounting for more deaths than any other cancer of the female reproductive system
- Lifetime risk is 1:72 or 1.4%
- Epithelial ovarian cancers are most common; ovarian tumors can also be due to germ cell tumors, sex-cord stromal tumors, or mixed cell types
- Metastatic ovarian tumors most commonly due to endometrial cancer, breast cancer, or Krukenberg tumors from the GI tract
- The risk of malignancy in an adnexal mass in a premenopausal woman is 7%, rising to 30% in postmenopausal women
- **FIGO Staging for Primary Carcinoma of the Ovary** (Table 3-22)

TABLE 3-22 FIGO STAGING FOR OVARIAN CANCER

FIGO Staging—Ovarian Cancer	
Stage I	**Tumor confined to ovaries**
IA	Tumor limited to 1 ovary; capsule intact, no tumor on surface, negative washings
IB	Tumor involves both ovaries (otherwise like IA)
IC	Tumor limited to 1 or both ovaries
IC1	Surgical spill
IC2	Capsule rupture before surgery or tumor on ovarian surface
IC3	Malignant cells in the ascites or peritoneal washings
Stage II	**Tumor involves 1 or both ovaries with pelvic extension (below the pelvic brim) or primary peritoneal cancer**
IIA	Extension and/or implant on uterus and/or tubes
IIB	Extension to other pelvic intraperitoneal tissues
Stage III	**Tumor involves 1 or both ovaries with cytologically or histologically confirmed spread to the peritoneum outside pelvis and/or metastasis to retroperitoneal lymph nodes**
IIIA	Positive retroperitoneal lymph nodes and /or microscopic metastasis beyond pelvis
IIIA1	Positive retroperitoneal lymph nodes only IIIA1(i): Metastasis ≤ 10 mm; IIIA1(ii): Metastasis > 10 mm
IIIA2	Microscopic, extrapelvic (above the brim) peritoneal involvement ± positive retroperitoneal lymph nodes
IIIB	Macroscopic, extrapelvic, peritoneal metastasis ≤ 2 cm ± positive retroperitoneal lymph nodes. Includes extension to capsule of liver/spleen
IIIC	Macroscopic, extrapelvic, peritoneal metastasis > 2 cm ± positive retroperitoneal lymph nodes. Includes extension to capsule of liver/spleen
Stage IV	**Distant metastasis excluding peritoneal metastasis**
IVA	Pleural effusion with positive cytology
IVB	Hepatic and/or splenic parenchymal metastasis, metastasis to extraabdominal organs (including inguinal lymph nodes and lymph nodes outside abdominal cavity)

Information reproduced, with permission granted by FIGO from Prat J; for the FIGO Committee on Gynecologic Oncology. FIGO Guidelines. Staging classification for cancer of the ovary, fallopian tube, and peritoneum. *Int J Gynecol Obstet* 2014;124:1-5.

Epithelial Ovarian Cancer (EOC)

Epidemiology

- 85–90% of ovarian cancers are EOCs
- Average age of diagnosis: Mid-50s; occurrence in women under 50 should raise suspicion of hereditary or familial disease
  - *BRCA*1 or *BRCA*2 (lifetime risk of 25–60% and 15–25%, respectively)
  - Lynch II Syndrome (Hereditary nonpolyposis colorectal cancer, HNPCC)

Risk Factors (Table 3-23)

TABLE 3-23 RISK FACTORS FOR OVARIAN CANCER AND ASSOCIATED RELATIVE RISKS

Risk Factor	Relative Risk
Two or three relatives with ovarian cancer	4.6
One first degree relative with ovarian cancer	3.1
Older age	3
Living in North America/Europe	2–5
Higher levels of education/income	1.5–2
White race	1.5
Nulligravity	2–3
Infertility	2–5
Early age at menarche	1.5
Late age at menopause	1.5–2
Perineal talc exposure	1.5–2
Past use of OCPs	0.65
History of hysterectomy	0.5–0.7
History of tubal ligation	0.59
Past pregnancy	0.5

Screening

- Currently, there is no screening test for ovarian cancer, as CA125 can be elevated in a multitude of benign conditions and in other types of cancer
- Therefore, routine screening is *not recommended* except in high-risk women who decline or defer definitive risk-reducing bilateral salpingo-oophorectomy (BSO)
  - Expert opinions recommend a 6-month interval between examinations until prophylactic BSO or hysterectomy/BSO can be performed
- Current recommendation for prophylactic oophorectomy: Perform at completion of childbearing or by age 40 in women with BRCA1 or BRCA2, or Lynch II syndrome

Types of EOC

- *Serous carcinoma*: Accounts for 75% of EOC; the histology resembles the lining of the fallopian tube; psammoma bodies are often seen. Usually high grade, but low-grade variant also possible
- *Mucinous tumors*: Account for 10% of EOC; largest EOCs (average diameter 18–20 cm), but remain confined to the ovaries longer than serous tumors. Histologically resemble endocervical epithelium
- *Endometrioid tumors*: Account for 10% of EOC; resemble endometrial cancer and may arise from endometriosis
- *Brenner tumors*: Benign or malignant; composed of transitional cells
- *Clear cell carcinoma*: Histologically similar to renal cell cancer, associated with hypercalcemia, hyperpyrexia, and VTE, and have early metastasis. Usually unilateral. Histologically both clear cells and hobnail cells (nuclei projected into apical cytoplasm) are seen
- *Mixed carcinomas*: Contain two or more distinct histologic types of cancer with each type involving at least 10% of the tumor; presence of a serous carcinoma or sarcoma gives a worse prognosis

Diagnosis

- *Symptoms* are often nonspecific: Abdominal discomfort and/or distention, bloating, constipation, fatigue, indigestion, urinary frequency, or dyspareunia. Late-stage disease may cause significant abdominal distention, early satiety, and nausea/vomiting due to ascites and bowel or omental metastases. Dyspnea may result from pleural effusions
- *CA125*: Elevated to >65 U/mL (normal is <35 U/mL) in **80%** of women with EOC; usually highest in women with serous tumors
  - CA125 is not specific for ovarian cancer. Can be increased in other malignancies (endometrial and pancreatic cancer), or in benign conditions (endometriosis, fibroids, or PID)
  - Measure baseline before surgery. If elevated pre-operatively, CA125 level can be followed during therapy to assess response
    - A plateau may indicate resistance
    - A rise may indicate recurrence before CT evidence of disease
- *Ultrasound*: Findings concerning for malignancy
  - Solid component, often nodular or papillary, or solid and cystic
  - Thick, enhancing septations (>3 mm), with flow seen on Doppler
  - Presence of ascites
  - Irregular shape
  - Peritoneal masses, enlarged nodes, or matted bowel
- *Radiographic* studies (CT, MRI) may demonstrate areas of metastatic spread; important for surgical planning. If no ascites or no pelvic mass, an extraovarian primary should be considered (breast, GI, pancreatobiliary)

Treatment

Surgery

- Surgical staging and primary surgical **cytoreduction**. Although "optimal" cytoreduction is defined as <1 cm residual disease, every increment below 1 cm results in improved outcomes
- **GOAL is NO residual disease!**
- Neoadjuvant chemotherapy (NACT) may be offered to poor surgical candidates or patients with unresectable disease (eg, diffuse mesenteric involvement). Followed by interval cytoreduction if possible

Surgical Staging (apparent early-stage disease)

- Obtain free fluid (ascites) or washings for cytologic evaluation
- Systematic exploration of all organs and surfaces—bowel, liver, gallbladder, diaphragms, mesentery, omentum, and peritoneum
- If no suspicious areas, take random biopsies from peritoneum of cul-de-sac, gutters, bladder, mesentery, diaphragm
- Omentectomy
- Pelvic and para-aortic lymphadenectomy
- Total Abdominal Hysterectomy (TAH) and BSO. (If fertility desired, can consider uterine and unilateral ovarian conservation in select patients)
- Appendectomy if suspect tumor involvement/mucinous histology
- *Can be performed via minimally invasive approach*

Surgical Cytoreduction (any gross extra-ovarian disease)

- Exploratory laparotomy
- TAH/BSO
- Resection of all visible disease: May include bowel resections, splenectomy, peritonectomy, diaphragm stripping/resection, liver wedge resection, etc
  - **MUST** vaccinate post-splenectomy patients with vaccines against encapsulated organisms (*Streptococcus pneumonia, Haemophilus influenzae*, and *Neisseria meningitidis*). If patients develop sepsis: Vancomycin, Ceftriaxone, and Levofloxacin are indicated
- *IF OPTIMAL RESULT IS NOT ACHIEVABLE, CLOSE PATIENT AND INITIATE NEOADJUVANT CHEMOTHERAPY*

Chemotherapy

- *First-line:* Platinum + Taxane combination therapy
  - GOG 111: IV Cisplatin/Taxol better than cisplatin/cyclophosphamide
  - GOG 157: 3 versus 6 cycles of IV chemo for early ovarian cancer. No statistically significant recurrence or survival benefit but increased toxicity with 6 cycles. However, post-hoc analysis showed statistically improved outcome for EOC but not other histologies with 6 cycles
  - GOG 158: IV carboplatin/paclitaxel (3-hour infusion) not inferior to cisplatin/paclitaxel (24-hour infusion) and *better toxicity profile*. Cisplatin associated with more neurotoxicity, nephrotoxicity, ototoxicity, and GI toxicity. Carboplatin associated with more myelosuppression
  - Dose Dense Taxol: Dose dense weekly paclitaxel with carboplatin improved progression-free survival (PFS) (28 versus 17 months) and overall survival (OS) (72.1% versus 65.1% at 3 years)

compared to conventional carboplatin/taxol. Similar toxicities between groups. Awaiting trials in non-Japanese patients before becoming standard of care
* *Stage III disease:* Intraperitoneal (IP) chemo more effective than IV chemo (*GOG 172*). Only 42% of patients completed 6 cycles of IP arm
  * PFS 18.3 months (IV) versus 23.8 months (IP)
  * OS 49.7 months (IV) versus 65.6 months (IP)
  * Increased GI, bone marrow, neurologic, and infectious toxicities with IP. IP arm with decreased quality of life (QOL) before cycle 4 and 3–6 weeks after, but no difference in QOL at 1 year
  * IP port may be placed at the time of surgery (if no bowel resection performed) or at the time of second-look procedure
  * Complications: Peritonitis and port catheter obstruction
* Bevacizumab: Angiogenesis inhibitor
  * Shows promise as newer targeted therapy (GOG218, ICON7)
* NACT: Chemotherapy before surgery
  * For patients with unresectable disease or poor candidates for cytoreduction
  * European RCT suggests that NACT followed by interval cytoreduction is not inferior as a treatment for bulky stage IIIC or IV ovarian cancer; however, outcomes poor in both arms

Recurrent Disease
* **Platinum sensitive** (>6 months disease free/platinum free)
  * Consider secondary cytoreduction: Ideal candidate has long platinum-free interval, no carcinomatosis, and resectable foci of disease
  * Retreat with platinum (Carboplatin-Gemcitabine, Carboplatin-Doxorubicin (*Doxil*), single agent Carboplatin)
* **Platinum resistant** (recurred within 6 months of last platinum therapy)
  * Chemotherapy options include Liposomal Doxil, Topotecan, Gemcitabine, Paclitaxel, Docetaxel, Vinorelbine, Pemetrexed, Etoposide, Altretamine
  * Noncytotoxic therapies: Bevacizumab, hormonal therapy [tamoxifen, letrozole (*Femara*), anastrozole (*Arimidex*)]
  * Clinical trials

Survival
* Stage Distribution and 5-Year Relative Survival by Stage at Diagnosis (Table 3-24)
* Survival Rates by Stage (SEER data from 1988–2001) (Table 3-25)

TABLE 3-24 STAGE DISTRIBUTION AND FIVE-YEAR RELATIVE SURVIVAL BY STAGE AT DIAGNOSIS: OVARIAN CANCER

Stage at Diagnosis	Stage Distribution (%)	Five-Year Relative Survival (%)
Localized	15	92.1
Regional (spread to regional lymph nodes)	19	73.2
Distant (metastasized)	60	28.3
Unknown (unstaged)	6	22.9

Data from SEER 18 2005-2011. http://seer.cancer.gov/statfacts/html/ovary.html. Accessed May 4, 2015.

TABLE 3-25 SURVIVAL RATES BY STAGE

Stage	One-Year Survival (%)	Five-Year Survival (%)
IA	98.9	94.0
IB	98.0	91.1
IC	92.4	79.8
IIA	96.4	76.4
IIB	88.3	66.9
IIC	80.4	57.0

(Continued)

TABLE 3-25 SURVIVAL RATES BY STAGE   (*Continued*)

Stage	One-Year Survival (%)	Five-Year Survival (%)
IIIA	86.4	45.3
IIIB	81.5	38.6
IIIC	82.2	35.2
IV	61.7	17.9

Hereditary Cancer Syndromes (Table 3-26)

TABLE 3-26 HEREDITARY CANCER SYNDROMES

Syndrome	Associated Cancers	Gene/Location	Other Features
Hereditary breast and ovarian cancer	Breast, ovary Pancreas, gastric, prostate, cervix, uterus	*BRCA1* *17q21*	AD; HR pathway; DNA double-strand repair
	Breast, ovary Pancreas, male breast, prostate, gastric, melanoma, GB, biliary	*BRCA2* *13q12*	AD: HR pathway: DNA double-strand repair
HNPCC	Colon, endometrial, bladder, ovary	*MLH1, MSH2, MSH6, PMS2,* or *EPCAM* Mismatch repair genes, Chromosome 7	AD; Recognize mismatched DNA and trigger excision/repair
Li–Fraumeni	Breast, sarcoma, leukemia, brain, adrenal, colorectal, pancreatic	*TP53* (and *CHEK2*) *17p13.1*	
Cowden	Breast, GI, endometrial, thyroid	*PTEN* *10q23*	AD; Multiple hamartoma syndrome; PTEN mutations
Ataxia telangiectasia	Breast, leukemia, lymphoma Pancreas, stomach cancers	*ATM* *11q22.3*	AR; cerebellar ataxia; dysarthria; endocrine dysfunction; immunodeficiency; telangiectasias
Multiple endocrine neoplasia (MEN) syndrome (type 2b)	*No increased breast cancer* Medullary thyroid cancer	*RET* *10q11.2*	AD; pheochromocytoma; hyperparathyroidism
Peutz–Jeghers	Breast, colon, pancreas, stomach, ovary (sex-cord stromal and granulosa-theca), adenoma malignum	*STK11* *19q13.3*	AD: Intestinal polyposis II (benign tumors of GI and gonads) Sex-cord stromal tumors with annular tubules (SCSTAT) Adenoma malignum cervix Granulosa-theca cell tumors

HR, homologous recombination; AD, autosomal dominant; AR, autosomal recessive; PTEN, phosphatase and tensin homolog gene.

Hereditary Nonpolyposis Colorectal Cancer (HNPCC)
• Also known as Lynch syndrome
• Risk of endometrial cancer in women with HNPCC is 27–41%
• Ovarian cancer risk is 3–14%

- Mutations in MSH2 and MLH1 account for about 90% of the heterozygous germline mutations
- Risks of ovarian cancer vary with mutation [MSH6 (71%), MSH2 (40%), MLH1 (27%)]
- In looking at all endometrial carcinomas, this accounts for 2–5%
  - Consider testing in young women, women with normal BMIs, and those with lower uterine segment involvement
- NCCN guidelines along with the Cancer Genetics Consortium recommends annual endometrial sampling starting at age 30-35, transvaginal ultrasound (for ovarian cancer screening, less for endometrial cancer screening), and colonoscopies every 1-2 years starting at age 20-25

BRCA1/BRCA2
- Autosomal dominant inheritance
- *BRCA1* (chromosome 17q21)
  - Breast cancer risk—60%
  - Ovarian cancer risk—59%
  - Earlier onset of ovarian cancer
- *BRCA2* (chromosome 13q12-13)
  - Breast cancer risk—55%
  - Ovarian cancer risk—16.5%
  - Higher risk of male breast cancer
- Genetic Testing Criteria: Number of affected relatives, degree of relativity between individual patient and affected family members, younger age at diagnosis, personal history of two breast cancer primaries, male breast cancer, and multiple primaries
- Strong association between BRCA mutations and diagnosis of triple negative breast cancer
- Risk-reducing BSO recommended in carriers between ages 35 and 40
  - Decreased Risk of *both* ovarian and breast cancer
- *Surveillance* with twice yearly ovarian cancer screening with transvaginal ultrasound and serum CA125 levels (from age 30 or 5–10 years prior to diagnosis of earliest family member)
- OCPs appear to reduce the risk of ovarian cancer

Germ Cell Tumors

- Derived from the primordial germ cells of the ovary
- Account for 20–25% of all ovarian tumors, but only 3% are malignant; account for less than 5% of all ovarian malignancies
- Usually seen between the ages of 10 and 30
- Symptoms: Abdominal enlargement and/or pain, precocious puberty, symptoms of pregnancy

Types of Germ Cell Tumors
- *Dysgerminoma*
  - 30–40% of non-EOCs
  - 75% occur in ages 10–30 (one-third of all ovarian malignancies in this age group)
  - Bilateral involvement in 10–15% of patients
  - Presentation usually is pain from rapid growth, torsion, or rupture
  - Histologically composed of undifferentiated germ cells; often syncytiotrophoblastic giant cells that produce LDH and placental alkaline phosphatase
- *Endodermal Sinus (Yolk Sac) Tumors*
  - Account for one-fifth of germ cell tumors
  - Average age at presentation is 18; one-third are premenopausal
  - Histologically resembles the endodermal sinuses of the rat yolk sac; derived from primitive yolk sac
  - Produces alpha feto protein (AFP)
  - Histology: Schiller–Duvall bodies
  - Adjuvant chemotherapy almost always indicated
- *Embryonal Carcinoma*
  - 4% of malignant germ cell tumors
  - Average age at diagnosis is 15
  - Aggressive tumor, with high number of mitotic figures on cytology
  - Multinucleated giant cells produce β-hCG, AFP
  - Presentation: Large pelvic mass. May involve precocious puberty, irregular bleeding, hirsutism, or amenorrhea as the tumor may secrete estrogen and/or androgens.
  - Pregnancy tests will be positive.
- *Polyembryoma*
  - Very rare! Usually associated with other germ cell elements
  - Composed of embryoid bodies that resemble normal embryos
  - AFP, β-hCG elevated

- *Immature Teratoma*
  - <1% of malignant germ cell tumors
  - Tissue from all three germ cell layers (ecto-, meso-, endoderm)
  - Graded by the number of neural elements, degree of differentiation, and presence of embryonal tissue
  - Tumor markers/hormonal elevations less likely to be increased because tumors have lost ability to secrete hormones. However, elevations of AFP, LDH, and β-hCG can occur

Treatment

- Surgery: As with EOCs, surgical treatment is dependent on stage of disease and desire for future fertility. Use EOC guidelines. Surgical staging should be performed in the same manner. Consider fertility conservation
- Chemotherapy: bleomycin, etoposide, cisplatin (BEP) is the treatment of choice, and generally gives good results. Other agents sometimes used include vinblastine, vincristine, actinomycin, and cyclophosphamide (*cytoxan*)
  - **Note:** No chemotherapy for stage IA dysgerminoma or stage IA grade 1 teratoma
- Radiation may be used for metastatic disease; dysgerminomas in particular are quite sensitive, and moderate dose radiation of 25–30 Gy in 20–25 fractions is usually sufficient

Sex-Cord Stromal Tumors

- Accounts for 5–8% of all primary ovarian neoplasms
- Usually derived from ovarian cell types, but on occasion testicular or mixed ovarian and testicular cell types occur
- Staging is according to FIGO guidelines for ovarian cancer
- Symptoms: Same as germ cell tumors (mass, precocious puberty, irregular menses/amenorrhea, virilization)

Types of Sex-Cord Stromal Tumors

- *Granulosa-stromal cell tumor*
  - 70% of sex-cord stromal tumors
  - Separated into adult (95%) versus juvenile type based on histology; adult type usually seen in postmenopausal women
    - Adult types possess **Call-Exner bodies** (round, pale cells with "coffee-bean" nuclei in rosettes around a central cavity)
  - Produce inhibin, Müllerian inhibiting substance (MIS). Inhibin can be used to assess response to treatment and as surveillance for recurrence. Tests for MIS not routinely available
  - Endometrial hyperplasia in approximately 20–25% of patients; 5–10% with endometrial cancer
- *Thecomas*
  - Usually benign fibromatous lesions of the stroma; presence of malignancy suggests a fibrosarcoma or diffuse granulosa cell tumor
  - Unilateral
  - Occur mostly in postmenopausal women
  - Usually present with abnormal uterine bleeding due to increased estrogen from theca cells. Endometrial hyperplasia occurs in 15%; carcinoma in 25%
- *Fibromas*
  - Solid tumors of the stroma. Usually benign and unilateral
  - Occur mostly in postmenopausal women
  - Seen in Meigs' syndrome (ovarian fibroma, **ascites**, pleural effusion); ascites thought to be related to secretion of vascular endothelial growth factors. Treatment is surgical excision; recurrence is rare
- *Sertoli–Leydig tumors*
  - Less than 0.5% of all ovarian tumors
  - Average age at diagnosis is 25
  - Presentation is with virilization in one-third of women, including amenorrhea, hirsutism, breast atrophy, acne, and clitoral enlargement; due to the secretion of androgens by tumor
- *Gynandroblastoma*
  - Rare tumor consisting of both Sertoli–Leydig and granulosa cells; at least 10% of tumor must be the minor component
  - May be associated with androgen and/or estrogen production
  - Usually benign; usually treat with unilateral salpingo-oophorectomy

Treatment

- Surgery is the primary treatment for most sex-cord stromal tumors; in most cases, they are confined to one or both ovaries at the time of diagnosis. The guidelines for EOCs can be used to determine appropriate treatment and staging options. In majority of patients (with stage I disease), long-term disease-free survival is 75–90%
- Chemotherapy is not generally recommended for stage I disease, given the good prognosis with surgery alone. However, postoperative chemotherapy has been shown to improve survival in some trials in patients with stages II–IV disease. Chemotherapy should include a platinum agent in combination with other agents such as BEP, Cytoxan, and/or doxorubicin

Markers
- Markers Secreted by Germ-Cell and Sex-Cord Stromal Tumors of the Ovary (Table 3-27)

TABLE 3-27 MARKERS SECRETED BY GERM-CELL AND SEX-CORD STROMAL TUMORS OF THE OVARY

Type	LDH	AFP	hCG	E2	Inhibin	Testosterone	Androgens	DHEA
Dysgerminoma	+	−	−	−	−	−	−	−
Embryonal	−	+/−	+/−	−	−	−	−	−
Immature teratoma	−	−	−	+/−	−	−	−	+/−
Choriocarcinoma	−	−	+	−	−	−	−	−
Endodermal sinus tumor	−	+	−	−	−	−	−	−
Thecoma-fibroma	−	−	−	−	−	−	−	−
Granulosa cell	−	−	−	+/−	+	−	−	−
Sertoli–Leydig	−	−	−	−	+/−	+	+	−
Gonadoblastoma	−	−	−	+/−	+/−	+/−	+/−	+/−

Pseudomyxoma Peritonei (PMP)

- Diffuse collections of gelatinous material
- Mucinous
- Informally referred to as "jelly belly"
- Usually originates from a cystadenoma of the **appendix,** occluding the lumen of the appendix, rupturing, and causing mucin-producing cells to seed the abdomen
- Increased abdominal girth is a common clinical finding
- CT findings similar in density to water, appears heterogenous
- Scalloping of the liver and spleen, mesentery is easily demonstrated. Calcifications are common

Treatment
- Cytoreductive surgery followed by EBRT, intraperitoneal radioisotopes, IP chemotherapy, and systemic chemotherapy

Survival rates with and without IP chemotherapy (Table 3-28)

TABLE 3-28 SURVIVAL RATES WITH AND WITHOUT IP CHEMOTHERAPY

	Five-Year Survival Rates %	
	Without IP Chemotherapy	With IP Chemotherapy
Disseminated peritoneal adenomucinosis (DPAM)	84	81
Peritoneal mucinous carcinomatosis (PMP)	7	59
Intermediate features	38	78

Data from Ronnett BM, Zahn cM, Kurman RJ, et al. Disseminated peritoneal adenomucinosis and peritoneal mucinous carcinomatosis. A clinicopathologic analysis of 109 cases with emphasis on distinguishing pathologic features, site of origin, prognosis, and relationship to "pseudomyxoma peritonei." Am J Surg Pathol. 1995;19: 1390–1408; chua tc, Moran BJ, Sugarbaker PH, et al. early- and long-term outcome data of patients with pseudomyxoma peritonei from appendiceal origin treated by a strategy of cytoreductive surgery and hyperthermic intraperitoneal chemotherapy. *J Clin Oncol.* 2012;30:2449–2456.

Borderline Tumors of Low Malignant Potential (aka Atypical Proliferative Tumors)

- Account for approximately 10–20% of EOCs and approximately 10% of ovarian malignancies
- Average age at diagnosis is 49, but this is skewed; the highest frequency occurs in the 15- to 29–year-old age group
- *BRCA*1 and *BRCA*2 do not confer an increased risk for these tumors

Diagnosis

- Patients usually present with an asymptomatic adnexal mass on pelvic CT or ultrasound; symptoms related only to the mass effect
- Ultrasound: Unilocular or complex mass; papillae are often seen
- Up to 50% have normal CA125, less than 25% have levels >100 U/mL

Staging

- Controversial, given good prognosis even with lymph node involvement (98% survival at 6.5 years according to recent retrospective study)
- However, staging does provide needed information in the 25% of patients with invasive disease on final path, so is often done
- Low possibility of invasive metastasis

Histologic Subtypes

- Serous
  - The majority of tumors
  - 75% are stage I
  - 25–50% are bilateral
  - Up to 25% of patients with an initial diagnosis of borderline will be upstaged to invasive cancer on final pathology
- Mucinous
  - Majority are stage I (>90%)
  - Less than 10% bilateral, except in endocervical type (up to 40% are bilateral)
  - Mucinous tumors of the ovary may actually be appendiceal in origin, and not borderline; important that appendix and bowel be examined in these cases

Treatment

- Because of excellent prognosis, treatment is generally surgery alone
- Can perform unilateral salpingo-oophorectomy, or even cystectomy, if patient desires fertility. But, cystectomy associated with recurrence of up to 30%
- If fertility-sparing treatment, obtain baseline CA125 levels and follow with serial TVUS
- For patients with higher stage disease or done with childbearing → hysterectomy-BSO
- If mucinous: Need abdominal exploration and appendectomy to rule out PMP
- Recurrence risk with conservative therapy is 9%; with radical surgery is 11.6%
- Post-op chemotherapy not shown to have significant survival benefit; not routinely used

Survival by Stage (Table 3-29)

TABLE 3-29 SURVIVAL BY STAGE FOR BORDERLINE TUMORS OF LOW MALIGNANT POTENTIAL

Stage	Five-Year Survival (%)	Ten-Year Survival (%)
I	99	97
II	98	90
III	96	88
IV	77	69

UTERINE CANCER

- Most common gynecologic cancer in the United States
- Abnormal uterine bleeding or spotting is frequently an early sign
- 40% more common in white than black women, but black women are two times more likely to die from the disease
- 69% of cases will be localized at the time of diagnosis

Risk Factors

- Age, increased estrogen exposure (PCOS, unopposed estrogen therapy, obesity, nulliparity), Tamoxifen
- HNPCC syndrome confers 39% risk of endometrial cancer by age 70
- Factors that decrease circulating estrogen, such as cigarette smoking and OCP use, decrease this risk
- Hyperplasia appears to be the precursor lesion

Classification

- Endometrioid: 75–80%
- Clear Cell: 1–5%
- Papillary Serous: 5–10%

- Mixed: Rare
- Sarcoma: 4-5%

Endometrial Carcinoma: Most common uterine malignancy (>90%); adenocarcinoma

- Type I:
  - Endometrioid histology
  - Associated with unopposed estrogen exposure
  - Preceded by endometrial hyperplasia
- Type II: Type II Endometrial Carcinoma (more aggressive)
  - *Serous carcinoma:* Resembles carcinoma of fallopian tube or ovary. Considered a high-grade lesion; often associated with LVSI, deep myometrial invasion. These tumors mimic the behavior of ovarian carcinoma, metastasize early and extensively.
  - *Clear cell carcinoma:* Tends to occur in older women, very aggressive. Also generally considered high grade
  - No known hormonal risk factors

Uterine Sarcoma: Comprise approximately 4% of uterine malignancies

Clinical Presentation/Evaluation of Uterine Sarcoma

- Vaginal bleeding (most common), pain, pelvic fullness, and foul vaginal discharge are common presenting symptoms
- Enlarged uterus, possible exophytic cervical mass on examination
- Endometrial biopsy may be negative if there is no endometrial involvement
- CT/MRI/ultrasound cannot reliably distinguish sarcoma/ leiomyoma/ carcinoma/ adenomyosis

GOG Classification

- Leiomyosarcoma
- Endometrial Stromal Sarcoma
- Mixed Homologous Müllerian Sarcoma—carcinosarcoma
- Mixed Heterologous Müllerian Sarcoma—carcinosarcoma
- Other

Leiomyosarcoma (LMS)

- Median age at presentation 43–53; premenopausal patients with better survival
- Hysterectomy performed for fibroids rarely demonstrates LMS (0.23%)
- Not hormonally responsive
- Have more than 10 mitoses/high power field (HPF), nuclear atypia, coagulative necrosis
- Consider adjuvant radiation therapy for locally advanced disease or systemic chemotherapy for advanced disease
- Gemcitabine/Docetaxel as first line adjuvant chemotherapy
- Doxorubicin also with high response rate

Endometrial Stromal Sarcoma (ESS)

- Resemble endometrial stromal cells that invade myometrium
- Generally low grade and highly hormonally responsive (menopause can be sufficient adjuvant treatment)

Carcinosarcoma (aka malignant mixed Müllerian tumors or MMMT)

- Most common uterine sarcoma; behavior mimics carcinomatous component
- Sarcomatous component resembles leiomyosarcoma, fibrosarcoma, malignant fibrous histiocytoma, (homologous); or rhabdomyosarcoma, chondrosarcoma, osteosarcoma, or liposarcoma (heterologous)
- Carcinosarcoma 5-year survival rate is 50% for early stage; 20% for advanced stage
- Surgically staged: TAH, BSO, washings, lymphadenectomy
- Extrauterine disease in 30% of patients
- Pelvic radiation provides local control but does not improve survival
- Chemotherapy with ifosfamide and paclitaxel results in improved response rate, overall survival, and progression-free survival but more neuropathy than ifosfamide alone
- Carboplatin/Taxol also acceptable regimen with less toxicity

Undifferentiated Endometrial Sarcoma

- Very aggressive, poor prognosis, and data are lacking
- Vascular invasion associated with worse 5-year survival (17% versus 83%)
- Ideal treatment not completely defined. After surgery, Carboplatin/Taxol ± pelvic radiation are reasonable
- Recurrences treated with carbo/taxol or doxorubicin or ifosfamide regimens

Endometrial Hyperplasia

- The progression of "untreated" endometrial hyperplasia over 10 years, with subsequent progression to malignancy, is illustrated in Table 3-30
- Prevalence of carcinoma in patients with a community hospital diagnosis of atypical hyperplasia with atypia has been shown to be 43%

TABLE 3-30 PROGRESSION OF UNTREATED ENDOMETRIAL HYPERPLASIA

Pathology	% Regressed	% Persisted	% Progressed to Cancer
Simple hyperplasia, no atypia	80	19	1
Complex hyperplasia, no atypia	79	17	3
Simple hyperplasia, with atypia	69	23	8
Complex hyperplasia, with atypia	57	14	29

Used with permission from Kurman RJ, Kaminski PF, norris HJ. the behavior of endometrial hyperplasia. A long-term study of "untreated" hyperplasia in 170 patients. *Cancer.* 1985;56:403–412.

Clinical Presentation/Evaluation of Endometrial Cancer

- Often presents as abnormal uterine bleeding or postmenopausal bleeding. *All* peri- or postmenopausal abnormal bleeding should be investigated.
  - 10% have cancer, 60–80% atrophy, 5–10% endometrial hyperplasia, 2–12% polyp, 15–25% hormone therapy
- Women on tamoxifen have an increased risk of developing endometrial pathology. Screening is not effective; ultrasound evaluation is limited since tamoxifen causes *subepithelial stromal hypertrophy;* increasing thickness of endometrial stripe. Any vaginal bleeding should trigger evaluation
- A prophylactic hysterectomy/BSO should be considered for women with HNPCC. If not, yearly endometrial biopsies and ultrasounds can be used for surveillance
- Appropriate evaluation for postmenopausal bleeding is much debated: Ultrasound and endometrial biopsy are the two main tools available. Numerous studies have attempted to determine which is superior
  - *Ultrasound measurement* of the endometrial stripe—cutoff of 5 mm
    - Positive predictive value of 9%; Negative predictive value of 99%
    - Sensitivity 90%, specificity 48% for endometrial cancer
    - Meta-analysis: the post-test probability of cancer after a pelvic ultrasound shows an endometrial stripe < 5 mm is 2.5%. If the stripe is > 5 mm, post-test probability of cancer is 32%
    - If ultrasound is first step, 50% of patients will require further evaluation
  - *Endometrial biopsy*
    - Specificity 98%; sensitivity 99%
    - False-negative rate is between 5% and 15%
    - Post-test probability of endometrial cancer is 82% if biopsy is positive and 0.9% if negative
    - "Insufficient sample" should trigger further evaluation (especially if large stripe); 20% will have pathology and 3% will have cancer
    - Atrophic endometrium *with* thickened stripe needs further workup
  - If bleeding persists or clinical suspicion is high, further evaluate with a D&C

Staging for Carcinoma of the Endometrium (surgical)

- Hysterectomy, BSO, pelvic and para-aortic lymphadenectomy
- Special considerations
  - Sentinel lymph node mapping
  - Cytoreduction if gross extrauterine disease
  - Radical hysterectomy if known cervical involvement
  - Omentectomy in high-grade histologies
- Extent of lymph node evaluation often determined intraoperatively
  - Presence of bulky, suspicious nodes
  - Frozen section showing high grade disease, deep invasion, or tumor size over 2 cm
  - Cytoreduction if gross extrauterine disease
- LVSI portends a 27% risk of positive pelvic nodes, and a 19% chance of positive para-aortic lymph nodes

FIGO Staging (revised in 2009)

- Endometrial Carcinoma (Table 3-31)
- Uterine Sarcoma (Table 3-32)
- Carcinosarcomas should be staged as carcinomas of the endometrium

TABLE 3-31 FIGO STAGING OF ENDOMETRIAL CARCINOMA

FIGO Staging—Endometrial Carcinoma	
Stage I	**Tumor confined to corpus uteri**
IA	Tumor limited to endometrium or invades less than one-half of myometrium
IB	Tumor invades one-half or more of the myometrium
Stage II	**Tumor in volves stromal connective tissue of the cervix but does not extend beyond uterus***
Stage III	**Disease outside of the uterus confined to pelvis or retroperitoneum**
IIIA	Tumor involves serosa and/or adnexa (direct extension or metastasis)[†]
IIIB	Vaginal involvement (direct extension or metastasis) or parametrial involvement[†]
IIIC	Metastases to pelvic and/or para-aortic lymph nodes[†]
IIIC1	Pelvic node involvement
IIIC2	Peri-aortic node involvement
Stage IV	**Tumor invades bladder and/or bowel mucosa, and/or distant metastases**
IVA	Tumor invades bladder mucosa and/or bowel
IVB	Distant metastasis (includes metastasis to inguinal lymph nodes, intraperitoneal disease, or lung, liver, or bone. It excludes metastasis to para-aortic lymph nodes, vagina, pelvic serosa, or adnexa)

*Endocervical glandular involvement considered stage I (no longer stage II).
[†]Positive cytology has to be reported separately without changing the stage.
Reproduced, with permission granted by FIGO, from FIGO Committee on Gynecologic Oncology. Revised FIGO staging for carcinoma of the vulva, cervix, and endometrium. *Int J Gynecol Obstet* 2009;105(2):103–4.

TABLE 3-32 FIGO STAGING OF UTERINE SARCOMA

FIGO Staging—Uterine Sarcoma	
Leiomyosarcomas and Endometrial Stromal Sarcoma	
Stage I	**Tumor limited to uterus**
IA	Tumor 5 cm or less in greatest dimension
IB	Tumor more than 5 cm
Stage II	**Tumor extends beyond uterus, within the pelvis**
IIA	Tumor involves adnexa
IIB	Tumor involves other pelvic tissues
Stage III	**Tumor infiltrates abdominal tissues (not just protruding into abdomen)**
IIIA	One site
IIIB	More than one site
IIIC	Regional lymph node metastasis
Stage IV	**Tumor invades bladder/rectum or distant metastasis**
IVA	Tumor invades bladder or rectum
IVB	Distant metastasis (excluding adnexa, pelvic, and abdominal tissues)

Note: Simultaneous tumors of the uterine corpus and ovary/pelvis in association with ovarian/pelvic endometriosis should be classified as independent primary tumors.
Reproduced, with permission granted by FIGO, from FIGO Committee on Gynecologic Oncology. Revised FIGO staging for carcinoma of the vulva, cervix, and endometrium. *Int J Gynecol Obstet* 2009;105(2):103–4.

Treatment

- Treatment is determined by stage, grade, histological type, and the patient's ability to tolerate further therapies
- **Low-risk diseases** (stage IA and IB grade 1 and 2; stage IA grade 3 without LVSI) do not require further treatment beyond surgery (using "old" staging)
- **High- to intermediate-risk disease:** Increased age, grade 2 and 3 diseases, LVSI, outer-third myometrial invasion. Adjuvant radiation therapy is recommended if age under 50 with 3 risk factors, age 50–70 with 2 risk factors, age over 70 with 1 risk factor
- While postoperative radiation (vaginal brachytherapy and/or pelvic EBRT) can significantly increase local control, it does not appear to impact survival, and can have significant toxicity
- *Stage II:* If cervical involvement is known preoperatively, a radical hysterectomy should be considered. If the diagnosis is made postoperatively, vaginal brachytherapy should be offered
- For stage III and IV cancers, optimal cytoreductive surgery has been shown to improve survival. Adjuvant chemotherapy after cytoreduction is advised; however, the optimal agent is unclear. Radiation Therapy—unclear
- Clear cell and serous carcinomas need adjuvant therapy regardless of stage. Despite therapy, these tumors are often very aggressive.
- *Women with very early endometrial cancer who wish to preserve their fertility can be treated with progesterone rather than surgery. D&C should be repeated every 3 months to assess response*

Prognosis

- Most significant factors: Stage, grade, depth of myometrial invasion
- Age, histological type, LVSI, and progesterone receptor activity also have prognostic significance
- Prognosis for the more aggressive histological types is less favorable. Even without myometrial invasion, 36% of uterine serous cancers will have positive lymph nodes.
- Five-year survival for stages I and II is 36%.
- **Clear cell cancer** has a 72% 5-year survival for stage I and a 60% 5-year survival for stage II. Overall 5-year disease free survival is 40%. Relapses tend to occur distally, often in the lungs, liver, or bones
- Better prognosis for uterine adenosarcomas (unless there is sarcomatous overgrowth or myometrial invasion)

Surveillance

- Examine every 3–6 months for 2 years, then yearly. If CA125 was elevated at the time of diagnosis, it can be followed at each visit
- Isolated vaginal recurrences can often be salvaged with surgery or vaginal radiation. Chemotherapy or progesterone can be tried for recurrence

Survival

- Stage Distribution and 5-Year Relative Survival by Stage at Diagnosis (Table 3-33)

TABLE 3-33 STAGE DISTRIBUTION AND FIVE-YEAR RELATIVE SURVIVAL BY STAGE AT DIAGNOSIS: ENDOMETRIAL CANCER

Stage at Diagnosis	Stage Distribution (%)	Five-Year Relative Survival (%)
Localized	67	95.3
Regional (spread to regional lymph nodes)	21	68.2
Distant (metastasized)	8	16.9
Unknown (unstaged)	4	48.5

Data from SEER 18 2005-2011. http://seer.cancer.gov/statfacts/html/corp.html. Accessed May 4, 2015.

VULVAR CANCER

- Fourth most common gynecologic cancer; 5% of malignancies of the female genital tract
- **Risk Factors:** Prior cervical cancer; immunodeficiency
  - Younger patient: Smoking, VIN or CIN, HPV
  - Older patient: Vulvar dystrophies
- **Clinical Manifestations:** Vulvar plaque, ulcer, or mass on the labia majora (perineum, clitoris, and mons are less frequent); pruritus is most common symptom
- **Diagnosis:** Biopsy center of the lesion; if clinical suspicion is high with no evident lesion; colposcopy
  - RULE WITH VULVAR LESIONS: BIOPSY, BIOPSY!
- **Squamous Cell Carcinoma:** 86.2% of vulvar cancer

FIGO Staging (revised in 2009)

• Table 3-34

TABLE 3-34 FIGO STAGING OF VULVAR CANCER

FIGO Staging—Vulvar Cancer	
Stage I	**Tumor confined to vulva**
IA	Lesions ≤2 cm in size, confined to vulva or perineum and with stromal invasion ≤1 mm*, no nodal metastasis
IB	Lesions >2 cm in size or with stromal invasion >1 mm*, confined to the vulva or perineum, with negative nodes
Stage II	**Tumor of any size with extension to adjacent perineal structures (one-third lower urethra, one-third lower vagina, anus) with negative nodes**
Stage III	**Tumor of any size with or without extension to adjacent perineal structures (one-third lower urethra, one-third lower vagina, anus) with positive inguinofemoral lymph nodes**
IIIA	One lymph node metastasis (≥5 mm), or One to two lymph node metastasis (<5 mm)
IIIB	Two or more lymph node metastases (≥5 mm), or Three or more lymph node metastases (<5 mm)
IIIC	Positive nodes with extracapsular spread
Stage IV	**Tumor invades other regional (two-thirds upper urethra, two-thirds upper vagina) or distant structures**
IVA	Tumor invades any of the following: Upper urethral and/or vaginal mucosa, bladder mucosa, rectal mucosa, or fixed to pelvic bone, or Fixed or ulcerated inguinofemoral lymph nodes
IVB	Any distant metastasis including pelvic lymph nodes

*The depth of invasion is defined as the measurement of the tumor from the epithelial-stromal junction of the adjacent most superficial dermal papilla to the deepest point of invasion.
Reproduced, with permission granted by FIGO, from FIGO Committee on Gynecologic Oncology. Revised FIGO staging for carcinoma of the vulva, cervix, and endometrium. *Int J Gynecol Obstet* 2009;105(2):103–4.

Survival

• Stage Distribution and 5-Year Relative Survival by Stage at Diagnosis (Table 3-35)

TABLE 3-35 STAGE DISTRIBUTION AND FIVE-YEAR RELATIVE SURVIVAL BY STAGE AT DIAGNOSIS: VULVAR CANCER

Stage at Diagnosis	Stage Distribution (%)	Five-Year Relative Survival (%)
Localized	59	85.8
Regional (spread to regional lymph nodes)	31	55.4
Distant (metastasized)	5	15.5
Unknown (unstaged)	5	49.3

Data from SEER 18 2005-2011. http://seer.cancer.gov/statfacts/html/vulva.html. Accessed May 4, 2015.

Treatment

• Treatment by tumor size (Table 3-36)
• Number of positive groin nodes is the best predictor of prognosis

Post-operative Care

• After radical vulvectomy with or without vulvar reconstruction, consider bed rest and/or no sitting for 3–5 days, VTE prophylaxis, physical therapy, suction drain in groin, low residue diet
• Complications: Seroma, DVT/PE, chronic lower extremity edema, recurrent lymphangitis, risk of significant groin-related complications as high as 50–60%
• Saphenous vein sparing decreases risk of infection following vulvectomy

TABLE 3-36 TREATMENT BY TUMOR SIZE

Tumor	Treatment
≤2 cm in diameter and ≤1 mm deep	Wide local excision with 1 cm margins if no LVSI
>2 cm in diameter or >1 mm deep	*If lateralized* (>2 cm from urethra, clitoris, posterior fourchette), radical local excision with ipsilateral lymphadenectomy • If all nodes negative → no further therapy • if (+) LN → dissect other groin LN. If >2 LN (+) → adjuvant radiation therapy *If <2 cm from midline* → radical local excision with bilateral groin lymphadenectomy. If >2 LN (+) → pelvic lymphadenectomy, radiate
Spread beyond vulva (urethra, vagina, anus, lymph nodes)	Standard of care is neoadjuvant chemo-RT in these patients; consider radical vulvectomy and inguinal lymphadenectomy or exenteration only if not a good candidate for chemo-radiation therapy

Nonsquamous Cell Vulvar Cancer

Melanoma: 4.8% of vulvar cancer; 3–7% of all melanomas in women
• Occurs in postmenopausal white women, median age 68 years
• Staging: Breslow's criteria (based on depth of lesion)
• *Treatment:* If <0.76 mm, treat with wide local excision (WLE) with 1 cm margins, if >0.76, treat with WLE plus bilateral groin lymphadenectomy

Bartholin's Gland Adenocarcinoma: 5% of vulvar cancers
• Enlargement of the gland in women over 40
• BIOPSY ALL BARTHOLIN'S LESIONS IN WOMEN OVER AGE 40
• Metastatic disease is common
• *Treatment:* Radical local excision and post-operative radiation therapy

Extramammary Paget's Disease: Less than 1% of vulvar cancers
• Similar in appearance to Paget's of the breast: Eczematoid appearance, well-demarcated, slightly raised edges, red background, usually multifocal, anywhere on the vulva
• 10–12% of patients with Paget's have invasive vulvar Paget's and 4–8% have underlying adenocarcinoma; 20–30% of patients have a noncontiguous carcinoma
• *Treatment:* WLE or vulvectomy depending on extent of disease
• 12–58% experience local recurrence

Basal Cell Carcinoma: 2% of vulvar cancers
• May be locally invasive but usually nonmetastasizing
• High incidence of antecedent or concomitant malignancy
• *Treatment:* Radical local excision without lymphadenectomy

Sarcoma: 1–2% of vulvar cancers
• *Treatment:* WLE, lymphatic metastasis uncommon

VAGINAL CANCER

• Approximately 1% of gynecologic cancers
• Primary vaginal cancer is rare but metastatic disease is not uncommon
• 3–7% of patients with vaginal intraepithelial neoplasia (VaIN) progress to invasive cancer

Risk Factors

• Same as cervical cancer (70% of biopsy specimens contain HPV 16/18)

Clinical Manifestations

• Majority present with vaginal bleeding
• Posterior wall of the upper one-third of the vagina is the most common site
• Affects ages 35–90. Over 50% of cases in women 70–90

Diagnosis

• Biopsy of lesion (mass, plaque, or ulcer)
  • Speculum can obscure visualization—inspect while removing!
  • 20% of vaginal tumors detected incidentally on pap for cervical cancer
  • Do vaginal colposcopy if abnormal pap without cervical explanation

Squamous Cell Cancer

• 85% of vaginal cancers
  • Nodular, ulcerative, indurated, endophytic, or exophytic lesions
  • Associated with HPV

Staging

• Staging is *clinical* (Table 3-37)
• Cancers in the upper third spread to pelvic, para-aortic lymph nodes
• Cancers in the lower third go to the inguinofemoral lymph nodes

TABLE 3-37 STAGING (CLINICAL)—VAGINAL CANCER

Stage	Description	Five-Year Survival (%)
I	Limited to vaginal mucosa	95
II	Parametrial invasion, not into pelvic wall	67
III	Tumor extends to pelvic wall; bones of pelvis	32
IVA	Bladder and/or rectum, outside of true pelvis	18
IVB	Distant metastasis	Almost 0

Treatment

• INDIVIDUALIZE (depending on proximity to bladder, urethra, rectum)
  • *Stage I:* Disease in upper part of vagina can usually be treated with radical surgery, most others are treated with radiation (7000 cGy) and brachytherapy; consider chemosensitization with cisplatin. Cancers in the lower one-third need the groin nodes to either be radiated or dissected
  • *Stages II–IV:* Radiation therapy
  • *Recurrent Disease:* May be candidate for pelvic exenteration

Miscellaneous

• *Adenocarcinoma:* Occurs in younger women, often with DES exposure. Treatment: Like cervical cancer [radical hysterectomy, pelvic lymphadenectomy, vaginectomy]. Five-year survival: Stage I 87%, stage II 76%, stage III 30%
• *Embryonal rhabdomyosarcoma* (sarcoma botryoides): Occurs in infants. Treatment: Chemotherapy [VAC (vincristine, actinomycin D, cyclophosphamide)], radiation, surgery
• *Melanoma:* <0.5% of vaginal cancers. Blue-black mass, usually in distal one-third of vagina. Aggressive. Five-year survival less than 20%

GESTATIONAL TROPHOBLASTIC DISEASE (GTD)/NEOPLASIA

Types

Complete Moles

• 46,XX
• Derived from empty ova and two sperm. No fetal parts or red blood cells. The villi are swollen
• 15% will invade locally after evacuation and 4% metastasize
• Incidence 1:1945 pregnancies
• Approximately 50% will have prominent theca lutein cysts
• Most common symptom is vaginal bleeding; 25% of patients measure size greater than dates (Table 3-38)

Partial Moles

• 69,XXY or 69,XXX
• Derived from one egg and two sperm. May have fetal parts and red blood cells. Persistent in 2–4% post-evacuation.
• Patients usually present with signs or symptoms of incomplete abortion (Table 3-38)

TABLE 3-38 FEATURES OF PARTIAL AND COMPLETE HYDATIDIFORM MOLES

	Partial Mole	Complete Mole
Karyotype	Usually 69,XXX or 69,XXY	46,XX or 46,XY
Pathology		
Fetus	Often present	Absent
Amnion, fetal red blood cells	Often present	Absent
Villous edema	Variable, focal	Diffuse
Trophoblastic proliferation	Variable, focal, slight to moderate	Diffuse, slight to severe
Clinical Presentation		
Diagnosis	Missed abortion	Molar gestation
Uterine size	Small for gestational age	50% larger for gestational age
Theca lutein cysts	Rare	25–30%
Medical complications	Rare	Frequent
Persistent trophoblastic disease	1–5%	15–20%

Used with permission from Cunningham F, et al. Gestational trophoblastic disease. In: Cunningham F, et al., eds. *Williams Obstetrics*, 23rd ed. New York, NY: McGraw-Hill; 2010.

Choriocarcinoma
- 3–7% of moles will develop into choriocarcinoma. 50% of choriocarcinoma follows moles, 25% follow normal pregnancy, and 25% follow miscarriages/terminations

Placental site trophoblastic tumors
- A rare variant of choriocarcinoma, β-hCG is not usually very elevated; human placental site lactogen (HPL) is elevated.
- Resistant to chemotherapy and requires hysterectomy

Evaluation

- After diagnosis, check quantitative β-hCG, chest xray, TFTs, CBC, PT/PTT, LFTs

Treatment

- D&C (but make sure to administer oxytocin; inform anesthesia that it is not a normal D&C, type and cross for 4 units). Remember RhoGAM as needed. Hysterectomy is appropriate treatment if no further childbearing is desired
- Follow β-hCG every week until negative three times, then every month for 6 months. Patients should be on birth control during this time (1 year)!
- For all further pregnancies: Early ultrasound, send placenta to pathology, check 6-week postpartum β-hCG. 1% risk of molar disease in future gestations after a molar pregnancy
- Invasive mole: About 15% of patients will have locally invasive disease after evacuation of a complete mole. Occurs rarely after other gestations

Follow-Up

- If after treatment for a mole, the β-hCG increases over 2 weeks, plateaus for 3 weeks, or increases after reaching 0, suspect persistent GTD
  - Persistent disease workup: β-hCG, LFTs, TFTs, renal assessment, CBC
  - Metastatic workup involves chest CT, abdomen/pelvis CT, CT or MRI of head

World Health Organization (WHO) Scoring System for Gestational Trophoblastic Tumors (Table 3-39)

- Risk according to Scoring System
  - Low risk: 0–4
  - Intermediate risk: 5–7
  - High risk: >8

TABLE 3-39 WHO SCORING SYSTEM FOR GESTATIONAL TROPHOBLASTIC TUMORS

Prognostic Factors	Points			
	0	1	2	4
Age	<39	≥39	–	–
Previous pregnancy	Mole	Abortion	Term	–
Interval (months)	<4	4–6	7–12	>12
β-hCG (mIU/mL)	<1 000	1 000–10 000	10 000–100 000	>100 000
ABO groups	–	O or A	B or AB	–
Largest tumor, including uterine (cm)	–	3-5	≥ 5	–
Site of metastases	Lungs, pelvis, vagina	Spleen, kidney	GI tract, liver	Brain
Number of metastases	–	1–3	4–8	>8
Prior chemotherapy	–	–	Single	Multiple

Treatment of Persistent GTD

Low risk
- Treat with single agent: Actinomycin D or Methotrexate (MTX)
- GOG 173: Randomized controlled trial of weekly MTX 30 mg/m² versus pulsed Actinomycin D. Biweekly dactinomycin regimen with higher complete response rate than weekly MTX
- Check β-hCG every month for 12 months then every 2 months for 12 months

High risk
- The best chemotherapy regimen is still unclear
  - EMA–CO regimen
    - Combination chemotherapy of 5 drugs (etoposide, MTX, dactinomycin, cyclophosphamide, vincristine)
    - Widely used as first line

CHEMOTHERAPY

- Mechanisms of chemotherapy agents (Table 3-40)
- Chemotherapy agents affect various stages of the cell cycle (Figure 3-4)
- Commonly used agents (Table 3-41)

TABLE 3-40 MECHANISMS OF CHEMOTHERAPY AGENTS

Chemotherapy Agent	Mechanism of Action
Alkylating agents (platinum, ifosfamide)	Disrupt DNA replication
Antimetabolites	Inhibit cell division or are incorporated into nuclear material
Plant alkaloids (taxanes)	Induce stable polymerization of microtubules → inhibit cell replication
Plank alkaloids (etoposide, topotecan)	Inhibit topoisomerase II → inhibit cell replication
Antitumor antibiotics	Various modes of action
Monoclonal antibodies (bevacizumab)	Antibody toward VEGF (vascular endothelial growth factor) inhibiting the binding of normal VEGF ligand to receptor, inhibiting angiogenesis

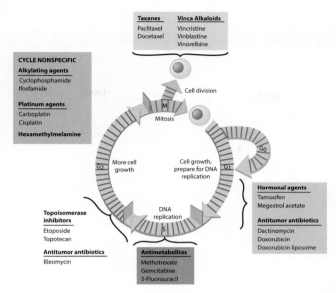

Figure 3-4 Chemotherapy agents and the cell cycle. (Used with permission from Hoffman BL, et al. Chapter 27. Principles of chemotherapy. In: Hoffman BL, et al., eds. *Williams Gynecology*, 2nd ed. New York, NY: McGraw-Hill; 2012.)

GYNECOLOGIC ONCOLOGY

TABLE 3-41 COMMONLY USED CHEMOTHERAPY AGENTS

Agent	Mechanism	Indications	Toxicity	Factoids
5-Fluorouracil	Antimetabolite	Vu, Va, C, Ov, potentiates RT	Myelosuppression, hyperpigmentation, stomatitis, emetogenic, acute cerebellar syndrome, cardiotoxic (MI, angina, arrhythmia)	
Bevacizumab (*Avastin*)	Monoclonal antibody	Ov, Ut	Hypertension, proteinuria; small risk of nasal or bowel perforations	
Bleomycin	Antitumor antibiotic	Ov, C	**Pulmonary fibrosis**, mucositis, alopecia, hypersensitization	Pulmonary fibrosis with over 283 mg/m²
Carboplatin	Alkylating-like agent	Ov, Ut, C	Myelosuppression (platelets), emetogenic, nephro-toxicity (decreases magnesium)	
Cisplatin	Alkylating-like agent	Ov, Ut, C, RT	**Nephrotoxicity** (magnesium loss), tinnitus, peripheral neuropathy, emetogenic, ocular toxicity, emetogenic	Less myelotoxic than carboplatin

(Continued)

TABLE 3-41　COMMONLY USED CHEMOTHERAPY AGENTS (*Continued*)

Agent	Mechanism	Indications	Toxicity	Factoids
Cytoxan cyclophos-phamide	Alkylating agent	Ov, Ut Sarc, C	Myelosuppression (leukocytes), hemorrhagic cystitis (pre-treat with Mesna), emetogenic, alopecia	
Dactinomycin	Antitumor antibiotic	Ov, Ut, germ cell	Emetogenic, mucositis, alopecia	
Docetaxel (*Taxotere*)	Plant alkaloid	Ov	Myelosuppression (neutropenia), alopecia, hypersensitization, stomatitis, emetogenic, paresthesias, arthralgias	
Doxorubicin (*Adriamycin*)	Antitumor antibiotic	Ov, Ut, Ut Sarc	**Cardiotoxic** (550 mg/m^2), myelosuppression, emetogenic, esophagitis, alopecia, cholestasis, hyperpigmentation	Red-orange urine, dexrazoxane cardioprotective
Etoposide	Plant alkaloid	Ov, GTD, germ cell	Myelosuppression, alopecia, emetogenic, chemical phlebitis	
Gemcitabine	Antimetabolite	Ov	Myelosuppression, hypersensitization, emetogenic	
Ifosfamide	Alkylating agent	Ov, Ut Sarc, C	Myelosuppression, **hemorrhagic cystitis** (from acrolein), emetogenic, alopecia, encephalopathy, nephrotoxic	Mesna protects bladder; treat encephalopathy with methylene blue
Liposomal doxorubicin (Doxil)	Antitumor antibiotic	Ov, Ut	Myelosuppression, **hand-foot syndrome (palmar-plantar erythrodyesthesias)**, hypersensitization	Less cardiotoxic than doxorubicin
Methotrexate	Antimetabolite	GTD	Myelosuppression, stomatitis, emetogenic, hepatitis, alopecia, decreases reflexes, peripheral neuropathy, nephrotoxic	Over 250 mg/m^2 give leucovorin-folic acid rescue
Paclitaxel (*Taxol*)	Plant alkaloid	Ov	Myelosuppression (leukocytes), alopecia, arthralgia, cardiotoxic (bradycardia, ventricular tachycardia), **hypersensitivity**, peripheral neuropathy, nausea/vomiting	Premedicate with dexamethasone, *Benadryl*, ranitidine (*Zantac*)
Topotecan	Topoisomerase inhibitor	Recurrent Ov	Myelosuppression (leukocytes), stomatitis, emetogenic, paresthesias	
PARP inhibitor (*Veliparib*)	Monoclonal	Recurrent Ov	Limited data on long-term toxicity	Beneficial in BRCA1/2 pts with recurrent ovarian CA

Vu, vulvar; Va, vaginal; C, cervical; Ov, ovarian; RT, radiation therapy; Ut, uterine; Sarc, sarcoma; GTD, gestational trophoblastic disease; PARP, poly ADP ribose polymerase.

Miscellaneous Information

- Neutropenia = absolute neutrophil count (ANC) < 500
- Patients at risk of being neutropenic for more than 7 days should be on antibiotic prophylaxis regardless of whether they are febrile
  - Prophylaxis: Ciprofloxacin 400 mg orally twice daily for 10 days
  - **Fever:** Piperacillin/tazobactam (*Zosyn*) 3.375 every 4 hours **or** cefepime 2 g IV every 8 hours INITIALLY then TAILOR based on culture
- *Pre-chemotherapy CBC goals*
  - WBC > 4.5; ANC > 1500
  - Hematocrit > 30%; Platelets > 100 000

Tumor Lysis Syndrome

- High potassium, uric acid, phosphate, low calcium
- Suspect when patients with a high tumor burden develop acute renal failure
- Treat with electrolyte correction, dialysis
- Prevent with allopurinol and uricase

Intraperitoneal Chemotherapy

- High cavity to plasma area under the curve ratio, high molecular weight, water insoluble equates to longer time in peritoneum
- Works by passive diffusion

Chemotherapy-Related Nausea/Vomiting

- Acute (within 24 hours)
- Delayed (after 24 hours)
- Anticipatory (a conditioned response after severe nausea and vomiting in the past)

First-Line Medications

- Ondansetron (*Zofran*) 4 mg IV/orally/oral disintegrating tablet (ODT) every 4 hours or 8 mg every 8 hours
- Promethazine (*Phenergan*) 12.5-25 mg orally/IM/IV every 4 hours/ per rectum every 12 hours
- Prochlorperazine (*Compazine*) 5–10 mg orally every 6 hours or 2.5–10 IM/IV every 3 hours, 25 mg per rectum every 12 hours
  - An extrapyramidal reaction (akathisia, parkinsonism, dystonia) can be seen with both Compazine and Phenergan. Treat with Benadryl
- Metoclopramide (*Reglan*) (5–10 mg orally/IV/IM every 6 hours) increases gastric emptying
  - Side effects include akathisia, dystonia, and tardive dyskinesia
- Serotonin antagonists (granisetron, dolasetron) are very effective but expensive
- Aprepitant 125 mg orally prior to chemotherapy (1 hour before) on day 1 in combination with serotonin agonist, 80 mg once daily on days 2 and 3 and combined with dexamethasone on day 4
- Lorazepam (*Ativan*) 0.5–1 mg every 6 hours. Works very well for chemotherapy-associated nausea and vomiting (and anxiety)

Moderate- to High-Risk Regimens

- Serotonin antagonist (ondansetron orally/IV—the two are equivalent) and dexamethasone 8 mg IV prior to chemotherapy. Then, dexamethasone 4–8 mg orally twice daily for 2 more days for delayed nausea

Extremely High-Risk Chemotherapy (especially cisplatin)

- Serotonin antagonist, dexamethasone 8 mg IV, and aprepitant 125 mg orally prior to chemotherapy. Then dexamethasone 8 mg orally daily for 3 days and aprepitant 80 mg orally daily for 2 days

Anticipatory Nausea

- Alprazolam (*Xanax*) 0.5–2 mg as needed.

Other options

- Scopolamine 1.5 mg transdermally every 72 hours
- Diphenhydramine (*Benadryl*) 25–50 mg orally every 6 hours or 10–50 IV
- Dimenhydrinate (*Dramamine*) 50 mg orally every 4 hours
- Corticosteroids are especially effective for chemotherapy-induced nausea
- Cannabinoids are modest antiemetics. Legal form = Dronabinol 5–10 mg orally every 6 hours
- Acupuncture

ANATOMY

Eight Avascular Planes/Potential Spaces of Pelvis

• Four are located in the midline and two along each pelvic sidewall (Figure 3-5)

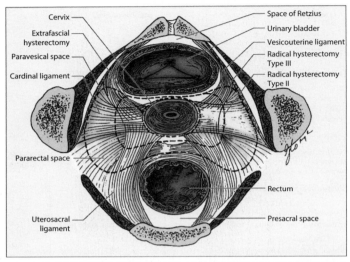

Retropubic	"Space of Retzius"
Vesicovaginal	Endopelvic fascia posteriorly, the detrusor muscle fibers anteriorly, and the vesicouterine webs laterally. Access to this space is achieved by exposing and separating the areolar tissue between the detrusor muscle fibers and the endopelvic fascia after incision of the peritoneum at the vesicouterine reflection. Development of this space allows direct access to the bladder, cervix, vagina, and distal ureters
Rectovaginal	Developed by dissecting between the longitudinal fibers of the rectum and the endopelvic fascia of the cervix and vagina. The lateral anatomic landmarks are the uterosacral ligaments. Development of this space exposes rectum, vagina, and posterior uterine supporting structures
Retrorectal	Presacral
Pararectal (2)	Internal iliac artery laterally; ureter medially; sacrum inferiorly
Paravesical (2)	Most inferior of the lateral avascular compartments. The landmarks include the external iliac vessels laterally and the obliterated hypogastric artery medially. After separation of these landmarks, continued dissection in a posterior, inferior, and slightly medial direction develops the paravesical avascular space down to the sacrum and to the levator muscles

Figure 3-5 Potential spaces of the pelvis. (Used with permission from Berek JS. *Berek & Novak's Gynecology*, 15th ed., Philadelphia, PA: Lippincott Williams & Wilkins: 2011.)

Branches of the Abdominal Aorta (Figure 3-6)

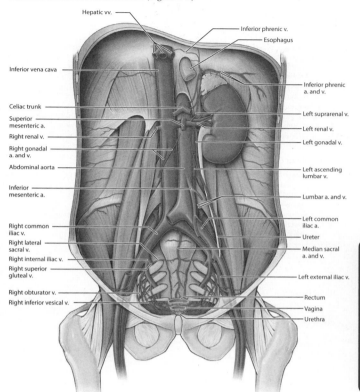

Figure 3-6 Branches of the abdominal aorta. (Used with permission from Morton DA, Foreman K, Albertine KH. Chapter 11. Posterior abdominal wall. In: Morton DA, Foreman K, Albertine KH., eds. *The Big Picture: Gross Anatomy.* New York, NY: McGraw-Hill; 2011.)

Omental Blood Supply

- Right
  - Right gastroepiploic
  - Gastroduodenal
  - Common hepatic
- Left
  - Left gastroepiploic
  - Splenic

Stomach Blood Supply

- Short gastric from splenic artery
- Right gastric from common hepatic
- Left gastric from celiac trunk

Celiac Trunk—three major branches

- **Left gastric**
  - **Esophageal** branches
  - Branches to left part of the lesser curvature of the stomach
- **Splenic**
  - Pancreatic branches
  - Short gastric: Supplies area of the fundus

- Left gastroepiploic: Passes into the greater omentum and supplies the left part of greater curvature of the stomach and eventually anastomoses with right gastroepiploic
- Splenic branches
- **Common hepatic**
- Proper hepatic
  - Right gastric artery [small vessel arising from the proper hepatic artery or left hepatic artery; may arise from the gastroduodenal, middle hepatic, or right hepatic artery→ enters the lesser omentum and anastomoses with the left gastric artery]
  - Terminates by forming right and left hepatic arteries
    - Cystic artery usually branches from right hepatic artery
- **Gastroduodenal** arteries
  - **Supraduodenal** artery(ies)
  - Terminates → **right gastroepiploic** artery, which enters the greater omentum and courses along the greater curvature of the stomach until it anastomoses with left gastroepiploic artery
  - The **superior pancreatoduodenal** artery, the other terminal branch, courses inferiorly between the second part of the duodenum, and the head of the pancreas, supplying both

Blood Supply to the Intestines (Figure 3-7)

- *Superior Mesenteric Artery*
  - Supplies the right colon, small bowel (injury can cause jejunal necrosis)
  - Inferior pancreaticoduodenal
  - Middle colic artery
  - Right colic artery
  - Ileocolic artery
  - Ileal/Jejunal arteries

- *Inferior Mesenteric Artery*
  - Supplies the large bowel
  - Left colic artery
  - Sigmoid artery
  - Continues as superior rectal artery
  - Collateral with internal iliac via middle/inferior rectal, hypogastric artery

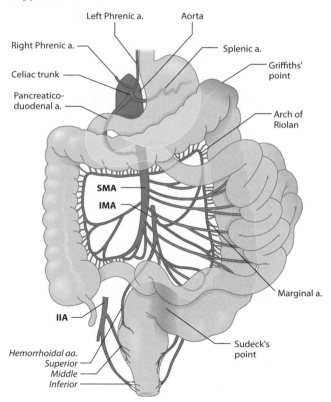

Figure 3-7 Blood supply to the intestines. (Used with permission from Gearhart SL. Chapter 298. Mesenteric vascular insufficiency. In: Longo DL, Fauci AS, et al., eds. *Harrison's Principles of Internal Medicine.* 18th ed. New York, NY: McGraw-Hill; 2012.)

Internal Iliac Artery Branches (Figure 3-8)

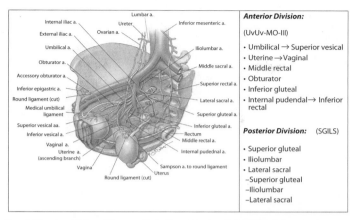

Anterior Division:

(UvUv-MO-III)

- Umbilical → Superior vesical
- Uterine → Vaginal
- Middle rectal
- Obturator
- Inferior gluteal
- Internal pudendal → Inferior rectal

Posterior Division: (SGILS)

- Superior gluteal
- Iliolumbar
- Lateral sacral
  - Superior gluteal
  - Iliolumbar
  - Lateral sacral

Figure 3-8 Branches of the internal iliac artery. (Used with permission from Hoffman BL, et al. Chapter 38. Anatomy. In: Hoffman BL, et al. eds. *Williams Gynecology*, 2nd ed. New York, NY: McGraw-Hill; 2012.)

Inguinal Canal

- Anterior wall: External abdominal oblique aponeurosis
- Floor: The inguinal ligament as the rolled under inferior edge of the external abdominal oblique aponeurosis, and the lacunar ligament medially
- Posterior wall: Transversalis fascia and parietal peritoneum
- Roof: No true roof, the internal oblique and transversus abdominis muscles arch over canal
- Superficial (external) ring: Triangular opening in external oblique aponeurosis
- Deep (internal) ring: Formed by an outpouching of transversalis fascia, lies superior to midpoint of the inguinal ligament, the inferior epigastric vessels lie medial to the ring

Inguinal or Hesselbach's Triangle

- Region on the inner, inferior portion of the abdominal wall
- The site of direct inguinal hernias
- The boundaries are
  - Inferior: Inguinal ligament
  - Medial: Lateral border of rectus abdominis muscle
  - Lateral: Inferior epigastric vessels
- Contents
  - Both sexes: Ilioinguinal nerve
  - Female: Round ligament of uterus
  - Male: Spermatic cord

Femoral Triangle Anatomy (Figure 3-9)

- Femoral Triangle
  - Superior: Inguinal ligament
  - Medial: Adductor longus
  - Lateral: Sartorius
  - Floor: Pectineus
  - Roof: Fascia lata
  - Contains femoral artery
- Femoral Artery Branches—Inguinal Canal
  - Superficial epigastric artery
  - Superficial iliac circumflex artery
  - Superficial external pudendal
  - Deep external pudendal

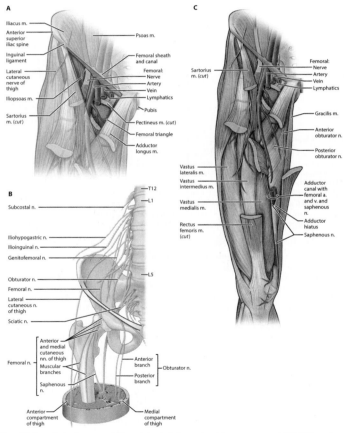

Figure 3-9 Femoral triangle anatomy. **A.** Femoral triangle. **B.** Innervation of the compartments of thigh. **C.** Femoral nerve. (Used with permission from Morton DA, Foreman K, Albertine KH. Chapter 36. Thigh. In: Morton DA, Foreman K, Albertine KH., eds. *The Big Picture: Gross Anatomy.* New York, NY: McGraw-Hill; 2011.)

Nerve Injuries: See Gynecology Section (Table 2-5)

Reproductive Endocrinology and Infertility

MENSTRUAL CYCLE

Figure 4-1

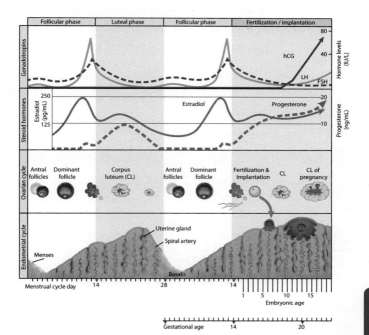

Figure 4-1 Changes in the ovarian follicle, endometrial thickness, and serum hormone levels during a 28-day menstrual cycle. P, progesterone; E₂, estradiol; LH, luteinizing hormone; FSH, follicle-stimulating hormone. (Used with permission from Hoffman BL, et al. Chapter 15. Reproductive endocrinology. In: Hoffman BL, et al., eds. Williams Gynecology. 2nd ed. New York, NY: McGraw-Hill; 2012)

INFERTILITY

Definitions

- **Infertility**: Inability to conceive after 1 year of frequent unprotected intercourse (evaluation recommended after 6 months if age is over 35)
- **Primary Infertility**: When a woman has never been pregnant
- **Secondary Infertility**: Infertility after a prior pregnancy

Statistics

- Affects 7% of married couples in which female partner is of reproductive age
- One-year prevalence of infertility is approximately 15%
- Infertility affects men and women equally
  - 20% of infertility cases can be attributed to male factors
  - 38% of infertility cases can be attributed to female factors

- 27% of infertility cases combined male/female
- 15% are unexplained
- Infertility and childlessness increase with age (Table 4-1)
- Risk of spontaneous abortion (SAB) also increases with age (Table 4-2)

TABLE 4-1 INFERTILITY INCREASES WITH AGE

Age Group	Percent Infertile	% Chance of Remaining Childless
20–24	7	6
25–29	9	9
30–34	15	15
35–39	22	30
40–44	29	64

Source: Data from Menken J, Trussell IJ, Larsen U. Age and infertility. Science. 1986;233:1389–1394.

TABLE 4-2 RISK OF SAB WITH INCREASED AGE

Maternal Age	Risk of SAB (%)
15–29	10
30–34	12
35–39	18
40–44	34
≥45	53

Source: Used with permission from Gindof PR, Jewelewicz R. Reproductive potential in the older woman. Fertil Steril. 1986; 46:989–1001.

Male Factor Infertility

- Incidence: 20%
- Etiology
  - *Hypothalamic pituitary disease (secondary hypogonadism)*: 1–2%
    - *Mechanism:* Deficiency of GnRH or gonadotropin
    - *Congenital:* Kallman syndrome, Prader–Willi syndrome
    - *Acquired:* Pituitary/Hypothalamic tumors, sarcoidosis, tuberculosis (TB), trauma, aneurysm, infarction, hyperprolactinemia, estrogen or cortisol excess, medications
    - *Systemic:* Chronic illness, nutritional deficiency, obesity
  - *Primary Hypogonadism*: 30–40%
    - *Congenital:* Klinefelter syndrome, cryptorchidism, androgen insensitivity
    - *Acquired:* Varicocele, orchitis, medication (alcohol, tetrahydrocannibol (THC), ketoconazole, spironolactone, histamine antagonists, calcium-channel blockers, steroids), environmental toxins, trauma, torsion, systemic illness (renal failure, cirrhosis, cancer, sickle cell)
  - *Post-testicular defects (disorders of sperm transport)*: 10–20%
    - *Congenital:* Absence of vas deferens (check for Cystic Fibrosis Transmembrane Conductance Regulator (CFTR) mutation)
    - *Acquired:* Infection, spinal cord disease, erectile dysfunction, premature ejaculation, retrograde ejaculation, vasectomy
    - *Obstruction:* Benign prostatic hyperplasia (BPH), infection, and scarring
  - *Unexplained:* 40–50%
- Evaluation: Semen analysis (Table 4-3)
  - Sample should be obtained after 2–3 days abstinence (no more than 7 days)
  - Sample must be received by the lab within 1–2 hours of collection
  - At least two samples should be collected 5–6 weeks apart

TABLE 4-3 SEMEN ANALYSIS PARAMETERS

Volume	≥1.5 mL
pH	≥7.2
Concentration	15×10^6 or more sperm/mL
Total #	39×10^6 or more spermatozoa/ejaculate
Motility	≥32% progressive motility or ≥40% total motility
Morphology	≥4% normal forms by strict criteria
Vitality	≥58% of sperm live
WBCs	White blood cells: <1 million/mL

Source: Used with permission from Cooper TG, Noonan E, von Eckardstein S, et al. World Health Organization reference values for human semen characteristics. *Hum Reprod Update.* 2010;16:231–245.

Female Factor Infertility

- Etiology

  - *Cervical* (3%)
    - *Common causes:* Cervical stenosis, hypoplastic endocervical canal, inhospitable cervical mucus (poorly estrogenized, *Clomid* can cause), infection
    - Evaluate using the post-coital test (PCT)

  - *Tubal* (23%)
    - *Common causes:* Pelvic inflammatory disease PID, endometriosis, pelvic adhesions, prior ectopic pregnancy, tubal surgery
      - Endometriosis accounts for approximately 9–15% of infertility
      - Tubal occlusion after one, two, and three episodes of salpingitis is 11, 23, and 54%, respectively
    - *Evaluation includes*
      - Document tubal patency using hysterosalpingogram (HSG)
      - Consider laparoscopy to rule out endometriosis, adhesions, etc

  - *Ovarian* (18%)
    - *Common causes:* Ovulatory dysfunction, endocrinopathies, decreased ovarian reserve, premature ovarian failure (POF) (also known as primary ovarian insufficiency)
    - The World Health Organization (WHO) classifies ovulatory disorders into three groups
      - *Class 1 (hypogonadotropic hypogonadal anovulation):* 5–10%
        Low or low-normal serum FSH and low serum estradiol due to decreased hypothalamic secretion of gonadotropin-releasing hormone (GnRH) or pituitary unresponsiveness to GnRH
      - *Class 2 (normogonadotropic normoestrogenic anovulation):* 70–85%
        May secrete normal amounts of gonadotropins and estrogen and may ovulate occasionally. However, FSH secretion during follicular phase is subnormal. Common cause: PCOS
      - *Class 3 (hypergonadotropic hypoestrogenic anovulation):* 10–30%
        Elevated FSH levels
        Primary causes: POF, ovarian resistance
    - *Hyperprolactinemia*
      - Anovulation secondary to hyperprolactinemia inhibits gonadotropin and estrogen secretion. May have regular anovulatory cycles, but many have oligomenorrhea or amenorrhea
      - Serum gonadotropin concentrations are usually normal
    - Document ovulation using basal body temperature (BBT), urinary LH kit, or midluteal serum progesterone (P4) level (10 days before expected menses, day 21 in a 28-day cycle, P4 level >3 ng/mL indicates ovulation)
    - Evaluate ovarian reserve if woman is over age 35
      - Day 2 or 3 FSH (values under 10 suggest adequate reserve)
      - Clomiphene citrate (*Clomid*) challenge test (CCCT): Measure day 3 FSH/Estradiol; patient takes 100 mg *Clomid* days 5–9, FSH/Estradiol measured day 10
        Normal if both FSH values <10 (or sum of day 3 and day 10 FSH <26 mIU/mL)
      - Anti-Müllerian Hormone (AMH): Produced by pre-antral and antral follicles, reflecting size of follicular pool. Consistent throughout cycle but may decrease in setting of hormonal contraception. (can be tested any day). AMH level >1 ng/mL suggests adequate ovarian reserve
      - Antral follicle count: Transvaginal ultrasound on cycles days 2–4 to measure follicles measuring 2–10 mm; >10 antral follicles suggests adequate ovarian reserve; 5–10 considered diminished ovarian reserve

- *Uterine* (2–3%)
  - *Common causes:* Filling defects (submucosal fibroid, uterine septum, synechiae, polyps, diethylstilbestrol (DES) exposure), Müllerian anomaly, luteal phase defect
  - *Evaluation includes*
    - HSG for filling defects
      - Uterine abnormality is not itself an indication for surgery
      - Proceed to surgery if submucous fibroid, septate uterus, or synechiae and patient has subfertility or recurrent loss
    - Saline infusion hysterography
      - Can be done in office
      - Higher sensitivity for small intracavitary lesions

- *Unexplained infertility* (25%)
  - Couples with unexplained infertility have no identifiable etiology of their infertility after comprehensive evaluation
  - Treatment strategies are empiric

Evaluation of Infertility

- *Semen analysis*
- *Hormone studies*
  - Clinical assessment of ovulation from menstrual history
  - If amenorrheic: Check FSH, prolactin, TSH; give progestin challenge
  - Progestin challenge test: *Provera* 10 mg for 5–7 days; withdrawal should induce menses; positive result suggests ovulatory dysfunction
  - If irregular menses: Check FSH, prolactin, TSH
  - If galactorrhea: Check prolactin, FSH
- *Postcoital test (PCT)*-**only if suspect cervical factor**
  - Assesses ability of sperm to travel through cervical mucus
  - Perform test 1–2 days before ovulation (about days 12–14 in a 28–30 day cycle), when cervical mucus becomes clear and thin
  - Mucus examined within 2–12 hours after intercourse
  - Normal test result usually defined as more than 5–10 progressively motile sperm per HPF (×400) and clear, acellular mucus with spinnbarkeit of 8 cm
- *BBT*
  - Test to confirm ovulation
  - Check oral temperature every morning at same time BEFORE GETTING OUT OF BED
  - Temperature rises about 0.4°F around the time of ovulation and lasts for >10 days
- *HSG*
  - Performed in follicular phase to minimize chance of interrupting a pregnancy
  - Premedicate with NSAIDs, but pain/cramping >24 hours later may still occur
  - Antibiotic prophylaxis (*Doxycycline* 100 mg orally twice daily for 5 days) if dilated tubes or history of PID
  - DO NOT PERFORM if suspicion of current infection
    - Types of contrast (iodine based): **Always ask about iodine allergy!!**
      - Water soluble (*Sinografin*): Advantages are high resorption, better contour for tubal mucosa. Disadvantage: Peritoneal irritation
- *Laparoscopy*
  - Diagnostic and therapeutic tool: Assesses peritoneal and tubal factors and allows for correction when possible
  - Performed in follicular phase to minimize disruption of a pregnancy
  - Chromopertubation: Injection of dye (indigo carmine) through tubes to document patency

Treatment of Infertility (based on the underlying cause)

Anovulation

Polycystic Ovary Syndrome (PCOS) (responsive to ovulation induction)
Agents used:

Clomiphene citrate (*Clomid*)

- *Mechanism of action:* Estrogen antagonist and agonist, results in increased FSH and LH release due to its anti-estrogen effects at level of the hypothalamus
- *Side effects:* Hot flushes, visual symptoms (blurry vision, scotomata), headaches, mood swings
- *Risks:* Approximately 10% risk of multiple gestation
- *Administration*
  - Begin on cycle days 2–5 at a dose of 50 mg every day for 5 days
  - If ovulation doesn't occur in first cycle, increase to 100 mg

- Advise intercourse every other day for 1 week beginning 5 days after last day of medications, or time intercourse based on ovulation predictor kit OR intrauterine insemination (IUI) just before ovulation
- Can also check 21-day serum progesterone level to confirm ovulation (ovulation if progesterone >3 ng/mL)
- After six unsuccessful cycles, consider new treatment

Letrozole (*Femara*) *(Ovulation induction is off-label use)*
- *Mechanism of action:* Aromatase inhibitor: decreases estrogen negative feedback at level of hypothalamus, results in increased FSH. As follicle develops, negative feedback usually results in monofollicular development
- *Administration:* Begin 2.5–7.5 mg on days 2–5 for 5 days
- *Side effects:* Edema, hot flashes, headaches
- Higher live-birth and ovulation rates with letrozole compared with clomiphene. May be a lower twin pregnancy rate. (NEJM 2014;371:119-29).

Glucophage (*Metformin*) or other insulin-sensitizing agents
- Insulin resistance commonly seen in women with PCOS
- Used alone or in combination with *Clomid* in women who are overweight and hyperandrogenic
- NIH multicenter trial: *Metformin* does not increase live birth rate

Gonadotropins [HMG (*human menopausal gonadotropins—LH/FSH mixture*) or recombinant FSH]
- Require close hormonal and sonographic monitoring
- Much more expensive than *Clomid*
- Carries a high risk of multiple gestation
- Follicular development must be monitored by ultrasound

Hypothalamic-pituitary axis dysregulation (WHO class 1)
- Causes: Excessive weight gain or loss, exercise, or emotional stress
- Address underlying problem by behavioral modification
  - If BMI >27 kg/m^2 and anovulatory infertility, advise weight loss
  - In obese women with PCOS, loss of 5–10% of body weight restores ovulation in 55–100% within 6 months
  - Anovulatory women with low BMI (<17 kg/m^2), eating disorders, or strenuous exercise regimens → advise weight gain

Hyperprolactinemia
- Treatment relies upon restoration of normal dopamine–prolactin balance
- Bromocriptine (dopamine agonist) inhibits pituitary prolactin
  - Starting dose is 2.5 mg at bedtime (per vagina if oral not tolerated)
  - Side effects: Nausea, diarrhea, dizziness, headache, postural hypotension
  - Success rate: 80% pregnancy rate
- Cabergoline may also be used with fewer side effects

Thyroid dysfunction
- Both hyperthyroid and hypothyroid can result in infertility

Uterine Factor
Filling Defects due to Uterine Fibroids or Uterine Septae
- *Uterine Fibroids:*
  - Mainstay of treatment is hysteroscopic resection
  - Pre-op treatment with GnRH may shrink myoma, but is controversial because it may also induce fibrous changes within the myoma
  - No size limit for hysteroscopic resection as long as cavity can be visualized and loop electrode safely placed around the lesion, but large fibroids may require an additional procedure
  - Long-term effects on placentation after resection are unknown
  - Abdominal myomectomy required for resection of intramural fibroids
  - Submucous myomas penetrating over 50% into myometrium should be removed abdominally
- *Uterine septae:*
  - Should be hysteroscopically resected if greater than 1 cm
  - May need to consider cesarean delivery if extensive resection

Tubal Factor

Endometriosis

- Requires surgical treatment, usually via laparoscopic resection or ablation
- Adhesiolysis improves possibility of conceiving
- If surgery fails to promote pregnancy, in vitro fertilization (IVF) may be required
- Treatment for patients not desiring fertility includes OCPs and/or GnRH agonists

Tubal Obstruction

- Surgical correction via tubal cannulation or microsurgical reanastomosis
- Most successful in distal tubal obstruction. Reconstruction of proximal tube not highly successful and the risk of ectopic pregnancy is high (about 20%)

Hydrosalpinx

- Salpingectomy improves outcome of IVF
- Proposed mechanism: Fluid in hydrosalpinx toxic to embryo or causes mechanical flushing of embryo out of uterus

ASSISTED REPRODUCTIVE TECHNOLOGY (ART)

Methods

Controlled Ovarian Hyperstimulation (COH)

Protocols

- *Antagonist protocol*
  - No medication prior to menses
  - Start gonadotropins cycle day 2
  - Add GnRH antagonist either cycle day 6 or when lead follicle is 14 mm
  - hCG trigger for ovulation
- *Oral contraceptives (OCPs)—GnRH analogues*
  - OCPs for 21 days, starting menstrual cycle day 1-3, followed by leuprolide (*Lupron*) 1 mg/day for 21 days
  - Stimulation with gonadotropins and leuprolide 0.5 mg/day
  - hCG trigger for ovulation when three follicles reach 18 mm
- *GnRH agonist long protocol*
  - Start leuprolide 1 mg/day for 21 days approximately 7 days after estimated ovulation of preceding cycle
  - Stimulation with gonadotropins and leuprolide 0.5 mg/day
  - hCG trigger for ovulation
- *Microdose GnRH Agonist Flare Protocol*
  - Mainly used for poor responders
  - OCPs for 21 days, starting menstrual cycle day 1-3
  - Stop OCPs for 3 days and then start leuprolide 0.04 mg every 12 hours for flare effect
  - 3 days after, start leuprolide
  - Begin ovarian stimulation with gonadotropins; continue leuprolide
  - hCG trigger for ovulation

Intrauterine Insemination (IUI)

- Indications: Male factor with more than 1 million motile sperm, cervical factor
- Consists of washing an ejaculated semen specimen to remove prostaglandins, concentrating sperm in small volume of culture media, and injecting sperm directly into upper uterine cavity
- Performed just prior to ovulation with natural cycle or with ovulation induction

In Vitro Fertilization—Embryo Transfer (IVF/ET)

- Indications: Tubal factor, severe endometriosis, ovarian failure (with donor egg), oligo-ovulation, unexplained infertility, severe male factor, HIV-positive sero-discordant couples, couples seeking preimplantation genetic diagnosis (PGD)
- Overall live birth rate: 36% (CDC, 2012)
- *Procedure*
  - Woman undergoes COH as above
  - Ultrasonographically guided aspiration of oocytes (retrieval)
  - Laboratory fertilization with prepared (washed) sperm
  - Embryo culture
  - Transcervical transfer of embryo(s) into uterus 2–6 days later

Intracytoplasmic Sperm Injection (ICSI) (live birth rate: 31%)

- Indication: Severe male factor with less than 1 million motile sperm
- May require testicular biopsy (by urologist) for sperm retrieval
- Ovarian stimulation and retrieval as above
- Followed by microscopic injection of single spermatozoon into each oocyte

Possible Complications of ART

Ovarian Hyperstimulation Syndrome (OHSS)

- Self-limiting in most cases but severe illness possible
- Rarely occurs if hCG withheld; more severe if pregnancy occurs
- Can prevent by stopping gonadotropins and awaiting reduction in estradiol before giving hCG, by canceling cycle, by using a *Lupron* trigger (in antagonist cycles) or freezing embryos
- *Medical treatment*
  - Maintain blood volume
  - Correct fluid/electrolyte balance (monitor strict ins and outs, daily weights)
  - Prevent thromboembolic events
  - Relieve secondary complications of ascites/hydrothorax
- *Surgical treatment*
  - Only if ovarian torsion, rupture, hemorrhage; relieve pulmonary symptoms

Ectopic Pregnancy (see GYNECOLOGY Section)

Heterotopic Pregnancy

- Simultaneous development of intra- and extrauterine pregnancies
- Incidence: Varying reports; approximately 1:3900 pregnancies overall to 1 in 100 ART pregnancies
- Majority of ectopics occur in fallopian tube (90%); however, can implant in cervix, ovary, cornua, abdomen, and cesarean scar
- Can be life-threatening and the diagnosis can be easily missed
- Risk factors: Ovulation induction, ART
- Ectopic usually treated surgically and intrauterine may continue normally
- Consider diagnosis in patient with a viable intrauterine pregnancy with significant abdominal pain (especially if ART, free fluid in pelvis, adnexal mass on sono, or rise in hCG after treatment)

Multiple Gestations

- High-order multiples (≥3 implanted embryos): Undesirable outcome of ART
- Multiples lead to increased risk of complications in both fetuses and mother
- ASRM/SART developed guidelines (Table 4-4) for determining appropriate number of cleavage-stage (usually 2–3 days after fertilization) embryos or blastocysts (usually 5–6 days after fertilization)

TABLE 4-4 2009 ASRM/SART GUIDELINES

	Recommended Limits on the Numbers of Embryos to Transfer			
	Age			
Prognosis	<35 years	35–37 years	38–40 years	41–42 years
Cleavage-stage embryos*				
Favorable[†]	1–2	2	3	5
All others	2	3	4	5
Blastocysts*				
Favorable[†]	1	2	2	3
All others	2	2	3	3

*See text for more complete explanations. Justification for transferring one additional embryo more than the recommended limits should be clearly documented in the patient's medical record.
[†]Favorable = first cycle of IVF, good embryo quality, excess embryos available for cryopreservation, or previous successful IVF cycle.
Source: Used with permission from Practice Committee of the American Society for Reproductive Medicine; Practice Committee of the Society for Assisted Reproductive Technology. Guidelines on number of embryos transferred. *Fertil Steril.* 2009;92:1518–1519.

PREIMPLANTATION GENETIC DIAGNOSIS (PGD) AND PREIMPLANTATION GENETIC SCREENING (PGS)

- Patients undergo COH ± oocyte retrieval and fertilization
- Biopsy and genetic analyses performed on one of the following:
  - 1–2 blastomeres of cleavage-stage (days 2–3) embryo
  - Trophectoderm tissue from blastocyst-stage (day 5) embryo
  - Polar body biopsy from metaphase II oocyte

- Testing performed
  - *Single-gene disorders: (use PCR for amplification)*
    - Screen for known hereditary disorder (eg, cystic fibrosis, Huntington's Disease)
    - Only unaffected embryos are transferred
  - *Aneuploidy testing (using FISH, single nucleotide polymorphism microarrays, or comparative genomic hybridization next-generation sequencing)*
    - Screen for aneuploidy or other chromosomal abnormalities
    - Offered to women with advanced maternal age, recurrent pregnancy loss, multiple IVF failures
    - Disadvantages: Mosaicism in embryo impairs accuracy
  - *Sibling human leukocyte antigen (HLA) matching*
    - Select for an embryo that is HLA-matched to a preexisting sibling with a potentially correctable genetic disorder
  - *Elective sex selection:* Ethically controversial

COMMON DISORDERS RELATED TO INFERTILITY

Polycystic Ovary Syndrome (PCOS)

- 74% of women with PCOS have infertility
- 80% with menstrual dysregulation

Diagnosis
- Rotterdam criteria (**need two out of three**)
  - Oligo- and/or anovulation
  - Clinical and/or biochemical signs of hyperandrogenism
  - Polycystic ovaries (by ultrasound) (Figure 4-2)
- Insulin resistance occurs in lean or obese
- Consider glucose tolerance test in PCOS patients who are obese and/or have a family history of type 2 diabetes

Treatment
- Depends on the woman's goals (desires fertility?)
- In obese women, weight loss can improve symptoms
- OCPs are first-line treatment

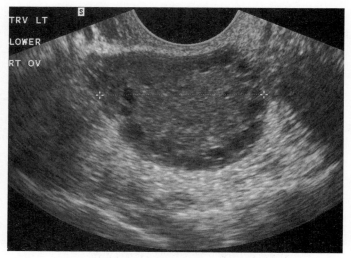

Figure 4-2 Ultrasound image of polycystic ovary. (Used with permission from Hoffman BL, et al. Chapter 17. Polycystic ovarian syndrome and hyperandrogenism. In: Hoffman BL, et al., eds. *Williams Gynecology*. 2nd ed. New York, NY: McGraw-Hill; 2012.)

- Drugs that reduce insulin levels can be effective in both obese and normal-weight women (ie, glucophage)
- *Hirsutism:* (see next section)
  - Hair growth may be slowed by administration of medication alone or in combination with mechanical hair removal
  - Treatment may also reduce acne
- *Endometrial protection*
  - Chronic anovulation is associated with increased risk of endometrial hyperplasia and cancer. Treat with OCPs or intermittent progestin
  - Progestin antagonizes endometrial proliferative effect of estrogen

Hirsutism

Definition

- Excessive and increased hair growth in women in locations where terminal hair normally is minimal or absent
- Hirsutism–androgen sensitive (male-pattern hair growth)
- Hypertrichosis–androgen insensitive
- Ferriman–Gallwey Scoring System (Figure 4-3)

Causes

- *Ovarian:* PCOS (testosterone produced by theca cells); Sertoli–Leydig tumor; insulin resistance syndromes (increased levels of androgen/insulin decreases sex hormone-binding globulin (SHBG) levels → increased free testosterone)
- *Adrenal:* Cancer (rule out if testosterone >200 ng/dL); hyperplasia; Cushing's syndrome
- Pregnancy (luteoma of pregnancy)
- Medications (eg, Danazol)
- Idiopathic

Workup

- *Initial labs:* Serum testosterone (T), 17 hydroxyprogesterone (17-OHP), progesterone, prolactin, TSH, dehydroepiandrosterone sulfate (DHEAS), FSH, estradiol (E2)
  - If total T >200 ng/dL → rule out ovarian androgen-secreting tumor
  - If DHEAS >700 μg/dL → rule out adrenal androgen-secreting tumor
  - If 17-OHP >200 ng/mL → rule out late onset congenital adrenal hyperplasia (must be in follicular phase: P4 must be less than 3 ng/dL)
  - If ↓E2 and ↓FSH → hypogonadotropic hypogonadism
  - If ↓E2 and ↑FSH → POF
  - If prolactin >30 ng/mL → prolactinemia
  - If TSH abnormal → further evaluate for thyroid disease
  - If hypertensive/examination suspicious (moon facies, buffalo hump, abdominal striae) → screen for Cushing's syndrome (below)
- **Cushing's Syndrome Workup**
  - Overnight dexamethasone suppression test (1 mg given at 11 PM then plasma cortisol drawn at 8 AM; <5 μg/dL rules out Cushing's syndrome)
  - If test is abnormal, establish diagnosis with 24-hour free urinary cortisol

Treatment Options

- <u>Hormonal:</u> Monophasic OCPs, *Depo-Provera*, leuprolide (LH suppression decreases testosterone production and increases testosterone clearance), flutamide, finasteride
- <u>Steroids:</u> Dexamethasone
- <u>Diuretic:</u> Spironolactone 100–200 mg daily (anti-androgen properties)
- <u>Cosmetic:</u> Mechanical hair removal (shaving, waxing, electrolysis, laser treatment) or medication eflornithine topical (*Vaniqa*)

Late-Onset Congenital Adrenal Hyperplasia (CAH)

- Most common: 21-hydroxylase deficiency (rarely 11β-hydroxylase and 3β-hydroxysteroid dehydrogenase deficiencies)
- 17-OHP >800 ng/dL is virtually diagnostic of late onset CAH
- If 17-OHP >200 ng/dL → adrenocorticotropic hormone (ACTH) stimulation test
- ACTH stim test: 250 μg IV ACTH → 17-OHP levels at time 0 and 1 hour

Galactorrhea

Definition

- Mammary secretion of a milky fluid, excluding breast feeding
  - Workup needed if nulliparous or if 12 months since childbirth/weaning

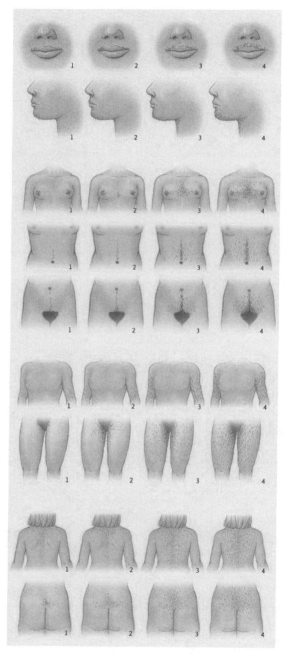

Figure 4-3 Ferriman–Gallwey scoring system for hirsutism. Hair growth is rated from 0 (no growth of terminal hair) to 4 (complete and heavy cover), in nine locations, giving a maximum score of 36. In Caucasian women, a score of 8 or higher is indicative of androgen excess. (Used with permission from Hoffman BL, et al. Chapter 17. Polycystic ovarian syndrome and hyperandrogenism. In: Hoffman BL, et al., eds. *Williams Gynecology*. 2nd ed. New York, NY: McGraw-Hill; 2012.)

- May be white or clear in color but also greenish or even bloody
- Bloody discharge suspicious for cancer and mammogram needed

Workup
- **Initial evaluation:** TSH, prolactin, progestin challenge (if amenorrhea)
- If elevated TSH → hypothyroid
- If withdrawal bleed and normal prolactin/TSH → anovulation
- If prolactin elevated after repeat testing → MRI of the brain

Primary Amenorrhea

Definition
- No period by age 14 without secondary sexual characteristics or no period by age 16 with or without secondary sexual characteristics
- **Initial evaluation:** hCG, check for signs of estrogen (breast development or serum E2), prolactin, thyroid function tests (TFTs), FSH, evaluate outflow tract (examination/pelvic sono)
  - If hypergonadotropic (increased FSH) → check karyotype
  - If hypogonadotropic (decreased FSH) → MRI
  - If hyperprolactinemia → MRI
  - If eugonadotropic (normal FSH) → rule out outflow tract defect

Secondary Amenorrhea

Definition
Absence of three cycles or 6 months in previously menstruating woman
- **Initial evaluation:** Pregnancy test, prolactin, TFTs, progestin challenge
  - Progestin challenge: 10 mg *Provera* for 5 days. Positive response is withdrawal bleed within 2–7 days after stopping *Provera*
  - If withdrawal bleed → anovulation (if prolactin, TSH normal)
  - If no withdrawal bleed → check FSH, pelvic sonogram
    - If FSH low/normal → hypothalamic
    - If FSH high → ovarian failure (consider karyotype)
  - If TFTs abnormal → further evaluate for thyroid disease
  - If prolactin elevated → prolactinemia workup (MRI if greater than 60 ng/mL)

Disorders due to Enzyme Deficiencies

- See Steroidogenesis Pathway (Figure 4-4)

Congenital Adrenal Hyperplasia (CAH)
- Due to 21-hydroxylase deficiency or 11β-hydroxylase deficiency (rare)
  - Autosomal recessive
  - Results in backup of androgen precursors and markedly reduced cortisol and aldosterone

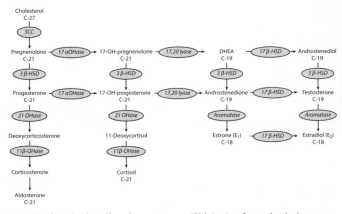

Figure 4-4 Steroidogenesis pathway. Blue ovals represent enzymes. "C" designation reflects number of carbon atoms. 3β-HSD = 3β-hydroxysteroid dehydrogenase; 11β-OHase = 11β-hydroxylase; 17αOHase = 17α-hydroxylase; 17β-HSD = 17β-hydroxysteroid dehydrogenase; 21OHase = 21-hydroxylase; DHEA = dehydroepiandrosterone; SCC = side-chain cleavage enzyme. (Used with permission from Hoffman BL, et al. Chapter 15. Reproductive endocrinology. In: Hoffman BL, et al., eds. Williams Gynecology, 2nd ed. New York, NY: McGraw-Hill; 2012.)

- Females may be born with masculinized external female genitalia
- Salt-wasting at birth may be life-threatening
- Late-Onset CAH (1:1000 births)—increased androgens present at puberty

5-alpha-reductase deficiency
- Inability to convert testosterone to more physiologically active dihydrotestosterone (DHT)
- XY individuals may be born with female external genitalia but then virilization occurs at puberty

17α-Hydroxylase deficiency
- Rare, presents with hypertension, hypokalemia, and hypogonadism
- XY individuals will have female genital, XX will have primary amenorrhea

NORMAL AND ABNORMAL PUBERTY

Normal Pubertal Development

- **Mechanism:** Leptin is proposed hormone responsible for initiation of puberty
  - Earlier onset of puberty in general population attributed to increased prevalence of childhood obesity
  - Leptin appears to aid in maturation of the GnRH pulse generator
- **Tanner stages:** System utilized to describe sequence of pubertal changes (Figure 4-5)
- **Thelarche:** Beginning of breast development (Tanner 2); usually first sign of puberty
- **Pubarche:** Minority of girls develop pubic hair as first sign of puberty
- **Peak height velocity**
  - Occurs approximately 0.5 years before menarche
  - 17–18% of adult height accrues during puberty
  - Limbs accelerate before the trunk
  - About half of total body calcium is laid down during puberty
- **Menarche**
  - Usually occurs 2.5 years after onset of puberty
  - Generally occurs at about age 12, with African-American girls experiencing menarche earlier than Hispanic and Caucasian girls
- **Weight changes**
  - Prior to age 16, increase in BMI generally due to fat-free mass
  - After age 16, increase in BMI due to increases in fat mass
  - Adolescent girls have greater proportion of adipose tissue distributed along the upper arms, thighs, and upper back

Precocious Puberty

- **Definition** (controversial)
  - Prior to age 6 in African-American girls; prior to age 7 in Caucasian girls
  - *Most pediatric endocrinologists in the United States use traditional threshold of 8 years old*
- **Types**
  - Central precocious puberty: Result of early but otherwise normal activation of hypothalamic-pituitary-gonadal function
    - 80–90% have no identifiable lesion (idiopathic)
  - Incomplete precocity (the early development of secondary sexual characteristics): A variant of normal puberty
    - Perform radiologic bone age to confirm that growth is not accelerated. If normal, no further testing required

Delayed Puberty

- **Definition:** Defined clinically by absence or incomplete development of secondary sexual characteristics by age at which 95% of children initiated sexual maturation; about age 12 for girls
- **Mechanism:** Inadequate gonadal steroid secretion
- **Causes**
  - *Primary hypogonadism*: Results from variety of causes of gonadal disease. Characterized by high serum levels of LH/FSH
  - *Secondary hypogonadism*: Results from diminished GnRH-induced gonadotropin secretion. Characterized by low or normal serum LH/FSH levels
    - Hypothalamic dysfunction (anatomic or functional)
    - Hypopituitarism
    - Hypothyroidism
    - Hyperprolactinemia

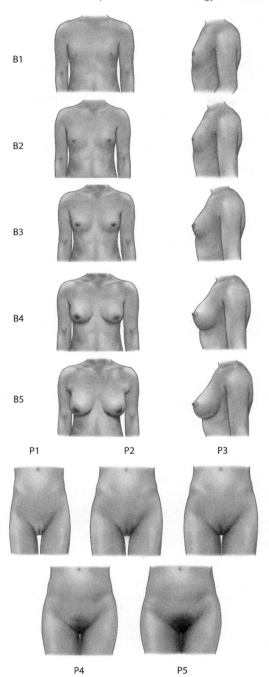

Figure 4-5 Tanner stages. (Used with permission from Hoffman BL, et al. Chapter 14. Pediatric gynecology. In: Hoffman BL, et al., eds. *Williams Gynecology*. 2nd ed. New York, NY: McGraw-Hill; 2012.)

CONGENITAL MÜLLERIAN ANOMALIES (FIGURE 4-6)

Prevalence

• Difficult to assess, about 0.16–10%. About 3% in women with repeated pregnancy loss

Mechanism

• At 6 weeks of development, male and female genital systems indistinguishable
• Two sets of ducts: Paramesonephric (Müllerian) and Mesonephric (Wolffian). In absence of testis-determining factor (Y chromosome), mesonephric ducts degenerate
• Paramesonephric ducts initially separated by septum. At 9 weeks, ducts fuse at inferior margin forming single lumen of the uterovaginal canal (fallopian tubes, uterus, upper two-thirds of vagina). *Note:* Urogenital sinus forms lower one-third of vagina
• Müllerian anomalies result from inappropriate fusion
• Patients with Müllerian anomalies therefore have normal ovaries and function

Septate Uterus (approximately 55%; most common)
• Results from partial or complete failure of resorption of the uterovaginal septum after fusion of the paramesonephric ducts
• Associated with poor reproductive outcomes: SABs (approximately 65%), preterm labor, breech
• Longitudinal vaginal septum may cause dyspareunia. Treat with hysteroscopic resection

Unicornuate Uterus (approximately 20%)
• Failure of development or migration of one Müllerian duct
• Associated with early SABs (41–62%), ectopic pregnancy, abnormal presentation, fetal growth restriction, preterm labor, endometriosis, infertility, chronic pain
• Rudimentary horn may be present. Most are asymptomatic because they are noncommunicating and endometrium is nonfunctional
• Urinary tract anomalies (usually kidney) more common in these patients (approximately 40%) than with other Müllerian duct anomalies

Uterus Didelphys (approximately 5%)
• Lack of fusion of the two Müllerian ducts causing duplication of corpus and cervix; no communication between duplicated endometrial cavities
• 75% have longitudinal vaginal septum
• One side is usually obstructed and symptomatic
  • Obstructed hemivagina: Treated with excision of vaginal septum
  • Can be associated with ipsilateral renal agenesis
• Pregnancy with increased SABs (32–52%), malpresentation, and preterm labor
• Treated by resection of the obstructed horn

Bicornuate Uterus (approximately 10%)
• Incomplete fusion of the two Müllerian ducts at the level of the fundus
  • Two symmetric cornua fused caudad, with communication of the two endometrial cavities
  • Single cervix with varying degrees of separation between the two uterine horns
• Little difficulty conceiving, but increased SABs (28–35%), preterm labor, breech presentation
• In select cases, may consider surgical reunification

Arcuate Uterus
• Mild indentation of the endometrium at the uterine fundus
• Results from almost complete resorption of the uterovaginal septum
• Normal external uterine contour
• Broad smooth indentation on fundal segment of endometrium

Mayer–Rokitansky–Küster–Hauser Syndrome
• Agenesis of the uterus and vagina
• One in 4000–10 000 newborn females
• Associated with normal karyotype and secondary sex characteristics
• <1% have a rudimentary uterine horn with functioning endometrium
• 15% have major urinary tract anomalies: Unilateral renal agenesis, unilateral or bilateral pelvic kidney, horseshoe kidney
• Approximately 25% with minor urinary tract abnormalities: Hydronephrosis, hydroureter, malrotation of kidneys, duplication of collecting system
• 5–10% associated with skeletal anomalies, generally spinal or middle ear
• Have normal external genitalia
• Presenting symptom is usually primary amenorrhea

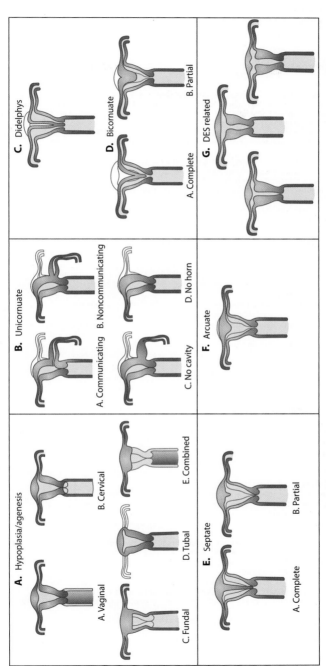

Figure 4-6 Classification of Müllerian anomalies according to ASRM classification system. (Used with permission from Reynolds R, Loar PV, III. Chapter 39. Gynecology. In: Doherty GM, ed. *CURRENT Diagnosis & Treatment: Surgery.* 13th ed. New York, NY: McGraw-Hill; 2010.)

- Ultrasound to confirm presence/absence of uterus
- MRI to evaluate extent of abnormalities; intravenous pyelogram to rule out urinary tract anomalies
- Remember: Do not confuse with complete androgen resistance syndrome (46 XY)

MENOPAUSE

Definitions

- ***Menopause:*** Final menstrual period, usually confirmed after no menses for 12 consecutive months (in absence of other obvious causes). Menopause is associated with reduced functioning of the ovaries due to aging, resulting in lower levels of estrogen and other hormones. It marks the permanent end of fertility
  - Menopause occurs, on average, at age 51, with normal range 43 to 57 years. Can also be induced by oophorectomy or iatrogenic ablation of ovarian function (chemotherapy, radiation)
  - **POF:** Loss of ovarian function before age 40 leading to permanent or transient amenorrhea
- In 2001 the Stages of Reproductive Aging Workshop (STRAW) divided normal female reproductive aging into stages (Figure 4-7)
  - Reproductive and post-reproductive life divided into several stages, with final menstrual period (FMP) serving as anchor
  - Five stages (−5 to −1) precede the FMP and two stages follow (+1 and +2)
  - *Menopausal transition:* Stages −2 to −1 (replaces term *perimenopause*)

Diagnosis

- Clinical diagnosis, without reliance on hormone measurements
  - When any doubt exists about the diagnosis of menopause, other causes of secondary amenorrhea must be ruled out
  - Lab tests should include serum pregnancy test and prolactin level
  - FDA: No scientific basis for using saliva testing to adjust hormone levels
- Vasomotor Symptoms
- About 80% of menopausal women experience hot flashes/flushes and night sweats
- Symptoms begin at an average of 2 years before the final menstrual period
- Risk Factors: Surgical menopause (up to 90% of women will have vasomotor symptoms), early menopause, low circulating levels of estradiol, smoking, and possibly low BMI
- Treatment of vasomotor symptoms
  - Needs to be tailored! Counsel patient on risks versus benefits of each treatment option

Mild Symptoms

- Lifestyle modifications: Lightweight cotton clothing, dressing in layers, fans/air conditioning, avoid hot foods/drinks, weight loss, exercise, smoking cessation
- Nonprescription remedies: Dietary isoflavones, black cohosh, vitamin E

Moderate to Severe Symptoms

- **Hormone Therapy (HT)** (Table 4-5)
  - *Recommended terminology*
    - EPT: Combined estrogen–progestogen therapy
    - ET: Estrogen therapy
    - HT: Hormone therapy (both ET and EPT)
  - The most effective therapy for vasomotor symptoms (75% effective)
  - Progestogen NEEDED to negate increased risk of endometrial cancer from systemic ET in women with a uterus
  - *Recommendation:* Lowest effective dose for the shortest time. Start at lowest dose and titrate up as needed
  - *Route:* No clear benefit of one route of administration versus another for systemic therapy. Transdermal may be associated with a lower risk of DVT than oral
  - **Local** ET is preferred when treating solely vaginal symptoms. Vaginal estrogen can also relieve urogenital atrophy symptoms
  - Reassess use of HT annually
  - *Discontinuance:* Many recommend considering discontinuing HT by 5 years. Symptom recurrence is similar when HT is tapered or abruptly stopped. No current recommendation as to how to discontinue therapy
  - OCPs can also be used during the menopausal transition to relieve vasomotor symptoms and as contraception
- If episodes of bleeding occur more often than every 21 days, last longer than 8 days, are very heavy, or occur after a 6-month interval of amenorrhea, evaluation of the endometrium must be undertaken to rule out neoplasm

Final Menstrual Period (FMP)

Stages:	-5	-4	-3	-2	-1	(0)	+1	+2
Terminology:	Reproductive			Menopausal Transition			Postmenopause	
	Early	Peak	Late	Early	Late*		Early*	Late
					Perimenopause			
Duration of Stage:	Variable			Variable			(a) 1 yr / (b) 4 yrs	Until demise
							Amen x 12 mos	None
Menstrual Cycles:	Variable to regular	Regular		Variable cycle length (>7 days different from normal)	≥2 Skipped cycles and an interval of amenorrhea (≥60 days)			
Endocrine:	Normal FSH		↑ FSH		↑ FSH			↑ FSH

*Stages most likely to be characterized by vasomotor symptoms   ↑ = elevated

Figure 4-7 Stages of female reproductive aging. (Used with permission from Hoffman BL, et al. Chapter 21. Menopausal transition. In: Hoffman BL, et al. eds. Williams Gynecology, 2nd ed. New York, NY: McGraw-Hill; 2012.)

TABLE 4-5 HORMONE THERAPY OPTIONS

Drug	Name	Comments
Oral Estrogens		
17β-estradiol*	Estrace, Gynodiol	0.5–2.0 mg daily
Conjugated estrogens	Premarin	0.3–1.25 mg daily
Synthetic conjugated estrogens	Cenestin, Enjuvia	0.3–1.25 mg daily
Esterified estrogens	Menest	0.3–2.5 mg daily
Estropipate (crystalline form of estrone)	Ogen, other generics	0.75 mg = 0.625 mg estrone
Transdermal Estrogen Preparations		
17β-estradiol*		
Patch	Alora, Climara, Estraderm, Estradot, Minivelle, VivelleDot, Menostar, Vivelle	Variable dosing; apply once or twice a week
Gel	Divigel, EstroGel, Elestrin	
Topical Emulsion	Estrasorb	Lotion packets
Spray	Evamist	
Vaginal Estrogen Products		
Creams		
17β-estradiol*	Estrace	Vulvovaginal atrophy
Conjugated estrogens	Premarin	Atrophic vaginitis, dyspareunia
Rings		
17β-estradiol*	Estring (90 days)	Mod to severe urogenital symptoms (PM atrophy)
Estradiol acetate*	Femring (90 days)	Vasomotor symptoms; releases systemic levels—if uterus, consider progesterone
Estradiol*	Vagifem	Tablet
Combination Estrogen–Progestogen Products		
Oral continuous—cyclic		
Conjugated estrogens (E) + medroxyprogesterone acetate (P)	Premphase	Varying dosages of E and P E days 1–14; E+P days 15–28
Oral continuous—combined		
Conjugated estrogens (E) + medroxyprogesterone acetate (P)	Prempro	Varying dosages of E and P
Ethinyl estradiol (E) + norethindrone acetate (P)	Femhrt	
17β-estradiol (E) + norethindrone acetate (P)	Activella	
17β-estradiol (E) + drospirenone (P)	Angeliq	
Oral intermittent—combined		
17β-estradiol (E) + norgestimate (P)	Prefest	E alone for 3 days, followed by E+P for 3 days, repeat

TABLE 4-5 HORMONE THERAPY OPTIONS (*Continued*)

Drug	Name	Comments
Transdermal continuous-combined		
17β-estradiol (E) norethindrone acetate (P)	CombiPatch	Varying dosages; twice weekly
17β-estradiol (E) + levonorgestrel (P)	Climara Pro	Varying dosages; once weekly
Oral Progestogens		
Medroxyprogesterone acetate	Provera	2.5–10 mg
Micronized progesterone*	Prometrium	100 mg daily continuously or 200 mg daily cyclically
Other Progesterones		
Levonorgestrel IUD	Mirena*	20 μg/day
Progesterone vaginal gel	Prochieve 4%, 8%	4% applicator = 45 mg

* "Bioidentical": Same structure as hormones produced in body.
For updates, see: http://www.menopause.org/docs/default-source/2014/nams-ht-tables.pdf

- **Alternatives to HT**
  - Selective serotonin and norepinephrine reuptake inhibitors (SSRI/SNRIs) (Table 4-6)
    - Effective in decreasing the frequency and severity of hot flashes by 50–60% compared to placebo
    - Need to be tapered when discontinuing
  - **Others**
    - Gabapentin (*Neurontin*) 900–2400 mg/day
      - Anticonvulsant; unknown mechanism for hot flashes
      - Reduces number and severity of hot flashes by 54%
      - Side effects: Somnolence, fatigue, dizziness, rash, palpitations, peripheral edema
    - Clonidine (0.05–0.15 mg/day). Limited efficacy/high toxicity
- **Herbal remedies**
  - Isoflavones (soy products): Weak estrogenic and anti-estrogenic activities
    - 80–120 mg/day
    - Data conflicting (may or may not be better than placebo). More long-term safety data on endometrial and breast cancer needed
  - Black cohosh 40–80 mg/day. Most randomized trials have shown mild or no improvement over placebo
- *Bioidentical hormones:* (compounded according to a health care provider's prescription)
  - May provide different doses, ingredients, and routes of administration that are not government approved
  - Have not been tested for efficacy or safety
  - Standardization and purity may be uncertain
  - The US FDA has ruled that compounding pharmacies have made claims about the safety and effectiveness of bioidentical hormones unsupported by clinical trial data and considered to be false and misleading

TABLE 4-6 ALTERNATIVES TO HT (SSRI/SNRI)

Venlafaxine ER (*Effexor EF*)	Effective at 75 mg/day
	Start 37.5 mg/day; slowly titrate
Paroxetine (*Brisdelle*)*	7.5 mg daily at bedtime
Fluoxetine (*Prozac*)	20 mg/day
Escitalopram (*Lexapro*)	10–20 mg/day
Citalopram (*Celexa*)	20 mg/day
Desvenlafaxine (*Pristiq*)	100 mg/day

*First FDA approved nonhormonal medication for vasomotor symptoms.

Women's Health Initiative (WHI) Key Points

- National Institutes of Health (NIH) study; established in 1991—included randomized clinical trial and observational arm
- Enrolled 161 808 PM women aged 50–79 (mean age 63)
- MAJOR CRITICISM was the mean age (remote from menopause onset!)
- Clinical trial enrolled 68 132 PM women, randomly assigned to receive HT or placebo. Primary outcome was coronary heart disease (CHD)
  - Two studies: (1) Estrogen + medroxyprogesterone 2.5 mg/day (*Prempro*; E+P) in women with uterus and (2) estrogen 0.625 mg/day (*Premarin*) in women without uterus
- In 2002, after 5 years, E+P arm stopped early because of increase in breast cancer cases with HT
  - During 1 year, among 10 000 PM women taking E+P, 38 diagnosed with breast cancer compared to 30:10 000 on placebo
- In 2004, the estrogen-alone study was stopped because of increased risk of stroke and no reduction in risk of CHD
- Fewer bone fractures and colon cancer cases in both hormone groups
- Secondary analysis of data showed that women who initiated HT closer to menopause had reduced CHD risk compared to women who initiated HT more distant from menopause
- Overall summary of effects of hormone therapy on event rates (see Figure 4-8)

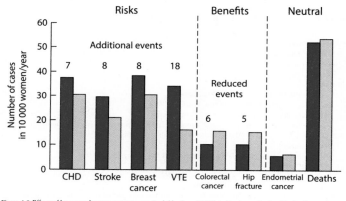

Figure 4-8 Effects of hormone therapy on event rates. Dark blue bars: E+P light blue bars: placebo. (Used with permission from Lindsay R, Cosman F. Chapter 425. Osteoporosis. In: Kasper D, et al., eds. *Harrison's Principles of Internal Medicine.* 19th ed. New York, NY: McGraw-Hill, 2015.)

OSTEOPOROSIS

- Silent disease until complicated by fractures
- Can be prevented, diagnosed, and treated before fractures occur
- Are effective treatments to decrease risk of further fractures after the first fracture
- Two million fractures per year attributed to osteoporosis
- Only 23% of women over 67 years old with an osteoporosis-related fracture receive either a bone mineral density (BMD) test or drug prescription for treatment in the 6 months following the fracture

Risk factors (Table 4-7)

TABLE 4-7 RISK FACTORS FOR OSTEOPOROSIS

• Family history of osteoporosis; low-trauma fracture in first-degree relative	• Alcohol abuse
• Body weight <127 pounds (BMI <20)	• History of previous fracture
• Smoking	• Diseases associated with osteoporosis
• Inadequate physical activity	• Early menopause, steroid use, Dilantin use
• Immobilization	• MANY MORE RISK FACTORS

Universal Recommendations

- Appropriate daily calcium intake (Table 4-8).
  - Supplements needed if diet sources not adequate. Average dietary calcium intake in adults over 50 is 600–700 mg daily. Intakes over 1200–1500 mg daily may increase risk of kidney stones, cardiovascular disease, and stroke (controversial literature)
  - Calcium is absorbed best when taken in amounts of 500–600 mg or less
  - Take most calcium supplements with food. **Except**—calcium citrate can absorb well when taken with or without food
- Appropriate daily vitamin D intake (Table 4-8)
  - There are two types of vitamin D supplements—vitamin D2 (ergocalciferol) and vitamin D3 (cholecalciferol). Both types are good for bone health
  - According to the Institute of Medicine (IOM), the safe upper limit of vitamin D is 4000 IU per day for most adults
- Regular weight-bearing and muscle-strengthening exercise
- Assess risk factors for falls and offer appropriate modifications
- Smoking cessation and avoidance of excessive alcohol intake (>2 drinks/day for women)
- Measure height annually

TABLE 4-8 CALCIUM AND VITAMIN D RECOMMENDATIONS (NATIONAL OSTEOPOROSIS FOUNDATION)

Children and Adolescents	Calcium (Daily)	Vitamin D (Daily)
1–3 years	700 mg	400 IU*
4–8 years	1000 mg	400 IU*
9–18 years	1300 mg	400 IU*
Adult Women		
19–50 years	1000 mg	400–800 IU**
51 years and over	1200 mg	800–1000 IU**
Pregnant and Breast-feeding Women		
18 years and under	1300 mg	400–800 IU
19 years and over	1000 mg	400–800 IU

*American Academy of Pediatrics recommendation.
**NIH recommends 600 IU for women under age 70; 800 IU over 70.
Sources: Data from http://ods.od.nih.gov/factsheets/Calcium-HealthProfessional/; http://ods.od.nih.gov/factsheets/VitaminD-QuickFacts/#h2

Bone Mineral Density (BMD) by Dual-Energy X-Ray Absorptiometry (DXA)

- Compares to two norms, "young normal" and "age-matched"
  - *T-score:* Compares to optimal BMD of a "young normal" adult (30 years) of same sex
  - *Z-score:* Compares BMD to expected BMD for patient's age, sex, and ethnicity
- Difference between patient's score and norm in standard deviations (SDs) above or below the mean
- At spine and hip, a decrease of 1 SD in BMD is associated with about a twofold increase in fracture risk

Indications for BMD Testing

- Women age 65 and older, regardless of clinical risk factors
- Younger PM or menopausal transition women with risk factors for fracture
- Adults who have a fracture after age 50
- Adults with condition (eg, rheumatoid arthritis) or taking a medication (glucocorticoids, daily dose ≥5 mg prednisone or equivalent for ≥3 months) associated with low bone mass/bone loss
- Limited to one BMD test every 2 years unless the patient has a medical condition that can result in rapid bone loss (ie, steroid treatment)

Vertebral Imaging

- Vertebral fracture is consistent with diagnosis of osteoporosis (even in absence of bone density diagnosis) and is an indication for treatment to reduce future fractures
- Most vertebral fractures are initially asymptomatic and are diagnosed by imaging
- Presence of a single vertebral fracture increases risk of subsequent fracture fivefold and risk of hip and other fractures two- to threefold

- Involves lateral thoracic and lumbar spine x-ray or lateral vertebral fracture assessment (available on most modern DXA machines). Can be performed at time of BMD test

Indications
- All women age ≥70 with T-score (spine, total hip, or femoral neck) ≤ −1.0
- Women age 65–69 with T-score ≤ −1.5 (spine, total hip, or femoral neck)
- PM *women with specific risk factors*
  - Low trauma fracture during adulthood (age 50)
  - Historical height loss of 1.5 in. or more (4 cm)
  - Prospective height loss of 0.8 in. or more (2 cm) during interval assessments
  - Recent or ongoing long-term glucocorticoid treatment
- If BMD testing not available, imaging may be considered based on age alone

WHO Fracture Risk Algorithm (FRAX®) (www.nof.org; www.shef.ac.uk/FRAX)

- Calculates the 10-year probability of a hip fracture and major osteoporotic fracture taking into account femoral neck BMD and risk factors
- Intended for PM women—not younger adults
- Not validated in patients currently or previously treated with medications for osteoporosis

Diagnosis of Osteoporosis (Table 4-9)

TABLE 4-9 DIAGNOSIS OF OSTEOPOROSIS

WHO Definition of Osteoporosis (Based on BMD of Lumbar Spine and Femoral Neck)	
Bone Classification	**T-Score**
Normal	Greater than or equal to −1
Osteopenia (low bone mass)	−1 to −2.5
Osteoporosis	Less than or equal to −2.5
Severe/Established osteoporosis	Less than or equal to −2.5 with one or more fractures

WHO classification is not for premenopausal women. Z-scores may be more appropriate.

Treatment of Osteoporosis

Who Should be Treated?
- PM women age ≥50 with the following should be considered for treatment:
  - A hip or vertebral fracture (clinically apparent or found on vertebral imaging)
  - T-score ≤−2.5 at femoral neck, total hip, or lumbar spine
  - Low bone mass (T-score between −1.0 and −2.5 at femoral neck or lumbar spine) and 10-year probability of hip fracture ≥3% or 10-year probability of major osteoporosis-related fracture ≥20% based on the US-adapted WHO algorithm

FDA-Approved Agents for Prevention and Treatment of Osteoporosis
- **Bisphosphonates**
  - Formulations
    - Alendronate (*Fosamax, Binosto*); Alendronate/Cholecalciferol (*Fosamax Plus D*)
      - Approved for prevention and treatment. Daily or weekly doses
      - Reduces spine and hip fractures by approximately 50% over 3 years if prior vertebral fracture or osteoporosis in hip
      - Reduces vertebral fractures by 48% over 3 years if no prior vertebral fracture
    - Risedronate (*Actonel, Atelvia*); Actonel + Calcium
      - Approved for prevention and treatment. Daily or weekly doses
      - Reduces vertebral fractures by 41–49% and non-vertebral fractures by 36% over 3 years, with significant risk reduction within 1 year in patients with prior vertebral fracture
    - Ibandronate (*Boniva*)
      - Approved for treatment
      - Reduces vertebral fractures by approximately 50% over 3 years, but no documentation of reduction in non-vertebral fractures
    - Zolendronic Acid (*Reclast*)
      - Approved for prevention and treatment
      - IV infusion once yearly (treatment); once every 2 years for prevention

- Reduces incidence of vertebral fractures by 70%, hip fractures by 41%, and non-vertebral fractures by 25% over 3 years in those with prevalent vertebral fractures and osteoporosis by BMD of hip
- Side Effects: Difficulty swallowing, esophagitis, gastric ulcer, visual disturbances (rare), osteonecrosis of jaw (very rare), may affect renal function. Long-term use may be linked to low-trauma atypical femur fractures
- **Estrogen agonist/antagonist**
  - Formulation
    - Raloxifene (*Evista*)
      - Approved for both prevention and treatment
      - Reduces risk of vertebral fractures by approximately 30% over 3 years if prior vertebral fracture and by approximately 55% if no prior fracture
      - Reduction in non-vertebral fractures has not been documented
      - Also indicated for reduction in risk of invasive breast cancer in PM women with osteoporosis
  - Side Effects: Increased risk of DVT; hot flashes; leg cramps
- **Hormone therapy**
  - Formulations
    - *Estrogen therapy or combined estrogen–progestogen therapy*
      - Approved for prevention of osteoporosis
      - WHI: 5 years of HT reduced risk of clinical vertebral fractures and hip fractures by 34% and other osteoporotic fractures by 23%
    - *Note:* FDA recommends that approved non-estrogen treatments be considered first
- **Calcitonin-Salmon**
  - Formulations
    - *Miacalcin, Fortical*
      - Approved for treatment of osteoporosis in women at least 5 years PM when alternative treatments are not suitable
      - Nasal spray or subcutaneous injection
      - Reduces vertebral fracture by approximately 30% in those with prior vertebral fractures
      - Has not been shown to reduce non-vertebral fractures
  - Side Effects: Rhinitis, epistaxis, or allergic reactions with nasal spray (especially if allergic to salmon). Possible increased risk of malignancies
- **Tissue-selective estrogen complex: Conjugated estrogens/bazedoxifene**
  - Conjugated estrogens paired with estrogen agonist/antagonist
  - Formulations
    - *Duavee*
      - Approved for prevention (and for moderate to severe vasomotor symptoms)
      - Bazedoxifene reduces risk of endometrial hyperplasia (don't need to take progestin)
      - Increases lumbar spine BMD and total hip BMD
    - *Notes:* Intended only for women who still have a uterus. Use for shortest duration and only after carefully considering non-estrogen alternatives
- **Parathyroid hormone**
  - Formulations
    - Teriparatide (*Fortéo*)
      - Approved for treatment
      - Anabolic agent
      - Reduces risk of vertebral fractures by approximately 65% and non-vertebral fractures by approximately 53% after an average of 18 months of therapy
      - Treatment should not exceed 18–24 months
  - Side Effects: Leg cramps, nausea, dizziness. Increased osteosarcoma in rats
- **Receptor activator of nuclear factor kappa-B ligand (RANKL) inhibitor**
  - Formulations
    - Denosumab (*Prolia*)
      - Approved for treatment in PM women at high risk of fracture
      - Reduces vertebral fractures by approximately 68%, hip fractures by approximately 40%, and non-vertebral fractures by approximately 20% over 3 years
      - Subcutaneous injection every 6 months
  - Side Effects: May cause hypocalcemia, cellulitis, rash. Rarely associated with osteonecrosis of jaw and development of atypical femur fractures

Duration of Treatment

- No pharmacologic treatment duration should be indefinite. Bisphosphonates may have residual effects that continue even after treatment is discontinued. Benefits of non-bisphosphonates rapidly disappear after discontinuation
- Evidence of efficacy for longer than 5 years is limited, but chances of serious side effects increases
- Treatment decisions must be individualized

SECTION 5

Urogynecology

NORMAL URINARY FUNCTION

Anatomy

- *Detrusor:* "Bladder muscle"—smooth muscle; innervation is parasympathetic (muscarinic acetylcholine—M2, M3; contraction) and sympathetic (β3-adrenergic receptors; detrusor inhibition or relaxation) (Figure 5-1)
- *Urethral sphincter*
  - Internal urethral sphincter (IUS): Smooth muscle; sympathetic (α1) innervation; muscarinic acetylcholine, α- and β-adrenergic receptors
  - External urethral sphincter (EUS): Striated muscle; somatic motor innervation via pudendal nerve (S2–S4); nicotinic acetylcholine receptors
  - Submucosal endovascular cushions
  - Surrounding tissue support—*hammock hypothesis*—the anterior vaginal wall with its attachment to the arcus tendineus of the pelvic fascia forms a hammock of tissue under the urethra and bladder neck that prevents urethral and bladder neck descent, such that the urethra compresses shut with increased intra-abdominal pressure

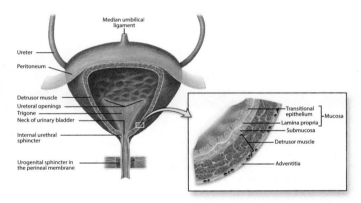

Figure 5-1 Anteroposterior view of bladder anatomy. (Used with permission from Hoffman BL, Schorge JO, Schaffer JI, Halvorson LM, Bradshaw KD, Cunningham F, Calver LE. Chapter 23. Urinary incontinence. In: Hoffman BL, Schorge JO, Schaffer JI, Halvorson LM, Bradshaw KD, Cunningham F, Calver LE, eds. *Williams Gynecology*. 2nd ed. New York, NY: McGraw-Hill; 2012.)

Physiology

- *Bladder filling* = SYMPATHETIC = "STORAGE"
  - *L1–L3* → lumbar sympathetic ganglia → forms *hypogastric nerve* to pelvis
  - Norepinephrine released → decreases smooth muscle tone in bladder
    - Relaxation of detrusor muscle: β3-adrenergic receptors in bladder stimulated (bladder fills)
    - Contraction of IUS: α-Adrenergic receptors in IUS stimulated (sphincter tightens)
      - Contraction of EUS by trained voluntary action (*pudendal nerve* originates from S2 to S4 to innervate EUS and perineal muscles—acetylcholine)
- *Micturition (emptying of bladder)* = PARASYMPATHETIC = "PEEING"
  - Full bladder sensed by mechano-receptors in bladder
  - *S2–S4* → sacral spinal cord → forms *pelvic nerve*
  - Stimulates bladder using acetylcholine and relaxes the urethra employing nitric oxide
    - Contraction of detrusor muscle: Muscarinic cholinergic (M3) receptors stimulated (bladder contracts)
    - Relaxation of IUS: M3 receptors stimulated (sphincter relaxes)
    - Relaxation of EUS by trained voluntary action (*pudendal nerve* originates from S2–S4—acetylcholine)

213

UROGYNECOLOGY

URINARY INCONTINENCE (UI)

Definition

Involuntary loss of urine. Prevalence in the United States is about 50% of adult women.

Types
- *Stress urinary incontinence (SUI):* Most common type (50–70% of UI)
  - Involuntary leakage during effort, exertion, sneezing, or coughing
  - Risk factors include age, parity, vaginal delivery
  - Leakage with stress test. Bladder capacity and post-void residual (PVR) normal (PVR generally considered normal if <150 cc or <1/3 void volume)
  - Urethral hypermobility (straining angle ≥30 degrees on Q-tip test) present in many women with SUI
  - *Urodynamic SUI:* During filling cystometry, involuntary urine leakage with increased intra-abdominal pressure and without detrusor contraction
- *Urge incontinence*
  - Leakage accompanied by or immediately preceded by urge to void
  - Typically results from sudden, involuntary detrusor contractions
  - Usually idiopathic; but can be from inflammation/irritation, calculi, neurologic disorders, outlet obstruction, increased urine output
  - *Urodynamics:* If detrusor contractions are seen on urodynamics, it is called Detrusor Overactivity (DO). Detrusor instability; small capacity bladder, normal PVR
- *Mixed urinary incontinence*
  - Combination of stress and urge incontinence
  - PVR within normal limits
  - Leakage with stress test, detrusor contractions on urodynamics
- *Functional incontinence* (Table 5-1)
  - Associated with cognitive, psychological, or physical impairments that interfere with appropriate toileting. May be transient.
- *Structural incontinence* (Table 5-1)

TABLE 5-1 CAUSES OF URINARY INCONTINENCE

Functional		Structural
D	Delirium or acute confusion	Upper motor neuron lesion
I	Infection (symptomatic UTI)	Overflow
A	Atrophic vaginitis or urethritis	Outlet obstruction
P	Pharmaceuticals	Bladder stone or tumor
P	Psychological (depression, behavioral disturbances)	Urinary fistula
E	Excess urine output (↑ intake, diuretics, CHF)	Urethral diverticulum
R	Restricted mobility	Ectopic ureters
S	Stool impaction	

Definitions of Lower Urinary Tract Symptoms (LUTS)

- *Urgency*: Complaint of sudden desire to pass urine, with or without urge urinary incontinence
- *Frequency*: The complaint of voiding too often (more than seven times in waking hours)
- *Nocturia*: The complaint of arousal from sleep to void one or more times per night
- *Nocturnal enuresis*: The complaint of urinary incontinence during sleep
- *The term "**overflow incontinence**" is **not** recommended by the International Continence Society (ICS)*

Workup of Urinary Incontinence

Basic Evaluation

History

- Frequency/amount of leakage, precipitating factors, impact of leakage on daily life, pad use, linkage to temporal events (childbirth, trauma, new medication, surgery, radiation therapy, medical conditions—eg, bronchitis, asthma), precipitants (eg, medications, caffeinated beverages, alcohol, physical activity, coughing, laughing, sound of water, placing hands in water), pelvic bulge/pressure, urinary urgency or frequency, nocturia, hematuria, recurrent UTIs, voiding problems, incontinence, defecating problems, effort maneuvers, interrupted voiding, incomplete emptying, straining to empty, bowel and sexual function (voiding, bowel control, and sexual function share sacral cord innervation; anal incontinence is more common in people with urinary incontinence). Urinary diary may be helpful (24 hours to 3 days)

Physical Examination

- *Pelvic examination*: For masses, pelvic organ prolapse (POP), vaginal atrophy
- *Cough stress test*: Ask patient to cough and look for leakage
- Palpate pelvic floor muscles (levator ani) for symmetry and bulk, and ability to voluntarily contract muscles
- *Cotton swab test*: Test of urethral hypermobility; place Q-tip in to level of vesical neck, measure change in axis with straining; >30 degrees is urethral hypermobility
- *Pelvic Organ Prolapse Quantification System (POP-Q)*, Figure 5-4
- *Neurologic tests*—The sacral reflexes (anal reflex and the bulbocavernosus reflex) should be assessed (pudendal nerve S2–S4). Anal reflex: stroke skin adjacent to anus; causes contraction of external anal sphincter. Bulbocavernosus reflex: tap or squeeze clitoris; causes contraction of the bulbocavernosus muscle and/or external anal sphincter
- *Post-void residual volume*: Passive or active; goal about 150 cc and <1/3 volume
- *Lab tests:* Urinalysis, urine culture, renal function tests, glucose, calcium

Further Evaluation

- *Urodynamic testing*: Combination of tests that involves simultaneous measurement of various physiologic parameters or urethral and bladder function during bladder filling and emptying
- Cystourethroscopy

STRESS URINARY INCONTINENCE (SUI)

Definition

Involuntary leakage during effort, exertion, sneezing, or coughing

Pathophysiology

- Leakage from urethra occurs when intravesical pressure exceeds urethral pressure
- Factors that affect urethral pressure: Bladder neck position, urethral sphincter muscle and nerve integrity, urethral smooth muscle and vascular plexuses, and surrounding tissue support

Mechanisms

- Urethral hypermobility: Poor urethral support; shown clinically by documenting movement of anterior vaginal wall during straining
- Intrinsic sphincter deficiency: Low-pressure urethra resulting from neurologic disease, radiation, scarring

Treatment

- Lifestyle Interventions: Weight loss, decreasing caffeine intake
- Pelvic Floor Muscle Training: Kegel exercises
- Medication: Goal to increase urinary sphincter tone
  - Imipramine 10–20 mg orally once daily to four times daily
- Devices: Pessaries and urethral inserts
- Surgery
  - Stabilize the urethra to prevent descent with increased abdominal pressure
  - Create a stable supportive layer for urethral compression

Surgical Approaches for SUI

Retropubic Suspension

- *Marshall–Marchetti–Krantz (MMK) vesicourethral suspension*
  - Sutures placed on each side of urethra through pubocervical fascia and fixed to periosteum of posterior pubic symphysis, suspending the fascia
  - Risk of periostitis and osteitis pubis
- *Burch Retropubic Urethropexy* (Figure 5-2)
  - Endopelvic fibromuscular tissue adjacent to mid and proximal urethra is attached to pectineal (Cooper's) ligaments on posterior surface of superior pubic ramus (rather than the periosteum of the pubic symphysis)
- *Similar cure rates*: 80–90% (1 year); 70–90% (5 years); >70% (10 years)

Midurethral Slings

- Emerging as procedure of choice for SUI
- Indication: SUI due to urethral hypermobility (± intrinsic sphincter deficiency)
- *Tension-free vaginal tape (TVT): Retropubic (Space of Retzius)* (Figure 5-3)
  - Acts as a "hammock" to support the bladder neck and urethra
  - Small mid-urethral incision two small suprapubic incisions
  - 85–94% cure rate
  - Bladder perforation rate 4.4–19% in patients with previous incontinence surgery; vascular injuries less than 1%

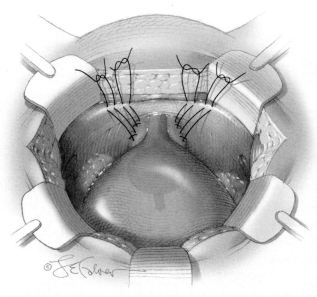

Figure 5-2 Burch colposuspension. (Used with permission from Hoffman BL, Schorge JO, Schaffer JI, Halvorson LM, Bradshaw KD, Cunningham F, Calver LE. Chapter 43. Surgeries for pelvic floor disorders. In: Hoffman BL, Schorge JO, Schaffer JI, Halvorson LM, Bradshaw KD, Cunningham F, Calver LE, eds. *Williams Gynecology*. 2nd ed. New York, NY: McGraw-Hill; 2012.)

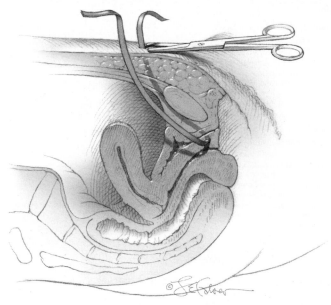

Figure 5-3 Tension-free vaginal tape. (Used with permission from Hoffman BL, Schorge JO, Schaffer JI, Halvorson LM, Bradshaw KD, Cunningham F, Calver LE. Chapter 43. Surgeries for pelvic floor disorders. In: Hoffman BL, Schorge JO, Schaffer JI, Halvorson LM, Bradshaw KD, Cunningham F, Calver LE, eds. *Williams Gynecology*. 2nd ed. New York, NY: McGraw-Hill; 2012.)

- *Transobturator Tape (TOT)*
  - Decreased risk of bladder injury (<0.1%), avoids retropubic Space of Retzius
  - In-to-out or out-to-in approach

Periurethral Injections
- Bulking agents (various options approved by the FDA)
- For patients with intrinsic sphincter deficiency without urethral hypermobility
- 50–60% report marked improvement; 20–30% cure
- Complications: Urinary retention, irritative voiding, 5% UTIs
- Limited duration, 50–90% effective at 6 months, poor long-term success rates, must repeat often

VOIDING TRIALS

- In general, always double-check with specific attending regarding preference on voiding trial protocol
- *Voiding trial procedure:* Remove Foley (or clamp suprapubic catheter) in AM. Patient is due to void within 4 hours. Perform straight catheterization (or unclamp suprapubic catheter) if there is no void in 4 hours or if the patient has pain (to avoid bladder overdistention and long-term urinary retention)
- *Goal:* Voided volume >200 cc; PVR <1/3 of voided volume OR PVR <100 cc with void >200 cc
- If patient "passes" two voiding trials, catheter may be left out
- If patient "fails," discharge with catheter in place/leg bag teaching OR teach catheter care or intermittent self-catheterization
- *Backfill bladder test:* Retrograde fill the bladder with 300–600 cc or to the point when patient has the urge to void, remove catheter, have patient void, measure amount voided. Passing is voiding ≥ to 2/3 of instilled volume. Repeat trial again
- If patient passes both trials, discharge to home without catheter
- If patient fails both trials, discharge to home with catheter or intermittent self-catheterization
- If patient passes one trial and fails one trial, inform attending who will make the final decision. Patients that fail voiding trials will need an appointment within 1 week to repeat the voiding trial

OVERACTIVE BLADDER

Definition

- Urgency with daytime frequency or nocturia with or without urge incontinence, in the absence of pathologic conditions
- Results from inappropriate contraction of the detrusor muscle (if demonstrated on urodynamic testing then it is called DO)
- Also referred to as idiopathic DO, detrusor instability, or unstable bladder

Treatment

Behavioral
- Timed voids with progressive increases in voiding interval
- Biofeedback ± Kegel exercises
- Functional electrical stimulation and weighted vaginal cones

Pharmacotherapy
- *Anticholinergic agents*
  - ACH: Primary neurotransmitter in detrusor contraction
  - Oxybutynin chloride (*Ditropan*) 2.5–5 mg orally three to four times daily; *Ditropan XL* 5–15 daily; patch
  - Tolterodine tartrate (*Detrol*) 1–2 mg orally twice daily; *Detrol LA* 2–4 mg orally daily
  - Other anticholinergic agents: Darifenacin, solifenacin, trospium
  - *Side Effects:* Dry mouth, dry eyes, blurred vision, gastroparesis, constipation, gastroesophageal reflux, somnolence. Contraindicated in narrow angle glaucoma
- *Tricyclic antidepressants*
  - Anticholinergic, alpha-adrenergic
  - Increases tone of urethra and bladder neck
  - Imipramine (*Tofranil*) 75 mg orally once daily
  - Doxepin (*Sinequan*) 50 mg orally at bedtime and 25 mg orally every morning—↓ nocturia and enuresis
  - *Side Effects:* Weakness, fatigue, fine tremors, orthostatic hypotension, arrhythmias
- *Vasopressin*
  - Useful in nocturnal enuresis in children and nocturia in adults; delays diuresis
  - Desmopressin (*DDAVP*)
  - *Side Effects:* (more common in elderly)—water retention and hyponatremia
  - Mirabegron (*Myrbetriq*): antispasmodic, beta3 agonist, relaxes the detrusor muscle and increases bladder capacity. Dosing is 25–50 mg orally daily. Check blood pressure 1–2 weeks after initiation, as can elevate blood pressure

Surgical

- Reserved for intractable cases
  - Sacral nerve root neuromodulation (*InterStim*)
    - 60–90% improvement in symptoms, 10–30% cure rate
    - Implantable battery that stimulates sacral spinal cord (pelvic nerve S3,4)
- Augmentation cystoplasty
- Urinary diversion via ileal conduit
- Intradetrusor onabotulinumtoxinA (*Botox*): 15–30 mg subepithelial injection, 40–80% success rates, durability 6–12 months; risks include long-term urinary retention, cystitis

PELVIC ORGAN PROLAPSE (POP)

- Pelvic organs supported by uterosacral/cardinal ligaments, levator ani, endopelvic fascia
- Includes anterior or posterior vaginal prolapse, apical prolapse, or enterocele
- Lifetime risk of surgery for POP/UI is 11% by age 80 years, with up to one-third representing repeat procedures

Risk Factors for POP

- Increasing age
- Obesity
- Higher parity (especially vaginal deliveries)
- Hysterectomy, especially if for prolapse
- Other POP/UI operations

Symptoms

- Pelvic pressure, heaviness
- SUI due to urethral hypermobility with weakened anterior wall support
- Voiding dysfunction due to urethral obstruction: Hesitancy, frequency, incomplete emptying
- Defecatory symptoms: Excessive straining, incomplete rectal emptying, need for perineal or vaginal pressure to accomplish defecation
- Altered sexual functioning or avoiding intercourse

Physical Examination

- Tongue depressor test for paravaginal defects: Place in lateral anterior vaginal sulcus, elevate → does defect resolve? If yes → paravaginal defect
- **Pelvic Organ Prolapse Quantification (POPQ) System** (Figure 5-4): Measure most advanced extent of prolapse (in cm) relative to the hymen of anterior vagina, cervix or vaginal apex, and posterior vagina
  - Clinical Stages of Prolapse (Table 5-2)
- **Pelvic Muscle Function:** With examiner's hands in vagina, then rectum, have patient squeeze like stopping urine stream, then like stopping defecation
  - Levator ani along pelvic sidewalls at 4 and 8 o'clock positions with fingers in vagina—can the patient localize these muscles, if so → Kegel exercises
  - Anal sphincter: Does the ring tighten circumferentially versus anterior sphincter defect? low resting tone? weak or absent voluntary contractions?

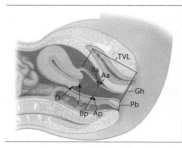

Aa: 3 cm proximal to the external urethral meatus = urethrovesical junction
Ba: Anterior vaginal wall, midpoint between Aa and anterior fornix (cuff)
Ap: 3 cm proximal to the hymen
Bp: Posterior vaginal wall, midpoint between Ap and posterior fornix (cuff)
C: Cervix or apex
D: Posterior fornix (no D point s/p hysterectomy)
Gh: Genital hiatus, middle of urethral meatus to posterior midline hymenal ring
Pb: Perineal body, posterior margin of genital hiatus to the middle anus
TVL: Total vaginal length

Figure 5-4 Pelvic organ prolapse quantification (POP-Q) system. (Used with permission from Hoffman BL, Schorge JO, Schaffer JI, Halvorson LM, Bradshaw KD, Cunningham F, Calver LE. Chapter 24. Pelvic organ prolapse. In: Hoffman BL, Schorge JO, Schaffer JI, Halvorson LM, Bradshaw KD, Cunningham F, Calver LE, eds. *Williams Gynecology*. 2nd ed. New York, NY: McGraw-Hill; 2012.)

TABLE 5-2 CLINICAL STAGES OF PELVIC ORGAN PROLAPSE

Stage 0	Perfect support. Apex can descend as far as 2 cm relative to TVL
Stage 1	All points <-1
Stage 2	Lowest point within 1 cm of the hymenal ring (between -1 and $+1$)
Stage 3	Lowest point >1 cm below hymenal ring, but less than TVL minus 2
Stage 4	Complete prolapse with lowest point between TVL and (TVL-2)

Bladder Testing

• Screening for UTI
• PVR urine volume (<50–100 cc normal as long as void >150 cc)
• Presence or absence of bladder sensation (by voided volume with sensation of fullness, by voiding diary, or by bladder filling)
  Looking for occult SUI; if found, consider incontinence procedure at time of prolapse surgery

Urodynamics

• Applicability to management decisions in POP is controversial

Management of POP

Observation (usually for asymptomatic patients)
• Offer information and reassurance that treatment is available when and if symptomatic
• Counsel that acute changes rarely occur in the setting of early prolapse
• Consider risk for persistent/recurrent UTI and possibly urosepsis if partial urinary retention; exposed vaginal epithelium at risk for erosion → reasons not to observe

Physical therapy for pelvic floor relaxation—Kegel exercises

Pessary use
• Decrease symptoms, delay or avoid surgery, potentially prevent worsening of prolapse
• Add local estrogen with pessary
• *Types of pessaries* (Figure 5-5)

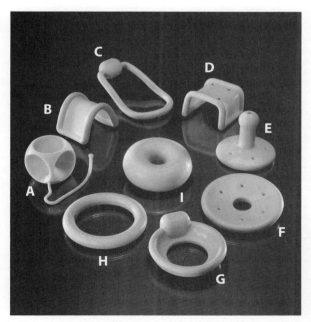

Figure 5-5 Pessary types. (Used with permission from Hoffman BL, Schorge JO, Schaffer JI, Halvorson LM, Bradshaw KD, Cunningham F, Calver LE. Chapter 24. Pelvic organ prolapse. In: Hoffman BL, Schorge JO, Schaffer JI, Halvorson LM, Bradshaw KD, Cunningham F, Calver LE, eds. *Williams Gynecology*. 2nd ed. New York, NY: McGraw-Hill; 2012.)

- *Unsuccessful fitting* associated with
  - Short vaginal length (<7 cm)
  - Wide introitus (four fingerbreadths)
  - Weak levator ani strength
- *Complications:* Rectovaginal/vesicovaginal fistulae, persistent vaginal erosions
- *Poor candidates:* Unable to clean, large genital hiatus, weak levator ani, vaginal erosions; but try with everyone
- *Care:* Remove nightly/weekly and replace in AM, or doctor removes every 3 months

Surgery

- Three groups of surgical procedures
  - *Restorative:* Use the patient's endogenous support structures
  - *Compensatory:* Attempt to replace deficient support with some type of graft, including synthetic, allogenic, xenogenic, or autologous material. Of note, the FDA Public Health Notification (July 2011) highlighted adverse events of transvaginal prolapse repair using mesh, including mesh erosion (10% within 12 months), pain, infection, urinary complaints, bleeding, and organ perforation
  - *Obliterative:* Close the vagina

Anterior Vaginal Repair

- *Anterior colporrhaphy:* Vaginal epithelium separated from underlying fibromuscular connective tissue, followed by midline plication of vaginal muscularis and pubocervical fascia with interrupted absorbable sutures, excision of excess epithelium, closure
  - 5 year success rate 30–40%
- *Site-specific defect repairs:* Isolated defects in the pubocervical fascia are identified and reapproximated, so that normal anatomy is restored
- *Paravaginal repair:* Reattaches anterior lateral vaginal sulcus to obturator internus muscle and fascia at level of the arcus tendineus fascia pelvis ("white line"), usually a bilateral procedure, via transvaginal or retropubic (abdominal or laparoscopic access)
  - 76–96% success rate

Posterior Vaginal Repair

- *Posterior colporrhaphy:* Separation of vaginal epithelium from underlying fibromuscular connective tissue (includes rectovaginal septum, in between the vaginal muscularis and the rectovaginal adventitia), followed by midline plication with interrupted sutures, excision of excess epithelium, and closure. A common complication is dyspareunia
- *Levator ani plication:* Controversial due to risk of dyspareunia
- *Perineorrhaphy:* Plicate transverse perineal, bulbocavernosus muscles; risk of dyspareunia
- *Site-specific defect repairs:* Isolated defects in the rectovaginal fascia are identified and reapproximated, so that normal anatomy is restored
- Complications: Mesh erosion, fistula, vascular injury, chronic pelvic pain, dyspareunia

Enterocele Repair

- *Moschowitz procedure (abdominal):* Concentric purse-string sutures around cul-de-sac (serosa of posterior vaginal wall, right pelvic side wall, serosa of sigmoid, left pelvic side wall)
- *McCall culdoplasty (vaginal):* Corrects enterocele at time of total vaginal hysterectomy (TVH)
- *Halban (abdominal):* Obliterates cul-de-sac using sutures between the uterosacral ligaments in the sagittal plane

Vaginal Apical Repair

- "Apical vaginal prolapse" = uterine prolapse and vaginal vault prolapse
- Usually perform a hysterectomy and a vaginal vault suspension procedure
- *Sacrospinous ligament suspension*
  - Suturing the vaginal apex (usually the right side) to the sacrospinous ligament (tendinous component of the coccygeus)
  - Place suture 2 fingerbreaths medial to ischial spine
  - High rates of subsequent anterior vaginal prolapse, perhaps due to pronounced posterior deviation of the vaginal axis (37%)
  - 63–97% success rates
  - Complications: Hemorrhage, nerve injury, buttock pain, SUI dyspareunia
- *Iliococcygeus*
  - Suturing of the vaginal apex to the iliococcygeus fascia below the ischial spine
- *Uterosacral ligament suspension*
  - Vaginal apex is sutured to uterosacral ligaments at the level of the ischial spines
  - 80–100% success rate
  - Complications: Ureteral kinking (remove offending suture); risk of ureteral injury up to 11%

Abdominal Apical Repair

- *Abdominal sacral colpopexy*
  - Replaces normal apical support with interposition of a suspensory bridge between the apical anterior and posterior vagina with the anterior sacral promontory
  - Cure rate: 78–100%
  - Complications: Hemorrhage middle sacral artery/venous plexus, 3–4% mesh erosion

Obliterative Procedures

- *Total colpectomy*
  - *Surgical removal of the vagina*: Vaginal epithelium removed and vault closed with purse strings in patient who has had hysterectomy
- *Partial colpocleisis, "LeFort"*
  - Closing off of the vaginal space—uterus left in place with lateral drainage channels for cervical secretions
  - Do pap, endometrial biopsy and transvaginal ultrasound, prior to procedure to exclude indication for hysterectomy
  - 86–100% cure rate; high satisfaction in well-counseled patients who desire no future vaginal coitus
  - *Complications:* Occult SUI; regret

ANATOMY

Anterior and Posterior Perineal Triangles (Figure 5-6)

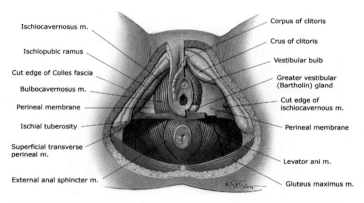

Figure 5-6 Anterior and posterior perineal triangles. Left: After removal of Colles fascia. Right: After removal of superficial perineal muscles. (Used with permission from Hoffman BL, Schorge JO, Schaffer JI, Halvorson LM, Bradshaw KD, Cunningham F, Calver LE. Chapter 38. Anatomy. In: Hoffman BL, Schorge JO, Schaffer JI, Halvorson LM, Bradshaw KD, Cunningham F, Calver LE, eds. *Williams Gynecology*. 2nd ed. New York, NY: McGraw-Hill; 2012.)

Connective Tissue and Surgical Spaces of the Pelvis (Figure 5-7)

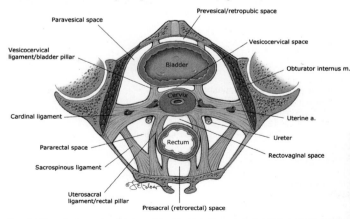

Figure 5-7 Connective tissue and surgical spaces of the pelvis. (Used with permission from Hoffman BL, Schorge JO, Schaffer JI, Halvorson LM, Bradshaw KD, Cunningham F, Calver LE. Chapter 38. Anatomy. In: Hoffman BL, Schorge JO, Schaffer JI, Halvorson LM, Bradshaw KD, Cunningham F, Calver LE, eds. *Williams Gynecology*. 2nd ed. New York, NY: McGraw-Hill; 2012.)

Anatomy of Presacral/Retrorectal Space

- Middle sacral artery
- Hypogastric plexus
- Venous plexus
- Anterior longitudinal ligament

Levator Ani

- Puborectalis
- Pubococcygeus
- Iliococcygeus

Superior View of Pelvic Floor and Pelvic Wall Muscles (Figure 5-8)

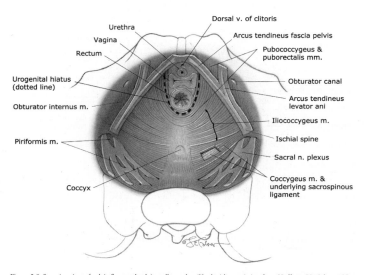

Figure 5-8 Superior view of pelvic floor and pelvic wall muscles. (Used with permission from Hoffman BL, Schorge JO, Schaffer JI, Halvorson LM, Bradshaw KD, Cunningham F, Calver LE. Chapter 38. Anatomy. In: Hoffman BL, Schorge JO, Schaffer JI, Halvorson LM, Bradshaw KD, Cunningham F, Calver LE, eds. *Williams Gynecology*. 2nd ed. New York, NY: McGraw-Hill; 2012.)

Pelvic Viscera and Connective Tissue Support (Figure 5-9)

Attachment of Rectovaginal Septum/Fascia

- SUPERIOR: Uterosacral/cardinal ligaments
- ANTERIOR: Levator ani/arcus tendineus fascia pelvis
- INFERIOR: Perineal body
- POSTERIOR/LATERAL: Arcus tendineus fascia, rectovaginalis

Attachment of Pubocervical Fascia

- LATERAL: Arcus tendineus fascia pelvis
- INFERIOR: Pubic symphysis
- SUPERIOR: Cervix/cardinal ligaments

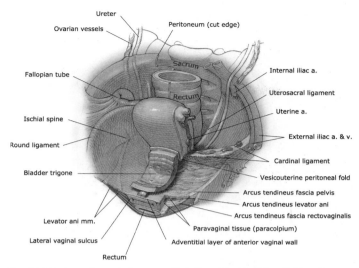

Figure 5-9 Pelvic viscera and connective tissue support. (Used with permission from Hoffman BL, Schorge JO, Schaffer JI, Halvorson LM, Bradshaw KD, Cunningham F, Calver LE. Chapter 38. Anatomy. In: Hoffman BL, Schorge JO, Schaffer JI, Halvorson LM, Bradshaw KD, Cunningham F, Calver LE, eds. *Williams Gynecology*. 2nd ed. New York, NY: McGraw-Hill; 2012.)

Delancey Levels of Support (Figure 5-10)

- *Upper Vertical Axis:* Cardinal and uterosacral ligaments
- *Horizontal Axis:* Ischial spine to posterior aspect of pubic symphysis
  - Paravaginal support of bladder
  - Upper two-thirds of vagina
  - Rectum
- *Lower Vertical Axis:* Perpendicular plane of levator hiatus, urogenital, anal triangles
  - Lower one-third of vagina, urethra, anal canal

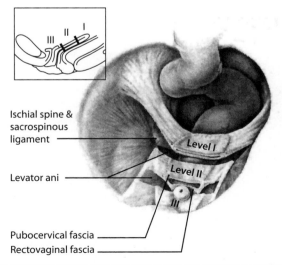

Figure 5-10 Delancey levels of support. (Used with permission from DeLancey, JO. Anatomie aspects of vaginal eversion after hysterectomy. *Am J Obstet Gynecol*. 1992;166(6):1717–1728.)

Index

Page numbers followed by f or t indicate figures or tables, respectively.